E DI

Peter Manu

The Pharmacotherapy of Common Functional Syndromes
Evidence-Based Guidelines for Primary Care Practice

Pre-publication
REVIEW . . .

"**C**hronic fatigue syndrome, fibromyalgia, irritable bowel syndrome, and premenstrual syndrome are conditions often associated with controversy and dispute, particularly when someone attempts to come up with an explanation as to what causes them. But, we all can be certain that taken together these are common disorders associated with considerable cost to the individual, family, and society, and that we know far too little about how to treat them.

Consequently, patients and doctors alike are surrounded by claims and counterclaims about the efficacy of treatments ranging from the sensible to the absurd. In this book, Peter Manu, a physician who has long specialized in these unpopular areas, brings some much needed rigor to the field.

Manu provides a careful, dispassionate, and accurate review of current treatments. Anyone who wishes to cut through the hype and come up with evidence, as opposed to simply putting a few keywords into a search engine, will welcome this book. Manu remains scrupulously guided by the evidence and follows the standard methodology of what we call on this side of the Atlantic 'evidence-based medicine.'

The book is therefore to be warmly welcomed. Where there is ignorance, Manu says so. Where there is uncertainty, he admits it. Sadly it is all too rare when he is able to clearly recommend a treatment of proven efficacy, but

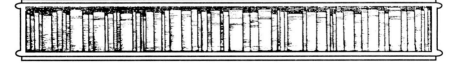

equally sad, none of these areas have ever attracted large-scale research or pharmaceutical funding commensurate with their personal and social importance.

I recommend this book to anyone who wants to find out more about the current state of evidence regarding the treatment of these four complex conditions. Clinicians who genuinely want to help their patients will want to refer to this book, while patients will use it to make sure they are protected from clinicians with less scrupulous motives."

Simon Wessely, MA
*Professor of Epidemiological
and Liaison Psychiatry,
Academic Department
of Psychological Medicine,
Guy's, King's, and St. Thomas's
School of Medicine
and Institute of Psychiatry,
London*

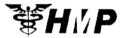

The Haworth Medical Press®
An Imprint of The Haworth Press, Inc.

The Pharmacotherapy of Common Functional Syndromes

Evidence-Based Guidelines for Primary Care Practice

THE HAWORTH PRESS
New, Recent, and Forthcoming Titles
of Related Interest

Betrayal by the Brain: The Neurologic Basis of Chronic Fatigue Syndrome, Fibromyalgia Syndrome, and Related Neural Network Disorders by Jay A. Goldstein

A Companion Volume to Dr. Jay A. Goldstein's Betrayal by the Brain: A Guide for Patients and Their Physicians by Katie Courmel

Chronic Fatigue Syndromes: The Limbic Hypothesis by Jay A. Goldstein

CFIDS, Fibromyalgia, and the Virus-Allergy Link: Hidden Viruses, Allergies, and Uncommon Fatigue/Pain Disorders by R. Bruce Duncan

Concise Encyclopedia of Chronic Fatigue Syndrome by Roberto Patarca-Montero

Health Care Resources on the Internet: A Guide for Librarians and Health Care Consumers edited by M. Sandra Wood

A Parents' Guide to CFIDS: How to Be an Advocate for Your Child with Chronic Fatigue Immune Dysfunction Syndrome by David S. Bell, Mary Z. Robinson, Jean Pollard, Tom Robinson, and Bonnie Floyd

The Love Drug: Marching to the Beat of Ecstasy by Richard S. Cohen

Drugs, the Brain, and Behavior: The Pharmacology of Abuse and Dependence by John Brick and Carlton K. Erickson

The Pharmacotherapy of Common Functional Syndromes
Evidence-Based Guidelines for Primary Care Practice

Peter Manu

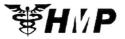

The Haworth Medical Press®
An Imprint of The Haworth Press, Inc.
New York • London • Oxford

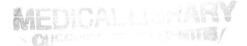
Published by

The Haworth Medical Press®, an imprint of The Haworth Press, Inc., 10 Alice Street, Binghamton, NY 13904-1580

Medicine is an ever-changing science. As new research and clinical experience broaden our knowledge, changes in treatment and drug therapy are required. While many suggestions for drug usages are made herein, the book is intended for educational purposes only, and the author, editor, and publisher do not accept liability in the event of negative consequences incurred as a result of information presented in this book. We do not claim that this information is necessarily accurate by the rigid, scientific standard applied for medical proof, and therefore make no warranty, expressed or implied, with respect to the material herein contained. Therefore the patient is urged to check the product information sheet included in the package of each drug he or she plans to administer to be certain the protocol followed is not in conflict with the manufacturer's inserts. When a discrepancy arises between these inserts and information in this book, the physician is encouraged to use his or her best professional judgement.

Cover design by Marylouise E. Doyle.

Library of Congress Cataloging-in-Publication Data

Manu, Peter, 1947-
    The pharmacotherapy of common functional syndromes : evidence-based guidelines for primary care practice / Peter Manu.
        p.   cm.
    Includes bibliographical references and index.
    ISBN 0-7890-0588-3 (hard : alk paper)—ISBN 0-7890-0589-1 (pbk. : alk paper)
    1. Syndromes—Chemotherapy. 2. Evidence-based medicine. 3. Primary care (Medicine) I. Title.
    [DNLM: 1. Fatigue Syndrome, Chronic—drug therapy. 2. Colonic Diseases, Functional—drug therapy. 3. Evidence-Based Medicine. 4. Fibromyalgia—drug therapy. 5. Premenstrual Syndrome—drug therapy. WB 146 M294p 2000]
    RC69 .M36 2000
    615.5'8—dc21   00-020078

CONTENTS

ABOUT THE AUTHOR

Dr. Peter Manu, certified by the American Board of Internal Medicine in 1980, is Director of Medical Services at Hillside Hospital, Long Island Jewish Medical Center, and Associate Professor at Albert Einstein College of Medicine. Previously he served on the faculties of the State University of New York at Syracuse and the University of Connecticut. His work on issues involving the interface of medicine and psychiatry has been published in journals including *Annals of Internal Medicine, American Journal of Medicine,* and *Journal of Affective Disorders.*

Introduction

As you set out for Ithaka
hope the voyage is a long one
full of adventure, full of discovery.

C. P. Cavafy, *Ithaka*

Functional somatic syndromes are illnesses characterized by constellations of symptoms, suffering, and disability that lack demonstrable structural abnormalities and cannot be explained by an evidence-based pathophysiologic mechanism (Manu, 1998; Barsky and Borus, 1999). The category is clearly dominated by chronic fatigue syndrome, fibromyalgia, irritable bowel syndrome, and premenstrual syndrome, well-defined conditions with a substantial prevalence in the community and among patients evaluated and treated by primary care practitioners. Other functional illnesses are managed predominantly within the confines of specialized practice, for instance, urology for interstitial cystitis; oral and maxillofacial surgery for temporomandibular pain syndrome; cardiology and gastroenterology for atypical (nonischemic) chest pain; neurology, neurosurgery, and orthopedics for repetitive strain injury and chronic whiplash; occupational medicine for sick building syndrome; and psychiatry for hyperventilation syndrome. Finally, a group of functional syndromes that includes multiple chemical sensitivities, Gulf War syndrome, and the illness alleged to follow silicone breast implants have only recently emerged and are still in search of validation and legitimacy.

The four common functional disorders (i.e., chronic fatigue syndrome, fibromyalgia, irritable bowel syndrome, and premenstrual syndrome) have been the focus of intense scientific efforts for decades, no doubt because their symptoms are experienced by a very large number of individuals and generate substantial suffering and expenditures. A conservative interpretation of data available in 1998 indicates that at least 10 percent of the U.S. adult population suffers from symptoms compatible with one of these four syndromes and that the direct and indirect health care costs exceed eight billion dollars annually in this country (Manu and Matthews, 1998; Abeles, 1998; Longstreth, 1998; Pearlstein, 1998). The 1966-1999 database maintained by the National Library of Medicine gives a sense of the magnitude of the research dedicated to these conditions by listing 8,808 publications, of which 3,047 report studies on irritable bowel syndrome, 2,096 on premenstrual syndrome, 1,943 on fibromyalgia, and 1,722 on chronic fatigue syndrome. This impressive body of work has been directed primarily at understanding the etiology of these syndromes, a meritorious and much needed enterprise that is in accordance with the accepted paradigm of scientific progress, which requires the definition of causality before testing therapeutic solutions. However, in this instance, the logic of science has poorly served the management of these syndromes, a process that is too often fastidious, frustrating, and fruitless. The lack of satisfaction that follows the failure of reassurance, explanation, and standard symptomatic treatment has been attributed to patients' tendency to enter a self-perpetuating cycle leading to symptom amplification; to their conviction that the illness will only worsen; to their belief that the functional syndrome is a potentially catastrophic disease; and to the consolidation of the "sick role" with all its implications regarding inappropriate utilization of medical resources, litigation, and disability (Barsky and Borus, 1999).

The burden of caring for patients with these common functional syndromes is placed squarely on the shoulders of primary care practitioners. Their first task is to search diligently for an organic explanation for the chief complaints and associated symptoms of these conditions. In addition, they must be able to detect somatic presentations of depressive and anxiety syndromes; to correct inappropriate disease conviction and avoidance behaviors; and to act as a gatekeeper for access to unnecessary testing (Sharpe, Bass, and Mayou, 1995). Nonetheless, their most important obligation to the patient is to treat the functional syndrome, to alleviate suffering and obtain the return to health and normal functioning in the context of a patient-provider relationship which has made the patient feel understood; has established the framework for a positive collaboration; has corrected the misconceptions about the illness; and has negotiated a justifiable plan of laboratory investigations and specialty consultations (Sharpe, Bass, and Mayou, 1995). For practical purposes physicians have adopted an empirical symptomatic approach to the drug therapy of these conditions. They use small doses of serotonergic antidepressants to treat the depressive features of chronic fatigue syndrome, nonsteroidal anti-inflammatory drugs for the cardinal symptom of fibromyalgia, or dietary fiber supplementation to correct the constipation reported by patients with irritable bowel syndrome. Given the multisymptomatic presentation of these syndromes, it is not unusual to find patients who have been prescribed up to a dozen different medicines. The physician's explanatory model is another source of therapeutic ideas, for instance, using fludrocortisone if chronic fatigue syndrome is considered related to autonomic disturbance, hypnotic agents if fibromyalgia is believed to be caused by a sleep disturbance, and progesterone or estrogen treatment if premenstrual syndrome is thought to represent a deficiency or "imbalance" of these hormones. Yet none of these treatments have had their effectiveness confirmed according to accepted scientific standards, most produce significant adverse reactions, and many prompt the patients to form unjustified beliefs about the etiology of their illness.

The time has come to transform the therapy of common functional syndromes into an evidence-based process. As in any other field of medicine, these decisions have been informed by a variety of sources and methods, including clinical impressions, uncontrolled studies, nonrandomized controlled comparisons, and randomized controlled trials (Sharpe et al., 1996). Clinical impressions and uncontrolled studies offer outcome data that cannot be distinguished from the placebo effect or the natural history of these syndromes. Nonrandomized controlled studies create the potential for comparing cohorts of patients with different clinical characteristics or prognostic factors. These are the reasons why the evidence must be sought in the randomized controlled therapeutic trials of these common functional syndromes. Overall, the literature catalogued by the National Library of Congress lists 183 trials: 69 for premenstrual syndrome, 53 for irritable bowel syndrome, 34 for fibromyalgia, and 34 for chronic fatigue syndrome. This evidence must be carefully evaluated according to a checklist that verifies the random assignment to treatment; the follow-up of all of the patients entered in the trial; the outcome evaluation of all the groups to which the patients were assigned; and the presence of an independent, blinded comparison of clinical improvement and adverse reactions observed after treatment with the supposedly active medicine and a suitable placebo using statistically sound methods (Oxman, Sackett, and Guyatt, 1993; Meade and Richardson, 1997). The study design must also provide concealment of randomization and blinding by keeping investigators unaware of the treatment group to which the patient will be randomly assigned and by masking the patients, care-givers, and research staff to treatment allocation for the entire duration of the trial (Meade and Richardson, 1997). While the evidence provided by well-designed controlled trials should help us determine what works best, applying the results to individual patients is reasonable only when the primary care physician is convinced that the trial has dealt with patients similar to those seen in his or her practice; that the treatment is feasible in the given setting and that there are no geographical or financial barriers to care; that the potential benefits are carefully weighed against the individualized risk for adverse reactions; and that the patient's values are compatible with the selected therapy (Glasziou et al., 1998).

This book presents the evidence generated by randomized controlled trials of drug therapy for common functional syndromes. The primary source was 183 published studies, out of which 153 met the requirements for methodological accuracy and clinical applicability outlined previously and include 21 controlled interventions in patients with chronic fatigue syndrome, 32 in fibromyalgia, 34 in irritable bowel syndrome, and 66 in premenstrual syndrome. In contrast with systematic reviews that contain only a brief description of the methodology and a summary of the results, this book is the first work that enables primary care physicians to access all of the facts needed to reach their own conclusions with regard to the risks and benefits of these pharmacological interventions. Each trial is described according to a sequence that defines the clinical setting and patients' recruitment, diagnostic criteria, reasons for exclusions, therapeutic and placebo interventions, baseline and outcome measurements, adverse reactions developed during the trial, reasons for withdrawal from the study, and the effect of therapy as compared with the placebo response.

The therapeutic focus of the book has prevented the inclusion of the epidemiological, biological, and clinical dimensions of the four syndromes, but recently published review articles or book chapters provide the necessary details regarding chronic fatigue syndrome (Demitrack, 1998; Komaroff and Buchwald, 1998; Manu and Matthews, 1998), fibromyalgia (Simms, 1998; Abeles, 1998; Goldenberg, 1999), irritable bowel (Drossman et al., 1997; Maxwell, Mendenhall, and Kumar, 1997; Longstreth, 1998), and premenstrual syndrome (Freeman and Halbreich, 1998; Pearlstein and Stone, 1998; Pearlstein, 1998). This book augments the description of pharmacological interventions recommended by these experts and uses prospective rules to structure the presentation of scientific evidence based on our conviction that primary care physicians must know which of the drug therapies studied in replicated trials are effective, controversial, or ineffective. The book identifies as *effective therapies* those demonstrated to be better than placebo for most of the clinical manifestations of the functional syndrome in at least two trials conducted by different research groups, or a clear preponderance of trials with positive results was required when the literature contained contradictory reports. *Controversial therapies* were those for which independent studies produced diametrically opposed outcomes and *ineffective therapies* were pharmacologic treatments shown to be similar to placebo in a definite majority of the available trials. Data generated in one-of-a-kind trials are described separately. For each of the four syndromes, the presentation of the evidence concludes with the practical framework for prescribing effective drug therapies and nonpharmacological interventions.

This work aims to be a therapeutic guide for internists, family practitioners, pediatricians, and gynecologists in their attempt to help patients with these disabling and vexing illnesses. The book is also intended to add precision to the management solutions offered by physicians practicing rheumatology, gastroenterology, physiatry, neurology, and psychiatry to whom these patients are often referred for expert consultation and to help clinical pharmacologists plan new drug trials. Last, but certainly not least, this book was written, with affection and respect, for the large number of patients with one or more of these syndromes who want to inform themselves and their families, avoid ineffective remedies, and create a science-based partnership with their physicians.

SECTION I:
CHRONIC FATIGUE SYNDROME

Chapter 1

Definition and Methodological Issues

The current definition of chronic fatigue syndrome (CFS) was developed by an international group of experts assembled at the initiative of investigators from the Division of Viral and Rickettsial Diseases, National Center for Infectious Diseases, Centers for Disease Control and Prevention, Atlanta, Georgia (Fukuda et al., 1994). The authors sought to develop a standard useful for accurate comparisons with control populations in cohort studies. The definition requires collection of data regarding history, physical examination, mental status evaluation, and screening laboratory tests. The history of present illness must include the physical and psychological symptoms and circumstances present at the onset of fatigue; inquiry into previously diagnosed psychiatric disorders or episodes of physical illness that have remained unexplained; a careful search for substance abuse or dependence; and a complete list of prescribed and over-the-counter medications, vitamins, food supplements, and adjustments in daily routines. The recommendations for mental status examination suggest focusing on symptoms of anxiety and depression as well as a thorough search for evidence of self-destructive behavior or psychomotor retardation. Formal psychiatric and/or neurologic evaluations must be obtained when symptoms suggestive of these disorders are identified during the initial evaluation. The designated battery of screening laboratory tests is restricted to the complete blood count, a standard chemistry profile, the determination of thyroid-stimulating hormone, and urinalysis. All other testing is to be performed only to exclude other diagnoses suggested by history and physical examination.

The diagnosis cannot be given in the presence of any active medical disorder known to be associated with persistent tiredness;

any previously diagnosed condition whose resolution has not been documented according to acceptable clinical standards and whose persistence may produce chronic fatigue; any type of substance abuse within two years prior to the onset of the fatigue illness and at any time during its course; and severe obesity, defined by a body mass index (weight in kilograms divided by the squared height in meters) greater than 45.

A positive diagnosis of chronic fatigue syndrome requires the presence of persisting or relapsing chronic fatigue (i.e., lasting longer than six months) that has been clinically evaluated as delineated previously and has remained unexplained. In addition, the clinician must document the presence of at least four of the following eight symptoms: impaired concentration or short-term memory severe enough to lead to "substantial" decrease in the level of occupation-al, social, and personal functioning; sore throat; painful cervical or axillary lymph nodes; muscle pain; joint pain at more than one location and without evidence of inflammatory signs; headaches new in type, severity, or pattern; unrefreshing sleep; and malaise lasting longer than 24 hours after exertion. The symptoms are counted toward a diagnosis of chronic fatigue syndrome only if they had been experienced after the onset of fatigue and have to occur concurrently with each other and with the symptom of fatigue in a persistent or recurrent fashion for six months or longer.

The definition has categorical rules with regard to the psychiatric disorders diagnosed during the evaluation process. On one hand, the authors specified a group of seven psychiatric disorders whose presence excludes a patient from being considered for the diagnosis of chronic fatigue syndrome: major depression with melancholic or psychotic features; bipolar disorders; anorexia nervosa; bulimia nervosa; delusional disorders of any subtype; schizophrenia of any subtype; and dementias of any subtype. On the other hand, the diagnosis of chronic fatigue syndrome is allowed in the presence of nonpsychotic or nonmelancholic depression, anxiety disorders of any type, and somatoform disorders of any type. Other diagnoses that do not exclude chronic fatigue syndrome are fibromyalgia, neurasthenia, and the functional somatic syndrome of multiple chemical sensitivities.

Some of the studies presented in this chapter have used a previous version of this definition to identify patients with chronic fatigue syndrome (Holmes et al., 1988) in which the patient had to have a minimum of eight out of eleven symptoms or at least six symptoms and two of three physical signs. The three symptoms dropped out of the revised definition (Fukuda et al., 1994) were fever, muscle weakness, and sudden onset of the fatigue illness; the three physical signs no longer required were low-grade fever, non-exudative pharyngitis, and enlarged or tender cervical or axillary lymph nodes. Another difference was the specification contained in the initial version (Holmes et al., 1988) that the degree of functional reduction be at least 50 percent in any one area of activity. A past history of psychiatric illness was considered to exclude chronic fatigue syndrome, but only if it had been present before the onset of fatigue. Investigators from Australia (Lloyd, Hickie, Boughton, et al., 1990) and the United Kingdom (Sharpe et al., 1991) have relied on their own definitions for this syndrome which are, however, comparable with the U.S. standard (Bates et al., 1994).

The methodological issues raised by the study of treatment approaches to chronic fatigue syndrome have received the attention of an interdisciplinary group of experts from Sydney, Australia (Wilson et al., 1994). After noting the paucity of placebo-controlled, double-blind trials in well-defined patient populations, the authors emphasized the critical need for such trials, given the fact that spontaneous remissions appear to be common, the patient samples are heterogenous, and the measured outcomes are by necessity of a subjective nature.

Chapter 2

Controversial Treatments

IMMUNOGLOBULIN INFUSIONS

The treatment of chronic fatigue syndrome with intravenous immunoglobulin has first been the object of two studies published simultaneously in the same journal in 1990 (Lloyd, Hickie, Wakefield, et al., 1990; Peterson et al., 1990). One group of investigators felt that "immunologic disturbances may be central to the pathogenesis of chronic fatigue syndrome" and that "immunomodulatory therapy has been demonstrated to be of use in a number of diseases featuring disordered immunoregulation" (Lloyd, Hickie, Wakefield, et al., 1990, p. 561), while the other group thought that immunoglobulin therapy "could correct an immunoregulatory defect" and "might contain neutralizing antibodies" against a viral infection involved in the causation of the syndrome (Peterson et al., 1990, p. 555). Considerable weight was given to the contemporary cross-sectional reports describing immunoglobulin G subclass deficiencies in individuals with this syndrome (Read et al., 1988; Linde, Hammarstrom, and Smith, 1988; Komaroff, Geiger, and Wormsely, 1988; Lloyd et al., 1989).

The first of these described a double-blind, placebo-controlled trial performed by an interdisciplinary group from Prince Henry and Prince of Wales Hospitals, Sydney, Australia (Lloyd, Hickie, Wakefield, et al., 1990). Patients were enrolled if they had a history of chronic and persistent exercise-worsened muscle fatigue requiring a prolonged recovery time, associated with other specified constitutional and neuropsychiatric symptoms for at least six months; frequent medical consultations and significant reduction in the ability to perform daily activities; and no previous immunologic therapy. Clinical examinations and extensive laboratory testing were employed to rule out infections, immunodeficiency-related disorders, and other conditions known to produce the main symptoms. All patients underwent a structured psychiatric evaluation and provided baseline self-assessments of their physical and psychological symptoms, quality of life, and functional status. The subjects were then randomly assigned to receive either intravenous placebo (10 percent maltose in water) or an equivalent volume of immunoglobulin solution containing 2 g/kg infused over 24 hours once a month for three months. The response to therapy was assessed three months after the last infusion.

Forty-nine patients (24 women) entered the trial. Their mean age was 36 years and the average duration of their fatigue syndrome was four years. An acute "viral-like" illness marked the onset in 76 percent of patients, but serologic diagnoses of acute infection were documented in only 10 percent of patients. Most patients (65 percent) were experiencing significant occupational disabilities and were unable to work or attend school. Seven patients met criteria for current major depression and 19 patients had psychometric scores consistent with mild depression. Laboratory evaluations indicated abnormal cell-mediated immunity in 82 percent of patients, as evidenced by T-cell lymphopenia and reduced delayed-type hypersensitivity responses to skin testing with seven different antigens. Sixty-two percent of the 23 patients assigned to the immunoglobulin arm of the study and 31 percent of the 26 patients assigned to receive placebo had evidence of decreased immunoglobulin subclasses. The two groups were otherwise similar with regard to demographic, clinical, and immunologic characteristics.

The study was completed by 47 of the 49 participants; two patients given immunoglobulin were withdrawn after developing abnormal liver function tests in one case and phlebitis in the other. Notable side effects included phlebitis, which occurred after 35 of the 65 immunoglobulin infusions (55 percent), but with only one of the placebo infusions. Fatigue, headache, and impairment of concentrating ability developed after 82 percent of immunoglobulin infusions and 24 percent of the placebo treatments. The adverse effects were typically noticed 12 to 24 hours after infusion and lasted up to ten days. The high prevalence of adverse effects, especially phlebitis, among patients receiving immunoglobulin infusions was acknowledged by the authors with the statement that "the patients and the investigators may have been partially unblinded by this differential" (Lloyd, Hickie, Wakefield, et al., 1990, p. 567).

At the completion of the trial, 43 percent of the immunoglobulin recipients, but only 11 percent of those receiving placebo, had a favorable response to treatment; the difference was statistically significant. Six of the immunoglobulin responders resumed full-time occupational activities. Among the immunoglobulin responders, the improvement was usually (80 percent) noted within three weeks of the first infusion, with gradual augmentation of the favorable effect after each subsequent treatment. Patients who improved were shown to have decreased psychological morbidity and a significant improvement in their measures of cell-mediated immunity. However, it is important to note that six of the ten immunoglobulin responders and all three placebo responders became disabled again and had considerable restoration of symptoms when evaluated three months later.

The second of the studies published in 1990 reported the results of a trial conducted at the Hennepin County Medical Center in Minneapolis, a major teaching affiliate of the University of Minnesota Medical School (Peterson et al., 1990). The patients recruited for the study met standard diagnostic criteria (Holmes et al., 1988). Extensive immunologic studies and assessments of the physical and social functioning, mental health and health perceptions were obtained prior to the start of the trial.

The study group comprised 30 patients (22 women). Their mean age was 40.6 years and the average duration of their fatigue illness was 3.8 years. With only one exception, the fatigue syndrome followed an acute "viral-like" illness. Most patients (77 percent) were highly educated, and a substantial proportion (43 percent) were vocationally disabled. In addition to fatigue, the most common symptoms were generalized muscle weakness (96 percent of patients), myalgias (96 percent), sleep disturbance (96 percent), headaches (93 percent), arthralgias (89 percent), forgetfulness (89 percent), and excessive irritability (89 percent). Baseline immunoglobulin G subclass concentrations were below the normal range in 43 percent of patients for subclass 1, 29 percent of patients for subclass 2, and 64 percent of patients for subclass 3. Other notable humoral immunity abnormalities included low levels of immunoglobulin A (21 percent of patients), low levels of immunoglobulin E (28 percent of patients), and high levels of immunoglobulin M (25 percent of patients). Cellular immunity abnormalities were detected in 18 percent of patients.

The 30 patients were randomly assigned to receive intravenous infusions of either immunoglobulin G (1g/kg body weight) prepared as a solution containing 50 mg/ml or placebo consisting of 1 percent albumin solution. The volume, color, viscosity, and rate of administration of the immunoglobulin and placebo infusions were identical. A total of six infusions were administered at intervals of 30 days. The immunoglobulin and placebo groups were well matched, the only exception being that of age, which averaged 45 years in the immunoglobulin group and 36 years in the placebo group.

One patient from each group was withdrawn because of adverse experiences. After five months of treatment, the symptoms of chronic fatigue syndrome improved in 20 percent of patients in both groups. Intragroup and intergroup comparisons failed to reveal statistically significant improvements for any of the symptoms assessed. With regard to functional status and well-being, the direct comparisons indicated significance for the improvement of social functioning in patients treated with placebo. Adverse effects were common and included headaches (77 percent), gastrointestinal complaints (60 percent), and fever (33 percent); only headaches were more prevalent in the immunoglobulin-treated group.

The contradictory results of these two clinical trials have been the object of a thoughtful editorial which pointed out that both of these patient populations failed to show improvement, as judged by the comparison of baseline and posttreatment scores of the quantitative self-assessment instruments (Straus, 1990). Neither study demonstrated any advantage over placebo beyond three months after completion of treatment. Finally, the occurrence of frequent adverse effects had the potential to unblind the Australian investigators and added a substantial burden of iatrogenic illness to individuals already debilitated by the fatigue syndrome. Moreover, toward the middle of the 1990s, one of the main justifications for such treatments weakened considerably after the publication of data showing no immunoglobulin subclass deficiency in chronic fatigue syndrome (Bennett et al., 1996). The authors, working at the Chronic Fatigue Syndrome Cooperative Research Center of the Brigham and Women's Hospital, Boston and Harvard Medical School, compared immunoglobulin subclass levels of 46 patients with those of a control group comprising 50 healthy subjects of similar age and gender distribution. The only significant difference was a higher average level of immunoglobulin subclass 1 among chronic fatigue syndrome patients. Nevertheless, the possibility that intravenous immunoglobulin may be effective in certain adult patients with chronic fatigue syndrome could not be entirely dismissed until investigators from Australia conducted a new trial that employed a much improved research methodology (Vollmer-Conna et al., 1997).

This time, the study's inception cohort consisted of 99 patients diagnosed with chronic fatigue syndrome at the Prince Henry Hospital, Sydney, and Woden Valley Hospital, Canberra. Exclusion criteria avoided a population overlap with the authors' previous trial of intravenous immunoglobulin. The patients enrolled in the trial were not receiving corticosteroids, nonsteroidal anti-inflammatory drugs, cholinesterase inhibitors, or immunomodulatory agents (e.g., levamisole and azathioprine), were not pregnant, and did not have a history of recent bronchial asthma. Outcome variables measured at baseline and every two weeks throughout the therapeutic trial included the investigator-rated ability to perform daily activities (Karnofsky et al., 1948), visual analog scales measuring the impact of physical and neuropsychological symptoms on quality of life, the number of hours of daily nonsedentary activity, a profile of mood states, and a subjective "energy" score. Cell-mediated immunity was assessed with T-cell subset analyses and delayed-type hypersensitivity skin testing.

The 99 patients studied (76 women) had a mean age of 40 years and an average duration of the chronic fatigue syndrome of six years. The onset of the syndrome correlated with an acute "viral-like" illness in 76 percent of patients, but only 23 percent had serologic confirmation of an infectious process (Epstein-Barr virus in 19 cases, cytomegalovirus in two patients, and toxoplasmosis and varicella virus in one case each). Delayed-type hypersensitivity skin responses were decreased or absent in 48 percent of patients. A substantial majority (72 percent) of the patients in this study cohort reported significant occupational disability, including housework and school.

A random procedure allocated 26 participants to receive placebo (1 percent albumin in 10 percent maltose in water) and 73 to receive immunoglobulin. Those assigned to the immunoglobulin arm of the study were given doses of 0.5 g/kg (22 patients), 1 g/kg (28 patients), and 2 g/kg (23 patients). The placebo and immunoglobulin solutions had an identical appearance and were infused over 24 hours at monthly intervals for three months. The placebo-treated group and the three immunoglobulin-treated groups were reasonably well matched with regard to demographic, clinical, and laboratory variables.

Three patients failed to complete the required series of immunoglobulin infusions because of severe side effects. New or worsened symptoms including tiredness, headaches, and cognitive dysfunction were reported by 88 percent of the patients treated with placebo, and by 76 percent of those receiving immunoglobulin infusions. Abnormalities in liver enzymes were relatively common, mild transient elevations of the serum alanine aminotransferase being recorded in 31 percent of the placebo recipients and 30 percent of patients treated with immunoglobulin. Postinfusion phlebitis occurred in 5 percent of patients.

Treatment with immunoglobulin was not better than placebo for any of the outcome variables measured three months after the last infusion. The investigator-rated performance scores and patient-rated "energy" scores improved significantly across the patient population regardless of the treatment received. Although a reduction in symptoms was noted, the amount of daily nonsedentary activities and the severity of perceived depression, confusion, and fatigue did not show significant changes compared with pretreatment benchmarks.

Intravenous immunoglobulin was also tested in a group of 71 adolescents aged 11 to 18 years who were selected from among 100 patients evaluated at the University of Melbourne Royal Children's Hospital, Victoria, Australia (Rowe, 1997). Performed with support from the drug's manufacturer, the study enrolled subjects who met standard diagnostic criteria (Fukuda et al., 1994), had neuropsychiatric impairment evidenced by new onset of difficulty with concentration or short-term memory, and had at least three of nine specified symptoms persistently or recurrently present during the course of their illness. The nine symptoms included six listed by the standard diagnostic criteria (i.e., myalgia, arthralgia, headache, sleep disturbance, lymphadenopathy, and pharyngitis) but also abdominal pain, nausea, and dizziness whose validity for diagnostic and classification purposes was not documented by the author. Psychometric testing was used to identify patients with major psychiatric disorders who were offered appropriate referral for specialized treatment, but were not excluded from the study. The size of the group was considered sufficient to support a projected functional improvement of 66 percent in the imunoglobulin group and 33 percent in the placebo group.

The patients were randomly assigned to intravenous therapy with immunoglobulin G (1 g/kg body weight) or placebo administered three times four weeks apart. The immunoglobulin G solution had a concentration of 6 percent in a 10 percent maltose in water solution. The placebo was a 1 percent albumin solution in a 10 percent maltose in water solution, identical in appearance to the immunoglobulin preparation. Infusions were started at a rate of 15 ml/hour and increased over one hour to a maximum of 160 ml/hour. Furosemide (40 mg orally) was given with infusion volumes exceeding 500 ml. Outcome measurements relied on the investigator's assessment of functional ability with regard to school or work attendance, proportion of school or work activities attempted, and proportion of other activities (e.g., sports) endeavored. Data collection relied on interviews with the subject and a parent, and on weekly activities logs kept by them. In addition, self-scored questionnaires were used to measure quality of life and general health as well as the presence and severity of anxiety and depression. The benchmark measures were the estimated premorbid levels of activity in each of these four domains. Comprehensive assessments of the immunological function were carried out at baseline, at the end of treatment, and three months later.

Seventy of the 71 patients completed the trial; one patient was lost to follow-up. The immunoglobulin (n = 36) and placebo (n = 34) groups were similar with respect to age, gender, duration of fatigue, and degree of functional impairment. Adverse effects were common during the three-month trial and included headache (69 percent in the immunoglobulin group versus 58 percent in the placebo group), fatigue (52 percent versus 46 percent), nausea (54 percent versus 30 percent), muscle pain (38 percent versus 39 percent), difficulty with concentration (26 percent versus 26 percent), abdominal pain (26 percent versus 14 percent), dizziness (15 percent versus 6 percent), swollen glands (13 percent versus 7 percent), and sore eyes (10 percent versus 2 percent). Of great interest is the fact that 64 percent of patients experienced severe headache after the first immunoglobulin infusion, while the corresponding proportion in the placebo group was only 20 percent, a statistically significant difference that may have "unblinded" this portion of the sample. This assumption is supported by the fact that the severity of the headache associated with the immunoglobulin infusion improved over the course of the trial (i.e., after the second and third administration of the drug), while the headache that followed the placebo injections did not change its intensity over time. Moreover, severity of headache was a sensitive (but not specific) predictor of clinical improvement.

Three months after the completion of the trial, the average functional improvement compared with the baseline value was significantly higher in the immunoglobulin-treated group than among the adolescents treated with placebo. A greater than 25 percent mean functional improvement of chronic fatigue syndrome that had been present for less than 15 months was observed in 70 percent of patients treated with immunoglobulin and 50 percent of those who had received placebo, a statistically insignificant difference. In those cases in which the duration of the fatigue syndrome exceeded 15 months, improvement was noted in 75 percent of the group treated with immunoglobulin and in 38 percent of the group treated with placebo, a difference that was statistically significant. Return to the premorbid functional status was observed in 25 percent of patients treated with immunoglobulin and 11 percent of those who had received placebo. For this difference our calculation obtains a $\chi^2 = 2.02$ (df = 1, p > 0.05), indicating lack of statistical significance. Immunologic and psychiatric measures did not indicate that immunoglobulin was superior to placebo in this trial.

HYDROCORTISONE

Based on limited research data suggesting that chronic fatigue syndrome is characterized by hypocortisolemia as the result of the impaired activation of the hypothalamic-pituitary-adrenal axis (Demitrack et al., 1991), a careful trial of hydrocortisone for the treatment of chronic fatigue syndrome was recently performed by investigators from the National Institutes of Health (McKenzie et al., 1998). The goal of the study was relatively modest; to seek amelioration of the fatigue syndrome by using low-dose hormonal supplementation (30 percent more than the expected daily physiologic output) administered at intervals designed to maintain the plasma cortisol levels and approximate their diurnal variation within the limits expected for healthy individuals. The candidates for the trial were patients 18 to 55 years of age who met standard criteria for the diagnosis of chronic fatigue syndrome (Fukuda et al., 1994). Eligibility criteria included the requirements for the rapid onset of the fatigue illness (six weeks or less), the absence of any chronic physical and psychiatric condition requiring continuous or intermittent drug therapy, or medical contraindications to the use of systemic corticosteroid treatment (e.g., peptic ulcer disease, arterial hypertension, diabetes mellitus, and untreated tuberculosis).

A total of 638 individuals complaining of chronic fatigue were referred to the National Institutes of Health for possible participation in the trial, and 70 of them constituted the study group. Of the other subjects, 151 could not be given a diagnosis of chronic fatigue syndrome, 186 could not discontinue other drug therapies, 61 had medical conditions (unspecified in the published report) that precluded their participation, 14 had contraindications to systemic corticosteroid use, and two were pregnant. In addition, 30 patients indicated that their chronic fatigue syndrome had a gradual onset exceeding six weeks in duration, and 109 eligible subjects declined participation for personal reasons.

The 70 patients were randomly assigned to receive either placebo or hydrocortisone tablets for 12 weeks; the daily dose of hydrocortisone was 16 mg/square meter of body surface, which translated into a 20-30 mg dose at 8 a.m. and 5 mg at 2 p.m. The demographic characteristics of the placebo and hydrocortisone groups were similar; average age around 37 years, average duration of illness four years, and clear-cut majority of white females with substantial occupational disability. The means for resting and stimulated serum cortisol levels as well as for urinary cortisol excretion were almost identical in the two groups. Self-rating and clinician-administered questionnaires confirmed the resemblance of the groups with regard to perceived wellness, level of activity, sickness impact, profile of mood states, depressive symptoms, and formal psychiatric diagnoses.

The trial was completed by 31 patients who took placebo and 32 patients assigned to the hydrocortisone arm of the investigation. Three patients from the placebo group and two patients from the hydrocortisone group withdrew because they felt that the therapy was exacerbating the symptoms of their chronic fatigue syndrome. One patient taking placebo developed a rash and one patient assigned to take hydrocortisone decided to pursue other therapeutic options; both were dropped from the study.

Adverse effects were reported by 31 of the 35 patients (89 percent) receiving hydrocortisone and 27 of the 35 subjects (77 percent) treated with placebo. Most important, at posttreatment testing, 12 of the 32 patients who completed the 12-week treatment with low-dose hydrocortisone, but none of the patients treated with placebo, were found to have subnormal cortisol response to adrenal stimulation with cosyntropin (synthetic ACTH). In five cases, the adrenal insufficiency was severe and required a tapering regimen of hydrocortisone supplementation. Other adverse effects significantly more common among patients treated with hydrocortisone were, as expected, increased appetite (49 percent versus 23 percent), increased weight (54 percent versus 23 percent), and difficulty sleeping (49 percent versus 23 percent).

Treatment with hydrocortisone was not better than placebo for any of the variables analyzed. A "wellness score" recorded on a single-item global scale indicated self-perceived improvement of 54 percent of placebo recipients and 67 percent of subjects treated with low-dose hydrocortisone. The severity of fatigue, degree of mental confusion, change in level of activity, and the composite sickness impact profile were little changed compared with baseline and remarkably similar for the two groups at the completion of the trial. The results raise substantial doubts about the validity of the construct (Demitrack et al., 1991) that formed the basis of this trial, a point supported by the fact the patients with the lowest adrenal reserve and cortisol levels were not the most symptomatic and did not show a more favorable response to treatment with hydrocortisone.

The efficacy of hydrocortisone for the alleviation of chronic fatigue syndrome was also evaluated by British investigators from London and Cambridge, England (Cleare et al., 1999). The initial sample consisted of 218 patients with chronic fatigue who had registered for care with academic outpatient clinics specializing in the evaluation and management of chronic fatigue syndrome. After a thorough clinical and laboratory evaluation the investigators identified a cohort of 32 patients that met standard diagnostic criteria for chronic fatigue syndrome (Fukuda et al., 1994); had been ill for more than eight years; had no concurrent psychiatric disorder; had no evidence of hypocortisolism or adrenal autoantibodies; and had no demonstrable medical disorders contraindicating treatment with hydrocortisone. The subjects (20 women and 12 men) had a mean age of 35 years. The onset of illness was considered by 19 patients (59 percent) to be related to an infection. A history of psychiatric disorder was recorded in nine cases (28 percent).

The trial required random assignment to treatment with hydrocortisone or placebo for 28 days, after which the subjects crossed over to the other treatment for an equal period of time. The first 16 patients entered in the trial were treated with a daily morning dose of 5 mg of hydrocortisone; the second group of 16 patients received 10 mg of hydrocortisone each day. Outcome measurements were based on data recorded at baseline and the end of each of the two treatment periods and consisted of a self-administered fatigue scale, a clinician-administered global improvement scale, and measures of disability and quality of life. The presence of treatment-induced adrenal insufficiency was evaluated with a standardized insulin stress test and 24-hour urinary free cortisol levels.

Adverse drug reactions were reported by two patients (6 percent) during the hydrocortisone phase of the trial and consisted of exacerbation of acne and nervousness. One patient had a fainting spell while being treated with placebo. None of the 32 patients withdrew from the study and the treatment with hydrocortisone did not have a measurable suppressive effect on the adrenal gland function.

Hydrocortisone was significantly better than placebo in reducing the self-scored severity of fatigue. This effect occurred with both dosages of hydrocortisone (5 and 10 mg daily) and was not affected by whether the hydrocortisone was the first or the second treatment during the trial. A clinically significant decrease in fatigue, i.e., a reduction of at least 30 percent in severity, was recorded for 11 patients (34 percent) after treatment with hydrocortisone but only in four patients (13 percent) at the end of the placebo phase of the trial, a statistically significant difference. In contrast, clinician evaluations using a global impression scale identified improvement in seven patients (21 percent) after hydrocortisone therapy and in two patients (6 percent) at the end of the placebo phase, a difference devoid of statistical significance. The severity of disability decreased only after treatment with hydrocortisone, but the quality of life measure did not indicate a significant improvement in functional activities. The modest clinical relevance and the potential lack of specificity justified the authors' conclusion that hydrocortisone should not be considered a treatment modality for chronic fatigue syndrome.

FISH AND PLANT OILS

A combination of concentrated fish oil and oil extracted from the seeds of evening primrose (*Oenothera* sp.) was tested as a therapeutic agent for patients with "postviral fatigue syndrome" by investigators from the University of Glasgow, Scotland and Scotia Pharmaceuticals, Guildford, Surrey, England, the product's manufacturer (Behan, Behan, and Horrobin, 1990). The study group comprised patients who had experienced overwhelming fatigue that was worsened by exercise, myalgias, cognitive dysfunction manifested as poor concentration and impaired short-term memory, depression, palpitations, shooting chest pains, and unsteadiness for at least one year. A febrile illness with upper respiratory or gastrointestinal symptoms was identified as the precipitating event in all cases. The type and number of symptoms included in this description are substantially different than the standard criteria for the diagnosis of chronic fatigue syndrome in the United States, as defined at the time of the study's publication (Holmes et al., 1988).

Sixty-three patients (36 women and 27 men) participated in the trial and were randomly assigned to receive capsules of either placebo, which consisted of 50 mg of linoleic acid in liquid paraffin and 10 international units of vitamin E as an antioxidant, or a mixture of fish oil and oil from seeds of evening primrose, which was known to contain 36 mg of gamma-linolenic acid, 17 mg of eicosapentanoic acid, 11 mg of docosahexanoic acid, 255 mg of linolenic acid, and 10 international units of vitamin E. The daily dose was eight capsules, and patients were instructed to swallow them whole. The authors indicate that ingested as intact capsules, the product did not produce potentially unblinding fishy taste or smell sensations. The investigators used two outcome measures, a symptom severity score, which combined self-assessed intensity of fatigue, myalgia, dizziness, poor concentration, and depression, and an overall appraisal regarding the status of the condition as better, worse, or unchanged. Data were obtained at baseline and after one and three months of treatment.

The combination of fish and plant oil was better than placebo with regard to both the overall change in condition and the severity of the symptoms selected as outcome variables. After one month of treatment, 74 percent of patients treated with the combination of organic oils felt that their condition had improved, as compared with 23 percent of the placebo-treated group. At the end of the three-month period, the proportion of patients feeling better overall increased to 85 percent in the group receiving the organic oils, but decreased to 17 percent in the placebo group. The global symptoms' severity score decreased after both the organic oils and the placebo treatments, but the difference between the magnitude of the changes indicate the statistical superiority of the organic oils. Compared with placebo, most improved were myalgia, fatigue, and dizziness. Laboratory investigations indicated that the concentration of phospholipids in the red cell membrane, which was decreased at baseline, returned to normal or near normal after treatment with the organic oils administered in this trial.

The authors did not identify the mechanism through which the organic oils with a high concentration of free fatty acids improved the symptoms of patients with chronic fatigue syndrome, and produced no direct evidence that the treatment reduced cytokine production or inhibited replication of viruses. Moreover, although recent research supports a role for free fatty acids in the symptomatic treatment of rheumatoid arthritis (Lau, Morley, and Belch, 1993; Zurier et al., 1996) mediated by a decrease in the concentration of proinflammatory prostaglandins and leukotrienes (Lau, Morley, and Belch, 1993), an active inflammatory process has not been demonstrated in patients with chronic fatigue syndrome.

The confirmation of the therapeutic role of essential fatty acids was attempted by investigators from the University of Sheffield, Northern General and Central Sheffield University Hospitals, Sheffield, United Kingdom (Warren, McKendrick, and Peet, 1999). The study group comprised 50 of 98 consecutive referrals to a regional infectious diseases clinic that were diagnosed as having chronic fatigue syndrome according to the British criteria (Sharpe et al., 1991). The eligible patients were randomly assigned to treatment with capsules containing placebo or the same preparation of evening primrose oil and concentrated fish oil as that used by Behan, Behan, and Horrobin, (1990). The placebo capsule contained sunflower oil, which included 335 mg of linoleic acid but no traceable amounts of eicosapentanoic and docosahexanoic acids. Both types of capsules were colored identically with a small quantity of riboflavine. The treatment consisted of one capsule four times daily for three months. Outcome measurements relied upon monthly self-assessments of physical symptoms (i.e., severity ratings for fatigue, myalgia, dizziness, difficulty with concentration, and depression) and depressive symptomatology.

The treatments were tolerated without any reported adverse effects. Five patients from each of the two treatment groups dropped out because of lack of change in their condition. The trial demonstrated no difference whatsoever between placebo and the combination of primrose and fish oils on the physical and depressive symptomatology of this population of patients with chronic fatigue syndrome.

Chapter 3

Ineffective Therapies

FLUOXETINE

Although selective serotonin reuptake inhibitors are probably commonly prescribed for patients with chronic fatigue syndrome, the two valid studies published thus far have shown the absence of demonstrable improvement (Vercoulen et al., 1996; Wearden et al., 1998). Both studies used fluoxetine, a phenylpropylamine-derivative with a *p*-trifluoromethyl substituent on the molecule, which is considered responsible for the drug's remarkable potency and selectivity for decreasing the reuptake of serotonin at the presynaptic neuronal membrane (American Hospital Formulary Service, 1997, p. 1694).

The first trial was conducted by a multidisciplinary group based in the outpatient clinic of the Department of General Internal Medicine, University Hospital, Nijmegen, Netherlands (Vercoulen et al., 1996). Patients were recruited in a manner that attempted to select equal numbers of subjects with and without a comorbid diagnosis of major depressive disorder. Depressed patients had to have a score of 16 or more on the Beck Depression Inventory (Beck et al., 1961), indicating moderate to severe depression, while nondepressed patients were required to have a score of ten or less on the same inventory, a finding consistent with the absence of depressive symptoms. The investigators were appropriately careful to exclude the symptoms of fatigue and lack of energy from among the symptoms counted toward the diagnosis of major depression as well as the calculation of the depression inventory score. All patients had a history of fatigue resulting in significant impairment of daily activities for at least one year. None of the patients had physical illnesses known to produce fatigue or psychiatric disorders other than major depression. Patients taking any psychotropic medications or receiving psychotherapy were not included in the trial.

Depressed and nondepressed patients with chronic fatigue syndrome were randomly assigned to take either placebo or 20 mg fluoxetine daily for eight weeks. Self-administered and objective measurements were performed during three 12-day periods: prior to starting the trial, prior to the end of the trial, and eight weeks after the completion of the trial. The variables recorded were the subjective feeling of fatigue, the severity of depression, the impact of the fatigue illness in major areas of daily functioning, physical activity as registered continuously by a motion-sensing device, quality and quantity of sleep, neuropsychological functioning (memory, concentration, speed of information processing, reaction time, and motor speed), the quality of social interactions, and the sense of control over symptoms. The type and severity of side effects experienced during placebo and fluoxetine were recorded after two weeks, six weeks, and eight weeks of treatment.

A total of 107 chronic fatigue syndrome patients started the trial; 48 patients had a comorbid diagnosis of major depressive disorder. Nine of the 54 patients (15 percent) assigned to the fluoxetine arm of the study stopped their participation because of new symptoms attributed to the drug. The side effects occurring in more than one patient each were skin reactions (three patients), nausea (two patients), and headache (two patients). Two patients assigned to the placebo arm of the study withdrew after developing similar side effects (skin reaction, headache). The 96 patients who completed the trial were divided into the following four groups: placebo/nondepressed (28 patients); placebo/depressed (23 patients); fluoxetine/nondepressed (28 patients); and fluoxetine/depressed (21 patients). These groups were similar with regard to age, predominance of females, duration of illness, and proportion of patients on sick leave or receiving long-term disability benefits. Compliance was assessed with plasma fluoxetine levels and was found to be perfect; the median concentration was 40 mg/liter, and no fluoxetine was detected in any of the patients in the placebo group.

None of the patients reported complete recovery at the end of the eight-week trial or at follow-up two months later. The proportion of patients who considered themselves to have improved at the end of the trial ranged from 5 percent in the fluoxetine/depressed group to 13 percent in the placebo/depressed group; the corresponding proportions at the two-month follow-up ranged from 7 percent in the placebo/nondepressed group to 21 percent in the fluoxetine/nondepressed group. The intergroup differences did not reach statistical significance. However, more patients given fluoxetine were likely to report feeling worse after treatment: 38 percent of patients in the fluoxetine/depressed group and 35 percent of patients in the fluoxetine/nondepressed group deteriorated as compared to 26 percent of the placebo/depressed patients and only 14 percent in the placebo/nondepressed group. None of the individual primary outcome measures improved after either fluoxetine or placebo treatments. At most, fluoxetine was demonstrated to produce a 3 percent improvement in fatigue and a 2 percent improvement in the severity of depression, a clinically meaningless change. The unexpected lack of improvement of depression was confirmed by subsequent analyses of the affective, cognitive, and somatic features of depression; taken separately, none of these subsets showed any significant change after treatment.

The disappointing performance of fluoxetine in chronic fatigue syndrome identified by the Dutch investigators was confirmed by researchers from the University of Manchester and Withington Hospital, Manchester and Royal Preston Hospital, Preston, United Kingdom (Wearden et al., 1998). The study was executed with limited technical support from the drug's manufacturer. The trial compared the effect of placebo to that of fluoxetine and graded exercise.

The study cohort was drawn from consecutive referrals for evaluation to the academic outpatient clinic from England and Wales. The diagnosis of chronic fatigue syndrome was established after a comprehensive clinical and laboratory evaluation according to the British research criteria (Sharpe et al., 1991), which required a chief complaint of fatigue of at least six months duration, significant impairment in at least three out of four principal areas of activity, and the absence of another medical cause of fatigue. Excluded from consideration were subjects with any one of a number of psychiatric conditions (schizophrenia, bipolar disorder, eating disorder, substance use disorder) or symptoms (suicidal ideation) and ischemic heart disease. Patients taking antidepressant drugs at the time of recruitment in the study underwent an appropriate washout period prior to taking the study medication. Overall, the authors screened 227 patients and found 165 to be eligible for the trial.

The pharmacologic component of the trial required the administration of 20 mg of fluoxetine daily for six months to 35 randomly selected patients and identical-looking placebo capsule to 34 subjects. With regard to physical activity, these patients were encouraged to do what they could when they felt able and to refrain from activity when they felt weary and in need of rest. A third group of patients ($n = 33$) received the same amount of fluoxetine and followed a daily exercise protocol designed to reach 75 percent of the subjects' tested functional maximum as measured by oxygen consumption. A fourth group ($n = 34$) was treated with graded exercise and placebo. Assessments and outcome measures included scales for the severity of fatigue; the degree of functional impairment and general well-being; the severity of anxiety and depression; muscle strength; and functional work capacity determined by oxygen utilization and carbon dioxide production under standard experimental conditions.

The trial was completed by 71 percent of the subjects. The dropout rate was 36 percent among patients assigned to receive fluoxetine and 24 percent among subjects treated with placebo. Nine (13 percent) of the 68 patients treated with fluoxetine and two (3 percent) of the 69 patients treated with placebo withdrew because of adverse effects of medication. Unfortunately, a description of the side effects leading to the discontinuation of the study medication was not provided in the report. The demographic and clinical characteristics of patients who completed the trial were similar to those who dropped out.

Placebo and fluoxetine groups were well matched with regard to gender distribution (proportion of women ranging from 67 percent to 79 percent), mean age (ranging from 38.2 to 40.4 years), and average duration of fatigue (ranging from 22 to 34 months). At baseline, the anxiety and depression scores, exercise tolerance, and self-perceived severity of fatigue were, on average, similar among the four treatment groups. More than 80 percent of patients in each group had to change occupation to accommodate the limitations imposed on them by their fatigue illness, 34 percent of patients had an active depressive disorder, 10 percent suffered from an anxiety disorder, and 2 percent were given the diagnosis of somatization disorder.

Fluoxetine had no effect on the subjective severity of fatigue or on the functional capacity measured objectively after 12 and 26 weeks of therapy. The drug led to a significant improvement in the depression scores after 12 weeks of treatment, but the effect was no longer detectable at the end of the 26-week trial. Analysis by intention-to-treat produced results similar to those observed among the subjects who completed the trial.

The lack of effect of selective serotonin reuptake inhibitors in patients with chronic fatigue syndrome is not surprising, because a serotonergic deficiency has never been demonstrated in this condition. Assessments of this nature are possible by performing a fenfluramine challenge, which promotes the release of serotonin from presynaptic nerve endings, prevents serotonin reuptake, and stimulates the postsynaptic serotonin receptors; the overall consequence in normal individuals is a substantial increase in central serotonin activity, which results in measurable increases of prolactin and cortisol levels, while in untreated depressed individuals these responses are attenuated or absent (Siever et al., 1984; O'Keane and Dinan, 1991; Cleare, Murray, and O'Keane, 1996). A recent study conducted at Dalhousie University, Halifax, Nova Scotia, has compared the response to *dl*-fenfluramine in patients with chronic fatigue syndrome (45 percent of whom had a past history or current diagnosis of major depression) and age- and gender-matched healthy control subjects (Yatham et al., 1995). Baseline and 60 mg oral fenfluramine-induced hormonal responses were similar in the patient and control groups. The severity of depression in the chronic fatigue syndrome group did not correlate with the hormonal responses to the fenfluramine administration. These findings were confirmed in a larger patient population by investigators from Maudsley Hospital and King's College Hospital, London (Cleare et al., 1995). The authors compared the response to the administration of 30 mg of fenfluramine in three groups: subjects with chronic fatigue syndrome, patients with major depression, and healthy control subjects matched with the other groups for age, gender, weight, and stage of menstrual cycle. Compared with the healthy control group, prolactin response to the serotonergic-activating challenge was significantly decreased among patients with major depression but increased in the chronic fatigue syndrome group. Conversely, cortisol levels increased in the major depression group and decreased in the chronic fatigue syndrome group as compared with the healthy control subjects. Finally, a recent report from the University Department of Psychiatry, Warneford and Littlemore Hospitals, Oxford, United Kingdom, has presented the results of *dl*-fenfluramine (30 mg orally) in ten men with chronic fatigue syndrome and a similar number of age-matched healthy volunteers. The prolactin response following the fenfluramine administration was significantly higher among the chronic fatigue syndrome patients. Together, these studies emphasize that serotonergic deficiency is not likely to be a contributor to the pathophysiology of chronic fatigue syndrome and that drugs designed to correct such a deficiency have no reasonable place in the management of these patients.

Chapter 4

Unreplicated Trials

PHENELZINE

The effect of phenelzine, a hydrazine derivative with a well-characterized inhibitory effect on monoamine oxidase leading to increased concentrations of serotonin, norepinephrine, and dopamine availability in the central nervous system (American Hospital Formulary Service, 1997, p. 1668), on the clinical manifestations of CFS was studied in a small placebo-controlled study conducted at the New Jersey Medical School in East Orange, New Jersey, with financial support from the drug's manufacturer (Natelson et al., 1996). The authors' working assumption at the onset of the trial was that CFS may represent a state of decreased sympathetic stimulation leading to the sensitization of the adrenergic receptors, which results in symptoms similar to those produced by the administration of reserpine, a potent sympathoblocking agent. Although the clinical uses of phenelzine have relied on its proven antidepressant effects, the study was designed to use phenelzine dosages (15 mg daily) "well below those used to treat depression" (Natelson et al., 1996, p. 226). In an independent verification of this statement, we were indeed able to confirm that published prospective trials have used daily dosages of phenelzine that ranged from 45 mg to 90 mg, and that higher doses work faster and are considerably more effective (Tyrer et al., 1980; Thase et al., 1992).

The study enrolled 24 patients who met the standard definition of the syndrome (Fukuda et al., 1994). At the time of the study, the subjects were followed at the university's specialized unit and had already had comprehensive evaluations that established the absence of "serious" psychiatric disorders. Care was taken to ensure that none of the subjects were pregnant and that all participants were willing and able to follow dietary and drug restrictions required during treatment with monoamine oxidase inhibitors. After enrollment, all subjects received placebo for two weeks, after which they were randomly assigned to the phenelzine or placebo groups. The phenelzine was administered at a dose of 15 mg every other day (alternating with placebo) for two weeks and 15 mg every day during the final two weeks of the trial. Measurements were performed using six standardized multitask instruments: a functional status questionnaire, a profile of mood status, a depression questionnaire, an illness severity scale, a fatigue severity scale, and a checklist recording the severity of symptoms. The instruments contained 20 separate tests which were administered at baseline, after the initial two-week period of treatment with placebo and then four weeks later at the completion of the trial.

Six patients were withdrawn before the end of the study; three subjects dropped out because of phenelzine-related side effects while taking the 15 mg daily dose, two patients withdrew during the placebo phase, and one patient was dropped out because of lack of compliance. The phenelzine group comprised nine women with an average age of 38 years, while the placebo group consisted of six women and three men with an average age of 31 years.

Phenelzine was no better than placebo on any of the variables tested individually. However, the authors indicate that a "pattern of improvement" was apparent from the fact that phenelzine-treated patients showed improvement on 11 of the 20 tests used, while for the placebo-treated patients, similar improvement was obtained for only five of the 20 measures. On the other hand, a plurality of placebo-treated patients indicated worsening on four tests; none of the tests used indicated posttreatment worsening in the phenelzine group. Depressive symptoms improved to a similar extent in both groups, supporting the study's hypothesis that the possible therapeutic effect of low dose phenelzine in chronic fatigue syndrome is not explained by its antidepressant properties.

SELEGILINE

The investigation of a possible role for monoamine oxidase inhibitors in the treatment of chronic fatigue syndrome was continued by the researchers based at the New Jersey Medical School with a clinical trial of low-dose selegiline performed with financial support from the drug's manufacturer (Natelson et al., 1998). Selegiline is a selective monoamine oxidase type B inhibitor used mostly as an antiparkinsonian agent, which also has antidepressant properties at dosages ranging from 30 to 60 mg daily (Mann et al., 1989; Sunderland et al., 1994). The study was designed as a single-blind trial; the patients were informed that for a portion of the six-week period of treatment they would receive placebo, but the duration and timing of the placebo administration was not disclosed.

A total of 25 patients were enrolled in the trial using diagnostic standards and inclusion and exclusion criteria identical to those employed in the clinical trial of phenelzine analyzed earlier in this chapter (Natelson et al., 1996). As in the phenelzine trial just described, six assessment vehicles with 19 individual tests were used to measure the presence and severity of fatigue and associated symptoms, the mental health, depressive symptomatology and mood states, and functional and disability status. All patients were given one placebo tablet twice daily during the first two weeks of the trial. During the third and fourth weeks of the study the patients took one 5 mg selegiline tablet and one placebo tablet each day. Finally, during the fifth and sixth week all patients were treated with 5 mg of selegiline twice daily. Outcome measurements were carried out at baseline, after the two-week placebo period and after the four-week escalating selegiline treatment period.

Only 19 of the 25 patients completed the trial; six patients dropped out before the end of the placebo period. The findings indicated selegiline-induced improvement in tension/anxiety, vigor, and sexual relations. However, these three variables stood among 12 unimproved variables on two of the instruments used (profile of mood states and functional status questionnaire). Moreover, none of the variables tested by the other four instruments showed a statistically significant therapeutic effect of selegiline. It was also clear that selegiline did not produce measurable changes in function. However, the authors claim to have detected a "pattern of improvement" in the fact that during the treatment with selegiline a plurality of patients had improved on 11 of the 19 tests used and appeared worse on one test, while treatment with placebo produced improvement for a similar plurality on only four tests and worsened the condition according to the results of six of the 19 tests. This "pattern of improvement" did not correlate with changes in the severity of depressive symptoms.

The analysis of these two research reports does not support a therapeutic role for low-dose monoamine inhibitors phenelzine or selegiline in patients with chronic fatigue syndrome. The patient populations were small and the issue of statistical power was not explicitly addressed. The selegiline study was not double-blinded and lacked a continuous placebo-control group. Most importantly, neither drug produced measurable improvements in the major clinical manifestations of the syndrome and did not lead to a change for the better in functional status. Finally, the "pattern of improvement" ostensibly identified by the authors for both drugs is meaningless because it took into account "any improvement at all." This defies basic rules of interpretation of evidence since it exaggerates the importance of marginal differences and affirms improvement despite any change in the clinical features of the syndrome and the burden of illness it creates.

POLY(I)-POLY(C12U)

Poly(I)-Poly(C12U) is described by its manufacturer as a specifically configured double-stranded ribonucleic acid (RNA) whose hypothetical utility in chronic fatigue syndrome is based on the compound's ability to restore 2-5A synthetase/Rnase L antiviral defense mechanism (Suhadolnik et al., 1994). At the time of this writing, the compound had not received the Food and Drug Administration's approval for marketing but is available for research and also for compassionate use on a cost-recovery basis. The only placebo-controlled trial of Poly(I)-Poly(C12U) was designed and paid for by its manufacturer and the list of authors of the published report included the codiscoverer of the compound and other employees of the manufacturing company who collaborated with clinical investigators from the University of Oregon in Portland, Oregon, and private practices located in Houston, Texas; Charlotte, North Carolina; and Incline Village, Nevada (Strayer et al., 1994).

The investigators recruited 92 subjects who fulfilled diagnostic criteria for chronic fatigue syndrome (Holmes et al., 1988) for at least one year prior to entry and were severely debilitated by their illness. A randomization process that stratified the patients according to their functional performance status was used to assign subjects to receive twice-weekly intravenous infusions of either Poly(I)-Poly(C12U) or an equivalent amount of saline for 24 consecutive weeks. In the first two weeks of treatment Poly(I)-Poly(C12U) was administered as a 200 mg dose; for the remainder of the trial the dose was increased to 400 mg. Baseline and outcome measures included assessments, made with well-validated instruments, of functional ability, cognitive deficits, and psychiatric symptoms as well as objective measurements of exercise tolerance. Concomitant medication use was carefully recorded throughout the trial.

The placebo and Poly(I)-Poly(C12U) groups were well-matched with regard to age, duration of the fatigue illness and degree of functional disability and cognitive dysfunction, number of symptoms of anxiety and depression, and prevalence of past history of depression and abnormalities on the magnetic resonance imaging of the brain. A substantial majority of patients (80 percent) indicated a sudden onset of their syndrome. Physical findings of cervical or axillary lymphadenopathy, nonexudative pharyngitis, and fever were present in most patients. The only notable difference between the groups was a higher number of women (85 percent versus 64 percent) assigned to receive placebo.

Eight (9 percent) patients (four from each group) withdrew prematurely from the trial; the reason was either the intensification of the chronic fatigue illness experience claimed by three patients assigned to receive placebo and one patient receiving Poly(I)-Poly(C12U) or a nonmedical reason. Twenty-three patients treated with Poly(I)-Poly (C12U) and 18 patients treated with placebo missed doses of medication, but in no case were the numbers of missed doses greater than six. Adverse effects were common; the 45 patients assigned to receive Poly(I)-Poly(C12U) reported 706 events as compared with 711 events reported by the 47 patients treated with placebo. Unfortunately, the list of adverse effects was not included in the publication. Mention is made of "several patients" who developed severe adverse effects during treatment with Poly(I)-Poly(C12U), but clinical data is provided only for two of these cases, indicating abdominal pain, tachycardia, and significant hepatic toxicity in one patient and localized areas of swelling and itching in another. Reports of flu-like symptoms, a known side effect of Poly(I)-Poly(C12U), were similarly prevalent in the two treatment groups.

Treatment with Poly(I)-Poly(C12U) was statistically better than placebo with regard to functional status, perceived cognitive dysfunction, and exercise tolerance. However, the clinical significance of some of these changes appears, at best, minimal. For example, exercise intensity increased 12 percent after 26 weeks of treatment with Poly(I)-Poly(C12U) and 6 percent after treatment with placebo, suggesting a drug-related net increase of only 6 percent, a change that is not likely to influence the daily activity level. The primary end point, i.e., the score on a standardized performance scale, increased by 20 percent in the group treated with Poly(I)-Poly(C12U) and remained unchanged in the placebo group. The authors describe the effect as "modest" but go on to indicate that in some patients the change may mean again being able to perform independently most of the activities of daily living.

NICOTINAMIDE ADENINE DINUCLEOTIDE

Nicotinamide, a water-soluble B complex vitamin, forms the structural basis of two coenzymes, nicotinamide adenine dinucleotide and nicotinamide dinucleotide phosphate with well-defined roles as hydrogen-carrier molecules necessary for glycogenolysis, cellular utilization of oxygen, and lipid metabolism (American Hospital Formulary Services, 1997, p. 2811). The therapeutic effects of the reduced form of nicotinamide adenine dinucleotide (NADH) have been tested in a sample of patients with chronic fatigue syndrome by a group of investigators from the Georgetown University School of Medicine in a collaboration that included financial support from the compound's manufacturer (Forsyth et al., 1999). The authors do not provide a plausible biological justification for the way in which NADH may affect the fatigue and cognitive dysfunction, except to state their belief that a depletion of cellular adenosine triphosphate may be the basic "metabolic lesion" in this condition.

Support for this belief is said to be provided by the authors' open-label trials of NADH in patients with Parkinson's disease (Birkmayer et al., 1989) and Alzheimer's dementia (Birkmayer, 1996), yet at least in Parkinson's disease double-blind testing has not confirmed that NADH is better than placebo (Dizdar, Kagedal, and Lindvall, 1994).

The authors recruited 35 patients who fulfilled the current diagnostic criteria of chronic fatigue syndrome (Fukuda et al., 1994) and also had at least two signs from among low-grade fever, nonexudative pharyngitis, and palpable or tender cervical or axillary lymph nodes. Patients treated with antidepressants, lithium, and neuroleptics were not included in the study group. Extensive testing was carried out to identify the presence of viral infections and immunologic dysfunction and to measure the oxidoreductase enzyme activity. After confirmation of eligibility, the subjects were randomly assigned to a four-week treatment period with a stabilized, orally absorbable preparation of NADH (10 mg daily) or placebo. This period was followed by a four-week washout interval, after which the patients were treated with the alternate agent for four weeks. The therapeutic effectiveness was judged on the basis of severity ratings generated by a 50-item questionnaire self-administered at baseline and after four, eight, and twelve weeks into the trial.

Two of the 35 initial participants were noncompliant with the study protocol and were withdrawn. With the exception of occasional reports of loss of appetite, heartburn, flatulence, and dry mouth and unpleasant taste, the treatments with NADH and placebo were well tolerated.

After the completion of the trial, data generated by nine (26 percent) patients treated concomitantly with psychotropic agents were not analyzed. Among the remaining 26 patients, improvement of the fatigue syndrome, defined as a modest 10 percent reduction of the global severity of symptoms, was recorded for 31 percent of subjects after treatment with NADH but in only 8 percent after the placebo phase of the study, a statistically significant difference. The response to treatment did not correlate with immunologic status or oxidoreductase activity.

MAGNESIUM

The effect of intramuscular injections of magnesium sulfate on the symptoms and general well-being of patients with chronic fatigue syndrome was studied by investigators affiliated with the Medical School, University of Southampton, Southampton General Hospital and the Centre for the Study of Complementary Medicine, Southampton, United Kingdom (Cox, Campbell, and Dowson, 1991). The authors hypothesized a beneficial role of magnesium based on three evidentiary sources: their knowledge of anecdotal clinical experiences; their view of chronic fatigue syndrome as a condition whose symptoms (e.g., anorexia, nausea, learning disability, personality changes, weakness, and myalgia) are similar to those of magnesium deficiency; and their pilot data indicating lower concentrations of red blood cell magnesium in patients with chronic fatigue syndrome as compared with healthy age- and sex-matched control subjects (average difference 0.1 mmol/l). The patients recruited for the trial fulfilled standard diagnostic criteria (Holmes et al., 1988) and were enrolled if their illness had a duration of between six and 18 months. The subjects were informed that they would be given either an "active" or an "alternative" treatment and then were randomly assigned to receive six weekly intramuscular injections of two cubic centimeters of a 50 percent solution of magnesium sulfate or sterile water. The patients had the option of receiving the second through the sixth injection from the investigators' assistants or from their general practitioner, but most chose the former. Main measurements performed at baseline and one week after the completion of the trial used a self-report instrument scoring the level of energy, severity of pain, sleep patterns, physical mobility, emotional reactions, and sense of social isolation.

A total of 38 patients were recruited and 34 were found eligible for the study and randomized to the two therapeutic arms of the trial. Two patients assigned to receive magnesium were withdrawn; one developed a generalized rash and the other could not obtain the full cooperation of his physician. Therefore, the trial was completed by 15 patients treated with injections of magnesium sulfate and 17 patients receiving intramuscular injections of sterile water. At baseline, the groups were similar with regard to demographic characteristics, average scores for the six clinical dimensions measured, and magnesium concentrations in plasma, red blood cells, and whole blood.

Twelve of the 15 patients (80 percent) treated with magnesium and three of the 17 subjects (18 percent) who received placebo considered themselves improved, a difference that reached statistical significance. The patients' perception was confirmed by findings indicating substantial improvement for three of the six dimensions assessed, i.e., level of energy, severity of pain, and emotional stability. The red blood cell concentration of magnesium increased by an average of 0.57 mmol/l in the group treated with weekly injection of magnesium, but decreased by an average of 0.018 mmol/l in the placebo group. The red blood cell magnesium levels were within the normal range in all of the patients treated with magnesium but in only one of the patients who had been treated with placebo.

The careful interpretation of these data findings is of utmost importance, because this is the first pharmacologic trial to claim unequivocal benefit for patients with chronic fatigue syndrome. The authors recognized that the small size of the patient population and the short duration of the clinical follow-up limited the strength of their findings. However, we are intrigued by the fact that the data have not stimulated efforts to duplicate the relatively straightforward and safe design of this trial. We can only speculate that this reluctance is based on data originating from four different laboratories showing that the concentration of magnesium is normal in patients with chronic fatigue syndrome (Gantz, 1991; Deulofeu et al., 1991; Clague, Edwards, and Jackson, 1992; Hinds et al., 1994). In addition, studies using intravenous loading with magnesium have been unable to demonstrate that chronic fatigue syndrome is a magnesium-deficient state (Clague, Edwards, and Jackson, 1992; Hinds et al., 1994). Moreover, it appears that the design of the study was faulty, because the intramuscular injections of magnesium sulfate were likely to produce significantly more pain than injections of sterile water. The 50 percent solution of magnesium sulfate has an osmolality of 2620 mOsm/kg by freezing point depression and 2875 mOsm/kg by vapor pressure (Trissel, 1990), i.e., about nine times greater than the osmolality of human biological fluids; in contrast, sterile water for injection contains no added buffer or any other type of solute (Abbott Laboratories, 1990). Experimental data have conclusively shown that hypertonic saline solutions produce significantly more pain than isotonic solutions, and that the difference between the two types of solutions is associated with an increase in the intramuscular concentration of magnesium (Graven-Nielsen et al., 1997). Thus, the design of the study conducted by Cox, Campbell, and Dowson (1991) had the obvious potential of unblinding the recipients to the fact that injections of hypertonic magnesium sulfate were pain-producing and therefore constituted the "active" treatment.

ACYCLOVIR

The antiviral drug acyclovir was tried for the treatment of chronic fatigue syndrome by a group of investigators from the National Institutes of Health and the Children's Hospital of Philadelphia, with partial financial support from the drug's manufacturer (Straus, Dale, Tobi, et al., 1988). The drug is the compound acycloguanosine, a synthetic analog of purine nucleoside derived from guanosine, which is effective against herpes viruses by inhibiting the viral DNA synthesis and subsequent replication of these intracellular infecting organisms (American Hospital Formulary Service, 1997, p. 2678). The study presented here was started in 1984 and completed in 1986, a period during which the Epstein-Barr virus was considered to have a major etiologic role in producing the prolonged illnesses later named chronic fatigue syndrome.

The authors chose acyclovir because it was a "safe drug that inhibits the replication of Epstein-Barr virus in vitro and in vivo" (Straus, Dale, Tobi, et al., 1988, p. 1693). The clinical data available at the time consisted of two publications reporting the drug's effect on symptoms and signs of acute infectious mononucleosis. In the first of these studies, ten patients with relatively severe infectious mononucleosis received a five-day course of acyclovir intravenously at eight-hour intervals to a total daily dosage of 1500 mg/square meter and ten patients were treated with placebo (Pagano, Sixbey, and Lin, 1983). The results showed that the administration of acyclovir temporarily interrupted virus excretion in the oropharynx and was associated with more rapid regain of weight, but did not affect the presence and severity of fever, lethargy, pharyngitis, lymphadenopathy, and splenomegaly. The second publication described 31 patients with infectious mononucleosis symptomatic for one week or less who were randomized to receive intravenous acyclovir (10 mg/kg) or placebo at eight-hour intervals for seven days (Andersson et al., 1986). Acyclovir reversibly inhibited the oropharyngeal shedding of the Epstein-Barr virus and improved the combined burden of fever, weight loss, tonsillar swelling, and pharyngitis. However, individual symptoms did not change significantly in the acyclovir-treated group.

For their study of acyclovir treatment of chronic fatigue syndrome the authors had access to patients with debilitating fatigue referred for evaluation to the National Institutes of Health. The 27 patients enrolled in the trial fulfilled standard diagnostic criteria (Holmes et al., 1988), had no other medical diagnosis, and had titers of antibodies to the early antigens of Epstein-Barr virus equal or greater than 1:40. These criteria were thought to identify a population in which a potentially active Epstein-Barr virus was likely to contribute to the mechanism and course of the syndrome.

The patients were randomly assigned to receive placebo or acyclovir. First, intravenous placebo or acyclovir 500 mg/square meter of body surface diluted in 150 ml of normal saline solution was infused over 60 minutes every eight hours for seven days. This phase was immediately followed by a 30-day period during which the patients took placebo or 800 mg acyclovir four times daily. After a six-week washout the participants received the alternate treatment. The patients recorded daily their oral temperature, levels of activity and energy, sense of wellness, and adverse effects. Once a week, the participants also completed a questionnaire assessing depression, anxiety, fatigue, vigor, confusion, and anger. Frequent urinalyses and hematologic and biochemical tests were used to detect signs of acyclovir toxicity.

The 27 patients (19 women and 8 men) had a mean age of 34 years and had been ill with chronic fatigue syndrome for an average of 6.8 years. All of the patients were well-educated white individuals described by the authors to be of "relatively high socioeconomic status." Twelve patients (44 percent) were vocationally disabled and ten (37 percent) were working part-time. In all cases, the fatigue syndrome followed an acute febrile illness; in six patients, this illness was heterophil-positive acute infectious mononucleosis. At entry into the trial, the group's most common symptoms other than fatigue were sore throat (96 percent), difficulty with concentration (93 percent), headache (89 percent) and tender lymph nodes (81 percent).

Side effects were common. Three patients developed acyclovir-induced renal failure and had to be withdrawn from the study. Data regarding this adverse outcome were published separately and indicated that the nephrotoxicity developed as a complication of the high-dose intravenous acyclovir administration (Sawyer et al., 1988). Despite precautions designed to avoid volume contraction in these cases, polarizing microscopy of the urinary sediments revealed leukocytes containing birefringent needle-shaped crystals. In the most severe case, the serum creatinine concentration reached a high of 8.6 mg/dl; a percutaneous renal biopsy showed foci of interstitial inflammation without tubular necrosis. All patients recovered and later received oral acyclovir without adverse effects. Compared with placebo, other adverse effects more common during the acyclovir trial were gastrointestinal symptoms (23 versus eight episodes), dizziness (seven versus three episodes), and headache (five versus one episode). Intravenous acyclovir was also associated with a significant increase in the erythrocyte sedimentation rate.

Of the 24 patients who completed the trial, four (17 percent) reported improvement that persisted for at least one year. This favorable change occurred during the placebo phase in three of these four subjects. Overall, 21 patients reported improvement during one treatment phase, but the proportion of patients feeling better during acyclovir therapy (46 percent) was similar to that produced by placebo (42 percent). With the four exceptions noted above, the improvement occurred during the first week of treatment and outlasted the treatment by only two to three weeks. The acyclovir therapy did not seem more useful in patients whose illness followed a well-documented episode of infectious mononucleosis. Titers of antibodies to the Epstein-Barr virus antigens generally decreased during the trial, but the changes were not correlated with type of treatment or the magnitude of clinical improvement. Levels of anxiety, depression, and confusion were significantly greater during the acyclovir treatment. Improvement, as reflected by higher wellness scores and decreased fatigue, was correlated significantly with positive mood changes (i.e., decreased depression, anxiety, and anger), but not with changes in body temperature.

The authors interpreted these unequivocally negative results to suggest that active replication of Epstein-Barr virus was not a major etiologic factor in chronic fatigue syndrome. However, this etiological inference is questionable given the fact that two recent studies have not been able to find an effect of acyclovir on patients with acute mononucleosis produced by this virus. In one of these trials, 120 patients were randomized to receive placebo or 600 mg of acyclovir five times daily for ten days (van der Horst et al., 1991). Compared with placebo, the severity and time to resolution of fever, need to rest in bed, lymphadenopathy, hepatosplenomegaly, atypical lymphocytes, and sense of well-being showed no significant difference in the acyclovir-treated group. Similarly, a trial involving 94 patients randomized to receive either placebo or a combination of acyclovir (800 mg five times daily) and weight-adjusted doses of prednisolone produced no significant effect with regard to duration of illness, sore throat, and number of days missed at school or work (Tynell et al., 1996). In any case, it appears that acyclovir is not indicated in the treatment of acute Epstein-Barr infection and it is certainly not a rational, effective, or safe treatment for chronic fatigue syndrome.

DIALYZABLE LEUKOCYTE EXTRACT (TRANSFER FACTOR)

Dialyzable leukocyte extract (transfer factor) is a constituent of white blood cells that has been tried for the treatment of chronic fatigue syndrome in a study conducted at the Prince Henry Hospital and the University of New South Wales, Sydney, Australia (Lloyd et al., 1993). The attempt was justified by the authors' belief that this extract is "capable of transferring delayed type hypersensitivity in humans" (p. 198) an effect with possible therapeutic importance given findings of impaired cell-mediated immunity in patients with chronic fatigue syndrome (Lloyd et al., 1989). Moreover, the agent was considered attractive on the basis of its relatively low cost, ease of administration by intramuscular injection, and small risk of major side effects. It is worth noting that as this study was planned, placebo-controlled clinical trials of nonspecific transfer factors had never been able to demonstrate effectiveness in other conditions associated with immunologic abnormalities such as atopic dermatitis (Hovmark and Ekre, 1978), lepromatous leprosy (Faber et al., 1979), Crohn's disease (Vicary, Chambers, and Dhillon, 1979), amyotrophic lateral sclerosis (Olarte et al., 1979), chronic mucocutaneous candidiasis (Mobacken et al., 1980), and malignant melanoma (Miller et al., 1988).

The clinical trial of dialyzable leukocyte extract was conducted according to a four-cell design that incorporated cognitive-behavioral therapy for half of the patients. To avoid the interpretative confusion that might result from two simultaneous therapeutic interventions, we will restrict the analysis to the evidence obtained from studying only patients given immunologic therapy or placebo.

The 47 participants suffered from persistent and disabling fatigue and were given a comprehensive medical, psychiatric, and laboratory evaluation. Criteria for enrollment were the absence of an alternative medical explanation for the fatigue illness and no prior immunologic therapy. Twenty-five patients were randomly assigned to receive a dialyzable leukocyte extract prepared for each patient from donor leukocytes. Donor leukocytes were obtained from either healthy family members living in the same household or from unrelated healthy individuals when family members were unavailable. All donors had normal results on tests of delayed-type hypersensitivity, no major medical illnesses in the past, and no history of symptoms compatible with chronic fatigue syndrome. Each treatment dose contained the extract obtained from 500 million leukocytes, more than half of which were mononuclear cells. Twenty patients were assigned to receive a placebo consisting of lyophilized normal saline. Treatment was administered intramuscularly from clouded vials every other week for a total of eight injections over a four-month period.

The treatment groups were similar with respect to age, gender distribution, duration of symptoms, ability to perform daily activities, severity of symptoms, and indices of cell-mediated immunity.

Physical capacity, symptoms, and the mood states scores for fatigue, vigor, depression, confusion, anger, and anxiety were recorded at biweekly intervals during the four-month trial period and for three months thereafter. Complete data sets were available for all except one patient in each group, who left the study without explanation.

One-third of patients in both groups reported improvements in the quantitative assessments of physical and psychological well-being. This symptomatic improvement correlated strongly only with the patients' conviction that they had received the leukocyte extract. In addition to being similar to the effect of placebo injections, the administration of dialyzable leukocyte extract was also clinically meaningless; three months after the therapeutic trial was completed, the number of daily nonsedentary hours had increased by only 12 minutes each day, and the index of participation in daily activities had improved by only 3 percent. The lymphocyte counts and the cutaneous responses to delayed hypersensitivity testing were not affected by the treatment with leukocyte dialyzable extract.

ALPHA INTERFERON

The interpretation of chronic fatigue syndrome as a condition produced or associated with immune dysfunction or persistent viral infection has led a group of investigators from the School of Medicine, University of California at Irvine, Orange, California, to study the therapeutic effect of alpha interferon in a double-blind crossover trial (See and Tilles, 1996). The drug is commercially available in the United States as a mixture of natural human interferons or, as was the case in this study, a single subtype preparation of recombinant DNA origin (American Hospital Formulary Service, 1997, p. 775). The authors' premise was debatable, given that careful research performed in Sweden (Linde et al., 1992) and Australia (Lloyd et al., 1994) had demonstrated normal levels of alpha interferon in sera obtained from patients with chronic fatigue syndrome.

The 30 subjects recruited for the study had no primary psychiatric illness and met standard diagnostic criteria for chronic fatigue syndrome (Holmes et al., 1988). Careful evaluations were carried out to ensure that there was no evidence of chronic infections (including acquired immune deficiency syndrome, tuberculosis, Lyme disease, and toxoplasmosis), rheumatologic, endocrinologic, and neurologic disorders. None of the patients had an immunoglobulin G deficient state and none had received treatment with intravenous immunogobulin, interferon, other cytokines, or corticosteroids during the year preceding the trial.

The subjects were randomly assigned to take alpha-2a interferon or placebo for 12 weeks and then crossed over, without an intervening washout period, to the alternative treatment. The treatment (three million units of interferon or sodium chloride 0.9 percent in solution) was administered by subcutaneous injection three times weekly. The patients were instructed to drink at least 450 ml water immediately after each injection and to take 650 mg of acetaminophen two hours later. Measurements were performed at baseline and at four-week intervals for seven months after the onset of the trial and included clinical assessments of ten main symptoms and signs of the fatigue illness as well as immunologic analyses of lymphocyte subsets, natural killer cell function, and lymphocyte proliferation. A cumulative quality-of-life score was calculated by taking into account individual ratings for each of the ten clinical variables (measured fever, fatigue, sore throat, lymphadenopathy, muscle aches, arthralgias, headaches, depression, difficulty with concentration, and insomnia).

The 30 participants had an age range of 22 to 58 and a mean age of 37 years. The group included 24 women and six men with an average duration of illness of 4.6 years. Adverse effects of interferon therapy were quite frequent (63 percent) and led to the withdrawal of four patients (13 percent). Two of these four patients developed neutropenia after eight and ten weeks of interferon therapy. A third patient dropped out because of increased fatigue after six weeks of treatment and one patient declined to continue the trial because of palpitations that occurred after one week of interferon injections. Adverse effects that did not preclude the completion of the trial included hair loss (30 percent of patients), significant flu-like symptoms at the onset of interferon therapy (13 percent) and diarrhea (7 percent).

The clinical variables rated by the 26 patients who completed the trial did not change after treatment with injectable interferon or placebo. However, interferon therapy appeared to improve the condition of the seven patients (27 percent) whose baseline evaluation indicated natural killer cell dysfunction. Nonetheless, the limited therapeutic benefit and the frequent and potentially serious adverse effects observed after three months of alpha-2a interferon injections does not justify the introduction of this therapeutic modality in clinical practice.

CYANOCOBALAMIN AND FOLIC ACID

Vitamins are often suggested for the treatment of chronic fatigue syndrome, despite a complete lack of evidence of their efficacy. In the only study that has focused on this type of treatment, a preparation for intramuscular administration containing cyanocobalamin (vitamin B12) and folic acid was used in a randomized, placebo-controlled, crossover trial involving 15 patients with chronic fatigue syndrome evaluated at the University of California Irvine Medical Center in Orange, California (Kaslow, Rucker, and Onishi, 1989). The diagnostic criteria required fatigue severe enough to reduce daily activities to less than 50 percent of premorbid levels for at least six months. In addition, the diagnosis required at least six of the following ten symptoms or signs: recurrent fever, nonexudative pharyngitis, painful cervical lymphadenopathy, myalgias, arthralgias, headaches, generalized weakness, sleep disturbance, prolonged postexercise tiredness, and neuropsychiatric disturbances (decreased libido, dizziness, impaired mentation or memory, or emotional lability). Extensive laboratory testing ruled out other medical causes of chronic fatigue in all patients. The outcome variables were measured using standardized questionnaires that assessed energy levels, overall symptoms, activities of daily living, and mental health.

At the onset of the trial, patients were randomized to receive either placebo or the vitamin treatment, which consisted of 220 micrograms of vitamin B12 and 0.8 mg of folic acid daily. Both treatments were self-administered as 2 ml intramuscular injections. After one week of treatment, the patients returned the empty syringes, completed a second set of evaluation questionnaires, and received the alternate preparation for the second week of the trial. After the second week, data were once again obtained and patients were offered a prescription for a two-week supply of the vitamin solution.

Fourteen patients completed the double-blind evaluation and 11 continued with the open-label trial and a fourth set of evaluation data. Treatment with placebo produced statistically significant improvement in the energy level, overall symptoms, and mental health. Vitamin administration produced significant improvement only with regard to the energy level. The differences between placebo and vitamins did not reach statistical significance for any of the four outcome variables recorded. During the open phase of the trial, the vitamin injections were followed by substantial improvement in all measures as compared to the baseline values.

TERFENADINE

The use of antihistamines in the empirical treatment of chronic fatigue syndrome has been advocated after the finding that a majority of 24 patients with this condition had a clinical history of atopy confirmed by epicutaneous skin testing (Straus, Dale, Wright, and Metcalfe, 1988). However, the efficacy of an antiallergic treatment modality has been tested only once, in a double-blind placebo controlled study of terfenadine conducted by investigators from the Hennepin County Medical Center, Minneapolis, with collaboration and support from the drug's manufacturer (Steinberg et al., 1996). The drug is a butyrophenone derivative with selective histamine-H1-receptor antagonist properties which does not readily cross the blood-brain barrier and thus is much less sedating than first-generation antihistamine compounds (American Hospital Formulary Service, 1997, p. 30). It is important to note that terfenadine was withdrawn from the U.S. market in 1998 when fexofenadine, its active and safer metabolite, became commercially available. Participation in the study was offered to patients entered in a regional research program, and 30 volunteers were enrolled after a thorough medical and psychiatric evaluation that satisfied standard diagnostic criteria (Holmes et al., 1988). Specific immunologic testing included puncture and intradermal skin tests for common indoor and outdoor inhaled allergens. The delayed-type hypersensitivity was assessed with a battery of five antigens, i.e., tetanus, mumps, *Candida albicans, Tricophyton mentagrophytes,* and tuberculin. Injections of codeine sulfate and histamine phosphate were used as positive puncture controls.

The thirty patients studied had a mean age of 36.2 years; 23 (77 percent) were women. A history of atopy was recorded in 73 percent of patients, manifested as allergic rhinitis, bronchial asthma, urticaria, atopic dermatitis, and food or drug allergy. All patients had positive reactions to the control injections and 53 percent reacted to one or more allergens. Positive responses were just as common for outdoor (40 percent) and indoor allergens (47 percent). Delayed-type sensitivity results indicate the expected high response rate to tetanus (97 percent) and mumps (83 percent). Only one patient had significant intradermal induration after tuberculin. Skin test reactivity was poorly correlated with a clinical history of atopy.

The patients were assigned to take either 60 mg of terfenadine or placebo twice daily for two months. They were instructed to refrain from taking antihistamines, tricyclic antidepressants, and ocular, nasal, or bronchial anti-inflammatory agents. The random assignment to the placebo and terfenadine arms of the study produced groups similar with respect to age, gender distribution, atopic history, and proportion of reactors to indoor and outdoor allergens. Baseline and outcome measurements included ratings of symptom severity, physical and social functioning, health perception, and mental health.

After eight weeks of treatment there were no detectable changes in any symptoms or self-assessed measures, of physical and social functioning, and mental health and health perception. For example, moderate to severe fatigue was reported by 71 percent of patients prior to starting therapy with terfenadine and by 86 percent of them within the last two weeks of the treatment period. Similarly, the frequency of myalgias changed from 57 percent to 64 percent and that of arthralgias from 43 percent to 57 percent. The subgroups with a history of atopy or positive skin reactions to indoor or outdoor allergens showed no differential changes from baseline during treatment with either antihistamine or placebo.

FLUDROCORTISONE

The effect of the mineralocorticoid analogue fludrocortisone in patients with chronic fatigue syndrome was recently tested by a group of experienced investigators from the Hennepin County Medical Center in Minneapolis, the major teaching affiliate of the University of Minnesota Medical School (Peterson et al., 1998). The postulated mechanism of action was the expansion of blood volume, which in turn was believed to treat neurally mediated hypotension, an abnormal cardiovascular reflex akin to vasodepressor or vasovagal syncope, which had been found on tilt-table testing among 22 of 23 patients with chronic fatigue syndrome evaluated at the Johns Hopkins University School of Medicine, Baltimore (Bou-Holaigh et al., 1995). The independent confirmation of the association between tilt-table-positive neurally mediated hypotension and chronic fatigue syndrome has been provided for only a minority (25 percent) of chronic fatigue syndrome patients (Freeman and Komaroff, 1997) and later work by the Johns Hopkins group concluded that the autonomic function did not differentiate chronic fatigue syndrome patients from healthy control subjects (Yataco et al., 1997).

In the Minnesota study, the subjects were recruited by invitation from among the 261 patients who had received the diagnosis of chronic fatigue syndrome (Holmes et al., 1988; Fukuda et al., 1994) through participation in two regional research programs. A total of 77 patients expressed interest in the study and 25 were enrolled. Forty-seven responders were considered ineligible because of insufficient severity of fatigue or current treatment with fludrocortisone, other corticosteroids, antihypertensive agents, antidepressants, and anxiolytic drugs.

Patients were randomly assigned to receive placebo or fludrocortisone acetate for six weeks, after which they entered a six-week washout period followed by six weeks on the opposite arm of the trial. The starting dose was one tablet of placebo or one tablet of 0.1 mg fludrocortisone acetate; patients were allowed to double the dose after the first week of treatment if their fatigue remained unchanged. The amount of salt in food was left to the discretion of the patient. Baseline and end-of-treatment measures included patients' ratings of the severity of their symptoms, level of postexertional fatigue, and functional and mood status. Objective measurements focused appropriately on the major physical and mental causes of disability by assessing the speed of cognitive processing and the exercise tolerance during treadmill walking. The sample size was adequate to detect a 30 percent change in the severity of illness and its functional impact.

The 25 subjects had a mean age of 40 years and had been experiencing the symptoms of chronic fatigue syndrome for an average of seven years. All patients were white and 76 percent of the group was female. On average, their fatigue was severe, as reflected in their inability to walk more than three blocks (less than 250 meters) without feeling worn out. Five patients withdrew from the study during the first phase of treatment; four of them (three of whom had been receiving fludrocortisone) gave as the reason for dropping out the worsening of fatigue, headache, or insomnia. Adverse effects were reported by eight of the remaining 20 patients (32 percent). Two patients dropped out during the placebo phase because of "racing pulse" and severe headache. Lack of improvement led to the doubling of the study medication by 11 subjects while taking placebo and eight subjects during treatment with fludrocortisone.

Fludrocortisone treatment did not improve any of the target symptoms (fatigue, distance before feeling exhausted, unrefreshing sleep, sore throat, painful lymph nodes, muscle pain, joint pain, forgetfulness, confusion, and depression) of this group of patients with chronic fatigue syndrome. Moreover, the fludrocortisone administration did not change the perceived severity of lightheadedness, the cardinal complaint of neurally transmitted hypotension. Placebo therapy was equally ineffectual; as a result, there were no outcome differences after fludrocortisone as compared with the postplacebo assessments. Similarly, the treatment with fludrocortisone or placebo did not improve the physical, social, and role functioning of these patients and their general well-being and level of energy. Objective measurements supported the futility of fludrocortisone therapy at this dosage; there were no changes in cognitive abilities tested and the variance in physical endurance was trivial, i.e., the treadmill time increased from an average of 19 minutes at baseline to 23 minutes after the completion of six weeks of treatment.

Chapter 5

Evidence-Based Therapy
of Chronic Fatigue Syndrome

Expert opinion regarding drug treatment of patients with chronic fatigue syndrome has been available for the past several years in the form of a booklet containing information for physicians compiled by the National Institute of Allergy and Infectious Diseases of the National Institutes of Health, Bethesda, Maryland (National Institute of Allergy and Infectious Diseases, 1996). The unnamed authors indicate that there are no specific drugs for the syndrome, and suggest symptomatic treatment with nonsteroidal anti-inflammatory agents to reduce the arthralgias, myalgias, and the feeling of feverishness that are often part of the clinical presentation of the syndrome. Small doses of tricyclic antidepressants and selective serotonin reuptake inhibitors are recommended in the booklet for the treatment of depression, pain, and sleep disturbance, and high-potency benzodiazepines are suggested for anxiety symptoms. However, these recommendations are not supported by data generated in controlled clinical trials.

From an evidence-based standpoint, all therapeutic agents tested in patients with chronic fatigue syndrome have failed to demonstrate their efficacy in replicated research studies. Even the glimmer of hope raised by some of the results of treatments with intravenous immunoglobulin infusions, low-dose glucocorticoids, and essential fatty acids does not withstand a careful assessment of methodological accuracy and clinical safety. The recognition of this reality has stimulated research efforts to organize controlled trials of the-nonpharmacological interventions of cognitive-behavioral therapy (Lloyd et al., 1993; Friedberg and Krupp, 1994; Sharpe et al., 1996; Deale et al., 1997) and graded aerobic exercise (Fulcher and White,

1997; Wearden et al., 1998). The experimental support for the potential benefit of these interventions is provided by work demonstrating that the physical fatigability and exercise capacity in chronic fatigue syndrome is not associated with psychopathology or with physiologic impairment of the cardiopulmonary system or skeletal muscles but correlated highly with exercise avoidance behavior leading to physical deconditioning (Fischler et al., 1997).

Of the two nonpharmacologic interventions, cognitive-behavior therapy has been more thoroughly studied, but has produced contradictory results. In the first trial, Australian investigators were unable to demonstrate improvement in global well-being, physical capacity, and functional status; when favorable changes occurred they were considered to be nonspecific and due to the propensity to remission that characterizes the natural history of this illness (Lloyd et al., 1993). Similar results were reported by investigators from the State University of New York at Stony Brook, who observed that cognitive-behavioral therapy did not change the severity of fatigue experienced by a group of patients with chronic fatigue syndrome, despite reduced depression-symptom scores; in contrast, in a control group of patients with primary depression, this therapy improved the severity of fatigue and fatigue-related thinking as it corrected the impact of depression and stress (Friedberg and Krupp, 1994). Positive results have been reported by a group of British clinicians from the King's College Hospital, London, who obtained improvement in at least three times as many patients treated according to a program of cognitive restructuring and graded activity than in a control group that had received relaxation therapy (Deale et al., 1997). A confirmation of these results was offered by a trial of cognitive behavior therapy conducted in Oxford, England, during which patients with chronic fatigue syndrome were helped to achieve gradual and consistent increases in activity by learning to try strategies other than avoidance (Sharpe et al., 1997).

Although it is clear that a decrease in avoidance behavior had greater impact on the outcome than changing the patients' beliefs about the etiology of their illness (Deale, Chalder, and Wessely, 1998), analysis of the data produced by these four trials suggests that the therapeutic agent may have been the increase in activity per se rather than the supportive, interpersonal, or psychodynamic dimensions of the cognitive-behavioral intervention. This impression is amplified by the results of trial performed at the National Sports Medicine Institute and St. Bartholomew's Hospital, London, in which patients with chronic fatigue syndrome without psychiatric disorders or sleep disturbance were randomly assigned to receive a 12-week program of either graded aerobic exercise or a combination of relaxation therapy and flexibility training (Fulcher and White, 1997). Analysis by intention to treat showed that the severity of fatigue, functional capacity, and fitness improved in 52 percent of patients enrolled in the aerobic exercise program as compared with 27 percent of the control group. Graded exercise was also effective when tested in a 28-week trial conducted at the Whitington Hospital by faculty members of the University of Manchester, United Kingdom (Wearden et al., 1998). Using a four-cell design that compared exercise with treatment with fluoxetine and placebo, the study showed that exercise was effective in reducing the severity of fatigue, improving functional work capacity, and favorably influencing the health perception of this group of patients with chronic fatigue syndrome. In all of these studies, and in additional research measuring immunological parameters (Lloyd et al., 1994; LaManca et al., 1999), graded aerobic exercise to exhaustion was well tolerated. Therefore, this review concludes that a prudent program of graded aerobic exercise offered in an environment capable of reducing the sufferer's avoidant behavior is the only evidence-based acceptable treatment for chronic fatigue syndrome.

SECTION II:
FIBROMYALGIA

Chapter 6

Definition and Methodological Issues

The current standard for the diagnosis of fibromyalgia was developed by a consortium of experts representing 16 clinical centers from the United States and Canada (Wolfe et al., 1990). Known as the American College of Rheumatology 1990 criteria for the classification of fibromyalgia, the definition was developed by comparing the clinical characteristics of patients considered to suffer from fibromyalgia with those of sex- and age-matched control subjects who had been diagnosed as having traditional musculoskeletal pain syndromes, such as rheumatoid arthritis and osteoarthritis. After a thorough statistical evaluation, data indicated maximal sensitivity (88 percent) and specificity (81 percent) for a set of two criteria: (1) history of widespread pain, and (2) pain at 11 of 18 musculoskeletal sites. Widespread pain, alone had a sensitivity of 98 percent but a low specificity of 31 percent, while tender points alone had a sensitivity of 90 percent and a specificity of 78 percent. The combination of the other three clinical features often reported in studies of patients with fibromyalgia, i.e., sleep disturbance, fatigue, and morning stiffness, had a sensitivity of 56 percent and specificity of 82 percent; a combination of any two of these three symptoms had a sensitivity of 81 percent and a specificity of 61 percent. The definition specified that the first criterion, widespread pain, is diagnosed when pain is present on both sides of the body, above and below the waist, and involving both axial and peripheral locations. The second criterion requires an examination during which the clinician attempts to determine by digital palpation whether there is tenderness at nine pairs of specified anatomic sites. Palpation must be performed with an approximate force of 4 kg and the maneuver is considered positive if the patient exhibits pain behavior or states that the palpation was "painful." The nine bilateral anatomic locations are: *occiput*, at the suboccipital muscle insertion; *low cervical*, at the anterior aspect of the intertransverse spaces of cervical verte-brae fifth through seven; *trapezius,* at the midpoint of the upper border; *supraspinatus,* at origins above the scapula spine near the medial border; *second rib,* at the second costochondral junction, just lateral to the junction on the upper surface; *lateral epicondyle,* two centimeters distal to the ulnar epicondyle; *gluteal,* in the anterior fold of muscle of the upper quadrant of buttock; *greater trochanter,* poste-rior to the trochanteric prominence; and *knee,* at the medial fat pad proximal to the joint line. The authors were careful to suggest that the elicited tenderness should be defined as absent, mild (complaint of pain without grimace, flinch, or body withdrawal), moderate (pain and flinch or grimace), or severe (pain and exaggerated body move-ment). The time-honored distinction between primary and secondary (i.e., occurring in patients with classical or definite rheumatoid ar-thritis, cervical or low back pain syndromes, and osteoarthritis of the knee or hand) was abolished, as the proposed criteria had similar diagnostic accuracy in both groups and the construct was considered valid independent of the presence of another rheumatologic disorder.

The American College of Rheumatology 1990 criteria replaced a number of other classification and diagnostic systems of fibromyal-gia, which have been used in some of the controlled drug trials reported here and which will be presented in details in the method-ological description and analysis of these reports.

Methodological issues regarding the credibility of data generated by the numerous controlled trials of pharmacological treatments for fibromyalgia have been well described by Simms (1994) and White and Harth (1996), who have pointed out that these studies did not use the same definition of a favorable response to therapy; did not rely on similar outcome measures; and did not have a sufficiently long follow-up period. A mathematically derived instrument has identified the clinician's global assessment score, the patient's self-rated quality of sleep, and the semiobjective tender point score as the combination of outcome measures that was best suited to identi-fy clinically meaningful differences between a potentially active drug and placebo (Simms, Felson, and Goldenberg, 1991). Its ap-plication to the analysis of published trials indicated that only a small percentage of patients have fulfilled all of the criteria for improvement.

Chapter 7

Effective Therapy

TRICYCLIC ANTIDEPRESSANTS

Amitriptyline

The treatment of fibromyalgia with amitriptyline, a dibenzocy-clohepten-derivative tricyclic antidepressant that enhances the effect of norepinephrine and serotonin on neurotransmission, has anticholinergic properties, and decreases the alpha wave activity of the brain (American Hospital Formulary Service, 1997, p. 675), has been the object of five controlled clinical trials conducted by investigators from the Boston area in the United States (Goldenberg, Felson, and Dinerman, 1986; Goldenberg et al., 1996), the provinces of Quebec and Ontario in Canada (Carette et al., 1986; Scudds et al., 1989, Carette et al., 1994), and Finland (Hannonen et al., 1998). The Canadian studies have provided high-quality data regarding the effectiveness of amitriptyline when used alone. In the United States, the trials have sought to evaluate also the potential advantages of combining the tricyclic agent with a nonsteroidal anti-inflammatory drug (Goldenberg, Felson, and Dinerman, 1986) or a selective serotonin-reuptake inhibitor (Goldenberg et al., 1996). Finally, the Finnish study compared the effectiveness of amitriptyline to that of moclobemide, a monoamine oxidase inhibitor (Hannonen et al., 1998).

The first publication from this body of work belongs to investigators from Laval University, Quebec City, University of Western Ontario, London, and University of Toronto, Toronto, Canada (Carette et al., 1986). The 70 patients enrolled in the double-blind, placebo-controlled trial were receiving care in the rheumatology outpatient clinics of these academic medical centers and had been diagnosed with primary fibrositis, a diagnosis compatible with the current definition of fibromyalgia because it required the presence of chronic widespread aching and local tenderness at 12 of 14 specified anatomic locations. In addition, all patients had symptoms of disturbed sleep, morning fatigue, and morning stiffness. Inclusion in the study group followed a physical and laboratory evaluation that ruled out other rheumatic disorders and confirmed the absence of inflammatory, infectious, neurologic, endocrinologic, and other musculoskeletal explanations of the symptoms. To avoid severe side effects, care was taken to exclude patients who had a history of glaucoma, urinary retention, ischemic heart disease, congestive heart failure, or arrhythmia. None of the patients participating in the trial had taken amitriptyline in the previous year.

The patients were randomly assigned to receive placebo or amitriptyline. The starting daily dose of amitriptyline was 10 mg; after one week the amount was increased to 25 mg daily for the second through the fourth week and then to 50 mg daily for five additional weeks. Adverse reactions prompted a decrease to the previous level of amitriptyline or placebo. The only other drug allowed was acetaminophen for pain, and each dose had to be recorded by the patient. The main measurements were carried out at baseline and after five and nine weeks of treatment. The patients provided data regarding the severity of pain during the previous week, sleep quality, duration of morning stiffness, and an overall assessment of their condition. Physicians used a standardized dolorimetric technique to measure point tenderness at specified anatomic sites and scored the overall status of the condition on a scale similar to that used by the patients.

Eleven of the 70 patients (16 percent) failed to complete the trial; seven of these patients had been assigned to take amitriptyline. Reasons for withdrawals were intolerable side effects (four patients) of amitriptyline-induced drowsiness and agitation, and placebo-induced drowsiness and gastrointestinal distress; lack of cooperation (four patients, three of whom were taking amitriptyline); intercurrent illnesses (two patients); and insufficient therapeutic effect (one patient taking amitriptyline). The 59 patients who completed the study were about equally divided among the amitriptyline group (27 patients) and placebo group (32 patients). Minor side effects were reported by 70 percent of patients on amitriptyline but only 12 percent of those receiving placebo; the severity of side effects required a decrease in the dose of amitriptyline in three cases. The potential unblinding effect of the difference in the proportion of minor side effects was duly acknowledged by the investigators. The amitriptyline and placebo groups were similar with regard to female predominance (93 percent versus 91 percent), age (42 versus 40 years), pain analog scores on 1-10 scale (6.3 versus 5.8), myalgic scores, and duration of morning stiffness. On average, the fibromyalgic symptoms had been present for six years in the amitriptyline-treated group and eight years in patients assigned to receive placebo.

Objectively measured tenderness showed substantial favorable changes in 22 percent of patients receiving amitriptyline and 15 percent of those treated with placebo. Compared with baseline, treatment with placebo improved pain and morning stiffness in 16 percent of patients, a statistically insignificant difference. Among amitriptyline-treated patients, 37 percent reported improvement (i.e., at least a 50 percent favorable change) in pain and morning stiffness, a significant change compared with baseline. Compared with placebo, amitriptyline was superior with regard to improved quality of sleep for the entire duration of the study (70 percent versus 40 percent). The overall assessment of the condition indicated a benefit of amitriptyline after five weeks of treatment, as shown by the fact that 77 percent of those taking amitriptyline but only 43 percent of patients treated with placebo assessed their disease as moderately to markedly improved. The difference in the rates of improvement lost statistical significance at the ninth-week measurement point, when 70 percent of the amitriptyline group and 50 percent of the placebo group reported feeling better. However, the magnitude of improvement was consistently higher among those treated with amitriptyline.

Confirmation of amitriptyline's efficacy in fibromyalgia was the aim of a second Canadian study (Scudds et al., 1989). Working at the University of Western Ontario in London, the investigators selected 39 subjects from among the fibrositis (fibromyalgia) patients receiving care through the university hospital's outpatient rheumatology unit. The diagnostic criteria and exclusionary rules were identical to those used by Carette et al. (1986).

The trial employed a double-blind crossover design. The subjects were randomly assigned to receive identical-looking capsules of amitriptyline or placebo for four consecutive weeks, then entered a two-week washout period, after which they took the alternative treatment for four weeks. The daily dose of amitriptyline was 10 mg in the first week, 25 mg in the second week, and 50 mg during the third and fourth weeks. Data were collected at baseline and four, six, and ten weeks after the onset of the trial. Measured variables included a total myalgic score assessed by standard dolorimetric testing of four predesignated fibromyalgic tender points; a pain threshold score reflecting dolorimetric results at four specified musculoskeletal sites that were not among the fibromyalgic point locations and were not tender at baseline; a pain tolerance score; a measure of the threshold for pain; a pain severity questionnaire; and the patient's global assessment of treatment effectiveness. The sample size was adequate to test the hypothesis that amitriptyline will improve pain scores by at least 50 percent and that the improvement obtained after placebo will be around 25 percent.

Three patients (8 percent) discontinued the trial medication and withdrew; two of them (one on placebo) had developed intolerable drowsiness and the third because of insufficient improvement while in the placebo phase of the study. No other side effects were reported. The 36 patients who completed the study had demographic and clinical characteristics similar to the population studied by Carette et al. (1986); preponderance of women (89 percent of the sample), mean age of 40 years, and an average duration of illness of five years.

Amitriptyline was found to be substantially better than placebo in decreasing the pain experienced by fibromyalgia subjects, a finding with statistical significance for objective (dolorimetric scores at tender point sites) as well as subjective measurements. Global assessments made by patients indicated that 20 patients (56 percent) felt moderately or markedly better after treatment with amitriptyline; in contrast, a similar level of improvement was reported by only three patients (8 percent) at the end of the placebo phase of the trial. A comparison of the 20 patients who improved on amitriptyline with the remaining 16 members of the study cohort revealed that patients who improved on amitriptyline had lower pain ratings at baseline and throughout the ten-week study period and that their pain threshold improved over time. The proportion of patients who rated their condition as worse was 25 percent after therapy with placebo but only 8 percent at the completion of the amitriptyline trial.

Canadian investigators have also attempted to determine whether the established therapeutic effectiveness of amitriptyline is maintained over time (Carette et al., 1994). The question was tested in a large trial involving patients referred from nine academic clinics and two private rheumatology practices. All patients fulfilled criteria for the diagnosis of fibromyalgia in accord with the definition formulated by the American College of Rheumatology (Wolfe et al., 1990); the physical and laboratory screening evaluations and the reasons for exclusion were identical to those employed in the previously described Canadian trials (Carette et al., 1986; Scudds et al., 1989). As in those trials, the only nonstudy medication allowed during the trial was acetaminophen.

Eighty-four patients were randomized to receive amitriptyline and 42 patients were assigned to treatment with placebo. The daily dosage of amitriptyline was 10 mg at bedtime in the first week, 25 mg for the following 11 weeks, and 50 mg for the final 12 weeks of the trial. The amitriptyline and placebo groups were similar with regard to age (44 versus 47 years), average duration of fibromyalgia (eight years in both groups), proportion of females (93 percent in both groups), proportion of patients not working because of fibromyalgia (25 percent versus 36 percent), educational levels, and marital status. The average number of tender points detected at baseline was 16 in both groups.

Measurements were carried out at baseline and monthly thereafter for the six-month duration of the trial, and care was taken to train all investigators to use the same data collection techniques. The patients were asked to rate six dimensions of their illness: intensity of pain, severity of fatigue, difficulty with sleep, feeling on awakening, morning stiffness, and global assessment of condition. Functional disability was assessed with well-validated instruments profiling the sickness impact on daily activities and on physical and psychosocial health. A standard personality inventory was completed at baseline to allow the classification of patients into one of three categories: normal, typical chronic pain profile, or psychological disturbance profile. Physicians measured tenderness at five pairs of specified anatomical sites to calculate a myalgic score and made a global assessment of condition at each visit. Treatment-related improvement was prospectively defined as at least 50 percent change in a majority of the following variables: pain, fatigue, sleep, global assessment as rated by patient or physician, and the total myalgic score.

Fourteen patients (17 percent) treated with amitriptyline and 14 patients (33 percent) receiving placebo withdrew from the study. Lack of response was given as the reason for dropping out by five patients (6 percent) from the amitriptyline group and seven (17 percent) from the placebo group. Adverse reactions produced by amitriptyline were invoked as reason for withdrawal by seven patients (8 percent) and consisted of excessive somnolence in four patients and abdominal pain, rash, and weight gain in one patient each. The frequency of side effect-related withdrawals in the placebo group was similar, involving two patients (5 percent; one patient developed excessive somnolence, the other complained of dizziness).

Amitriptyline was statistically better than placebo after one month of treatment, with 21 percent of patients given the active drug but none of the placebo recipients found to show significant improvement as prospectively defined by the investigators. After three months in the trial, the difference lost its significance, with 18 percent of amitriptyline-treated patients and 13 percent of those taking placebo indicating persistent favorable changes. A trend (just short of statistical significance) toward a superior effect was identified at the six-month evaluation; the proportions of patients reporting improvement were 36 percent in the amitriptyline group and 19 percent in the group treated with placebo. Compared with the baseline scores, amitriptyline therapy significantly improved the severity of pain, quality of sleep, the level of fatigue, and the global assessments of the condition made by patients and physicians at all of the six monthly evaluations required by the trial. The sickness impact profile evaluation after six months substantiated the overall improvement produced by amitriptyline as compared with the baseline status, but the placebo treatment had a similarly favorable effect. A normal personality profile (as opposite to a "chronic pain profile" or "psychologically disturbed profile") and a higher level of education were the only predictor variables of the amitriptyline-induced improvement after one month of treatment, but not after three or six months into the trial.

The two U.S. studies of therapeutic effectiveness of amitriptyline in patients with fibromyalgia were conducted, a decade apart, by investigators from the Boston area. In the first trial, the investigators carried out their research at the Multipurpose Arthritis Center, Boston University (Goldenberg, Felson, and Dinerman, 1986). The diagnosis of fibromyalgia was based on the presence of at least six "typical" tender points in the context of an illness producing generalized aches or prominent stiffness involving at least three anatomic sites for at least three months. In addition, the diagnosis required at least three of the following eight features: chronic headache, irritable bowel syndrome, fatigue, anxiety, poor sleep, numbness, subjective swelling, and modulation of symptoms by physical activity, weather, or stress. Exclusion criteria were a history of cardiac arrhythmia or peptic ulcer disease. Prior to enrollment, the patients underwent evaluations confirming the absence of other causes of their symptoms and had all their analgesic, anti-inflammatory, or psychotropic medications discontinued. Other than the study medications, the only other drug allowed was acetaminophen at a dose of 650 mg every four hours as needed for relief of pain. The study cohort comprised 62 patients (95 percent females) with a mean age of 44 years and mean duration of chronic pain illness of 3.5 years. In addition to pain symptoms, most patients were also experiencing at baseline symptoms of fatigue (95 percent), morning stiffness (95 percent), sleep disturbance (73 percent), numbness (73 percent), and subjective swelling (73 percent). Each patient had at least six tender fibromyalgic points.

The study compared treatment with low-dose amitriptyline alone (25 mg at bedtime) with a combination of amitriptyline (25 mg at bedtime) and the anti-inflammatory drug naproxen (500 mg twice daily). Control treatments were placebo and naproxen alone (500 mg twice daily). Random assignment to one of the four treatment groups was performed with appropriate precautions that ensured balanced distribution according to main demographic and clinical features. The groups were similar with respect to duration of fibromyalgia and prevalence of sleep disturbance and morning tiredness. Main outcome measures consisted of patients' ratings of pain or stiffness, fatigue, quality of sleep, and the global assessment of illness and physicians' tender point examinations and global assessments of illness. Data were collected at baseline and two, four, and six weeks into the trial.

Fifty-eight of the 62 patients who entered the study completed the trial. One patient dropped out from each treatment group. The dropout from the group assigned to receive amitriptyline and naproxen withdrew because of excessive daytime somnolence and headache. The dropout assigned to receive placebo developed significant epigastric discomfort. The remaining two dropouts failed to return for follow-up assessments. Adverse effects were also reported by eight patients who completed the trial, bringing the frequency of treatment-related complications to 10 of 62 cases (16 percent). Four patients given amitriptyline complained of dry mouth and two patients each from the groups given naproxen or placebo reported dyspepsia and diarrhea.

The patients treated with amitriptyline (alone or in combination with naproxen) had outcome measures clearly superior to those receiving naproxen alone or placebo. Highly significant levels of improvement were noted for the global assessments of status made by patients and physicians, as well as for the severity of pain, fatigue, and sleep disturbance and the total myalgic score. The favorable effect of amitriptyline-containing regimens increased over the duration of the trial. The study found no relationship between response and the baseline severity of sleep disturbance or morning tiredness, suggesting that the hypnotic property of the tricyclic antidepressant agent did not form the basis for its beneficial effect. Statistical evaluation of drug synergy indicated that the addition of naproxen did not increase the efficacy of amitriptyline in patients with fibromyalgia.

The second U.S. trial of amitriptyline in fibromyalgia was conducted by investigators from the Newton-Wellesley Hospital, Newton, and New England Medical Center, Tufts University, Boston, Massachusetts (Goldenberg et al., 1996). The design of this placebo-

controlled study allowed the assessment of the effect of amitriptyline alone and in combination with fluoxetine, a selective serotonin
reuptake inhibitor. The patients enrolled in the trial had been evaluated by the senior author and given the diagnosis of fibromyalgia
according to the 1990 American College of Rheumatology classification criteria (Wolfe et al., 1990). Exclusion criteria were current or
past history of systemic illness; age younger than 18 or older than 60;
pain severity less than 30 on a 0-100 analog scale; and significant
depressive symptoms. The study cohort comprised 31 patients with a
mean age of 43 years and a mean duration of fibromyalgia symptoms
of six years. All patients were white and 90 percent were female.
Eleven patients (36 percent) were not working because of illness-
related disability.

The study was designed as a randomized, double-blind, crossover
sequence of four six-week trials, during which the patients took
placebo in the morning and 25 mg of amitriptyline at bedtime; 20 mg
of fluoxetine in the morning and 25 mg of amitriptyline at bedtime;
20 mg of fluoxetine in the morning and placebo at bedtime; and
placebo in the morning and at bedtime. The treatments were separated by washout periods lasting two weeks. Main measurements
included the patient's assessments on visual analog scales of global
well-being, pain, fatigue, sleep disturbance, and feeling refreshed
upon awakening. In addition, the subjects completed a depression
inventory and a fibromyalgia impact questionnaire to measure
physical functioning and work status as well as anxiety, depression,
sleep, pain, fatigue, and stiffness (Burckhardt, Clark, and Bennett,
1991). Physicians' measurements included tender point evaluation
and the assessment of global well-being. All measurements were
obtained at baseline and at the beginning and end of each treatment
phase.

Twelve patients (39 percent) withdrew before the end of the
study, in three cases after developing adverse effects produced by
the combination of amitriptyline and fluoxetine. Data collected
from the remaining 19 patients indicated that amitriptyline alone
and the combination of amitriptyline and fluoxetine were significantly superior to placebo with regard to patients' ratings of global
well-being, severity of pain, and degree of sleep disturbance. The
same variable pointed out than the combination of amitriptyline and

fluoxetine performed better than either drug alone. Patients' ratings for depressive symptoms, fatigue, and feeling refreshed after awakening, as well as the physicians' ratings of global well-being, did not differ between the amitriptyline and placebo treatment phases. The fibromyalgia impact scores improved in 63 percent of patients during the amitriptyline and fluoxetine treatment phase, 24 percent of patients taking amitriptyline alone, and 5 percent of patients during the placebo treatment phase. Despite changes in the perceived severity of pain and overall well-being, the tender points assessment showed little change compared with baseline.

The latest attempt to characterize the therapeutic impact of amitriptyline in fibromyalgia was a double-blind, placebo comparison of this tricyclic agent with moclobemide, a reversible inhibitor of monoamine oxidase not available at this time in the U.S.; the research was carried out at Tampere University Hospital, Tampere; Rheumatism Foundation Hospital, Heinola; and Central Hospital, Jyvaskyla, Finland (Hannonen et al., 1998). The authors recruited the potential participants for the trial from their outpatient practices and from a register of patients with fibromyalgia. Inclusion in the study required the confirmation of standard diagnostic criteria (Wolfe et al., 1990); at least moderate severity of symptoms recorded on three of four dimensional scales measuring general health, disability, sleep quality, and fatigue; the absence of any psychiatric disorder within the past six months as demonstrated by a highly structured clinical interview; and the absence of any significant physical illness, pregnancy or breast-feeding, or laboratory abnormalities. Of 184 subjects screened, 130 were found eligible for the trial and were randomly assigned to treatment with amitriptyline (n = 42), moclobemide (n = 43), or placebo (n = 45). The trial started with a two-week, single-blind, placebo run-in phase. This was followed by treatment with moclobemide (150 mg) morning and afternoon plus one placebo capsule in the evening; one placebo capsule morning and afternoon and one amitriptyline (12.5 mg) capsule in the evening; or three capsules of placebo daily. The treatment was continued for 12 weeks and only paracetamol tablets were allowed for analgesia. Patients were allowed to increase the moclobemide and amitriptyline dosages by one capsule after two weeks and again after six weeks of treatment. Outcome data were generated by self-scored dimensional scales and by clinical assessments of global change in condition and number of tender points.

The study was completed by 32 of the 42 patients (76 percent) in the amitriptyline group. Five patients (12 percent) discontinued their participation after developing adverse drug reactions, but no clinical details are presented with the exception of a case of vasovagal reaction requiring hospitalization. The proportion of withdrawals due to side effects was similar in the moclobemide (14 percent) and placebo (11 percent) groups.

Amitriptyline was statistically better than both moclobemide and placebo with regard to global improvement, which was noted in 74 percent of patients treated with the tricyclic agent, 54 percent of patients who received treatment with moclobemide, and 49 percent of the placebo-treated group. Amitriptyline was the only therapy leading to substantial improvement in the level of energy and emotional control, and the only agent producing a positive change in occupational, social, and family functioning. Amitriptyline and moclobemide were similar with regard to the ability to decrease the severity of pain and number of tender points at a level significantly lower than that recorded at baseline.

Dothiepin

Dothiepin, a tricyclic antidepressant compound similar in structure to amitriptyline, has been tested for effectiveness in fibromyalgia in a treatment trial conducted by investigators from the Rheumatology Service, L. Sacco Hospital, Milan, Italy, in collaboration with researchers employed by the drug's manufacturer (Caruso et al., 1987). The 60 subjects recruited for the study were diagnosed with fibromyalgia according to the clinical standards of the investigators, but no details were provided. The participants were randomly assigned to receive dothiepin (75 mg each evening) or identical-looking and tasting placebo tablets for eight weeks. The effect of treatment was assessed after two, four, and eight weeks using the patients' and physicians' global judgment with regard to change in condition, the pain response at 40 specified anatomic sites, and the patients' visual analog quantitation of the severity of their musculoskeletal pain.

The two treatment groups were similar with regard to all baseline demographic and clinical variables. Most patients were middle-aged females (mean age 46 years, proportion of women 85 percent) who had had the symptoms of fibromyalgia for an average of six years. The subjective severity of pain and the response to the examination of tender points were identical in the two groups. Adverse drug effects were reported by 18 of the 30 patients (60 percent) treated with dothiepin, the most common being drowsiness (40 percent), weakness (10 percent), and dry mouth (10 percent). The incidence of adverse effects in the placebo-treated group was significantly lower (20 percent). However, the number of subjects who withdrew from the study because of the perceived severity of treatment-related effects was similar in the two groups, i.e., three of the patients assigned to receive dothiepin and four of those treated with placebo. Another patient treated with dothiepin could not discontinue previously prescribed anxiolytic therapy and dropped out of the study. Thus, the trial was completed by 26 patients from each of the two treatment groups.

Compared with placebo, the eight-week treatment with dothiepin led to a significant reduction in the subjective assessment of the severity of pain, as well as in the pain response elicited by physical examination of specified musculoskeletal areas. The favorable change was also reflected in both patients' and physicians' global impression. A placebo effect was not demonstrated for any of the intermediate and final outcome measurements performed. A careful analysis of data indicates that the pain symptoms increased in severity during the last four weeks of treatment with placebo.

Chapter 8

Controversial Therapies

CYCLOBENZAPRINE

Four studies (Bennett et al., 1988; Quimby et al., 1989; Reynolds et al., 1991; Carette et al., 1994) have attempted to demonstrate that the tricyclic agent cyclobenzaprine is better than placebo in producing symptom relief for patients with fibromyalgia. Although the agent's chemical structure is similar to that of amitriptyline, it lacks meaningful antidepressant effect and is generally used as a muscle relaxant in combination with a nonsteroidal anti-inflammatory drug for short-term therapy of acute musculoskeletal disorders with pain and spasm (Basmajian, 1989; Borenstein, Lacks, and Wiesel, 1990). Cyclobenzaprine was believed to produce its muscle relaxant effect by activating neurons from locus ceruleus to increase output of noradrenaline in the ventral horn leading to inhibitory action of noradrenaline on the effector alpha motoneurons (Commissiong et al., 1981). However, recent research has contradicted this mechanism and has suggested that cyclobenzaprine acts as a serotonin receptor antagonist and that the muscle relaxation is actually due to the inhibition of the serotonergic descending system in the spinal cord (Kobayashi, Hasegawa, and Ono, 1996). The "central" explanation for the favorable effect of cyclobenzaprine in fibromyalgia is also, albeit indirectly, supported by the disappointing performance of chlormezanone, a primarily "peripheral" muscle relaxant (Pattrick, Swanell, and Doherty, 1993), which will be described elsewhere in this presentation.

The first clinical trial of cyclobenzaprine included patients receiving rheumatological care in outpatient settings at the Oregon Health Sciences University, Portland, and the Center for Arthritis and Back Pain, Philadelphia (Bennett et al., 1988). Criteria for the diagnosis of fibromyalgia (fibrositis) differed moderately from the standard affirmed later by the American College of Rheumatology (Wolfe et al., 1990); that is, the patients had to have at least seven tender points at 16 specified anatomical locations, increased tension in the muscles of neck and shoulders, sleep disturbance described as fatigue upon arising, and early morning worsening of aching and stiffness. In addition, the diagnosis required at least two of the following features: dermatographism, exacerbation of symptoms by emotional stress or strenuous exercise, weather-related changes in symptoms, and temporary relief of symptoms with heat applications. Patients with significant physical and psychiatric disorders, manipulative behavior, or pending litigation were not eligible for the trial. Care was also taken to prevent the inclusion of patients with evidence of glaucoma, urinary retention, recurrent urinary tract infections, and pregnancy or likelihood of pregnancy. The only concomitant therapy allowed was fixed doses of nonsteroidal anti-inflammatory agents.

The design was a placebo-controlled double-blind trial that assigned the patients to receive either placebo or 10 mg cyclobenzaprine tablets. The initial dose was one tablet at night, but if symptoms did not improve the patients had the option of increasing the dose during the first two weeks of treatment to a maximum of four tablets each day administered at equal intervals during the day and evening. Baseline and outcome measures provided by patients included weekly assessments of severity of pain and duration of morning stiffness. The physician-investigators recorded the number and degree of tenderness at the 16 anatomical locations used to define the condition in this study. They also scored a global measure of musculoskeletal pain and the overall response to treatment at the completion of the trial. Statistical analyses were performed with help from the research unit of the drug's manufacturer.

A total of 120 patients (116 females) were entered in the study. Fifty-three patients (44 percent) were given the diagnosis of primary fibrositis and 67 (56 percent) were considered to have fibrositis secondary to arthritis or trauma. Fifty-eight patients were assigned to receive placebo and 62 were treated with cyclobenzaprine. The demographic and clinical features of the patients receiving placebo and cyclobenzaprine were similar; a mean age of 49 years, an average of four months since diagnosis, an average of seven hours of morning stiffness and eight hours of fatigue daily, and 13 tender points. Past trauma with possible etiologic significance was recorded in slightly more than half the sample and osteoarthritis was diagnosed in a quarter of the patients in each group.

The daily dosage of 10 mg of cyclobenzaprine was maintained by 21 percent of patients; 34 percent of patients increased their dose to 20 mg, 23 percent to 30 mg, and 21 percent ended up taking 40 mg of cyclobenzaprine daily. Forty patients (65 percent) treated with cyclobenzaprine and 23 (40 percent) of those receiving placebo completed the study. Lack of response was invoked as the reason for withdrawal by 33 patients (57 percent) on placebo, but only by ten patients (16 percent) taking cyclobenzaprine, a clinically and statistically significant difference. Adverse reaction led to the withdrawal of 8 percent of the cyclobenzaprine group and 5 percent of patients treated with placebo. Serious events occurred in three patients taking cyclobenzaprine and consisted of recurrence of angina pectoris, severe gastric burning, and severe depression in one patient each. Treatment with cyclobenzaprine was associated significantly more often with dry mouth (57 percent versus 17 percent) and drowsiness (34 percent versus 17 percent) starting in the first two weeks of treatment, but the intensity of these adverse reactions was usually mild or moderate and their incidence did not increase over time. Clinically insignificant weight increase (range 1-4 lb.) and tachycardia were recorded consistently only among patients taking cyclobenzaprine.

Cyclobenzaprine therapy was superior to placebo with regard to patients' report of improved pain severity and quality of sleep. Improvement in fatigue was also noted, but did not persist through the last month of the 12-week trial. Compared with placebo, the change in the duration of morning stiffness did not reach significance. All four variables (pain, sleep, fatigue, and stiffness) appeared significantly improved at the end of the trial when compared with the baseline values. In contrast, only one variable (sleep quality) improved over baseline value in the placebo-receiving group. The number of tender musculoskeletal points was consistently lower in the cyclobenzaprine-treated group, and the difference against placebo reached significance after two weeks and was maintained after four weeks of treatment. Physicians' assessments of muscle tightness and global severity of musculoskeletal pain indicated an advantage for cyclobenzaprine that was more marked among patients with primary rather than secondary fibrositis. Overall, the blinded evaluation of treatment efficacy identified improvement of 54 percent of patients treated with cyclobenzaprine and 35 percent of those receiving placebo, a difference with statistical significance.

The second trial of cyclobenzaprine for the treatment of fibromyalgia enrolled patients from a private rheumatology practice in Bangor, Maine, with assistance from the Department of Psychology, University of Maine, Orono, and partial funding provided by the drug's manufacturer (Quimby et al., 1989). The study cohort was assembled over an eighteen-month period and included female patients given the diagnosis of fibromyalgia according to a set of criteria which consisted of persistent aches and stiffness at three or more sites, normal laboratory and radiologic findings, and the presence of a specified number of tender points and symptoms, e.g., five tender points and three symptoms from a list that included poor sleep, general fatigue, aggravation of symptoms by anxiety and stress, modulation of symptoms by physical activity or weather, chronic headaches, irritable bowel syndrome, and numbness, as suggested by a controlled investigation of criteria for the diagnosis of "primary fibrositis" (Yunus et al., 1981). Exclusion criteria were identical to those used by Bennett et al. (1988).

The design of the trial required all patients to enter a two-week washout for analgesics (not including nonsteroidal anti-inflammatory agents used for conditions other than fibromyalgia, which were allowed at fixed dosages), muscle relaxants, antidepressants, and anticholinergic drugs. The 45 patients found eligible for the trial were then randomly assigned to receive cyclobenzaprine (23 patients) or an identical-looking placebo (22 patients). Again similar to the trial conducted by Bennett et al. (1988), the initial dose of cyclobenzaprine was 10 mg, but the patients had the option of increasing the daily amount by 10 mg every week to a maximum of 40 mg/day, which was taken in divided doses of 10 mg in the morning and 30 mg at bedtime. Comprehensive baseline evaluations measured tender points, depressive symptoms, physical symptoms, emotional and cognitive response to pain, and pain tolerance to electric shock, immersion in ice water, and pressure dolorimeter. Outcome measures after six weeks of treatment included patients' ratings of change in muscle pain, musculoskeletal stiffness and aching, severity of fatigue and quality of sleep, and patients' and physicians' assessment of overall improvement.

Five patients (two taking cyclobenzaprine and three taking placebo) were withdrawn from the trial. One patient developed severe dizziness while taking cyclobenzaprine and two patients on placebo were withdrawn because they had to take analgesics to relieve musculoskeletal discomfort. The 40 patients who completed the trial had a mean age of 45 years, a mean duration of their pain syndrome of 11 years, and an average of seven tender points. Patients treated with cyclobenzaprine were similar to those receiving placebo in all demographic and clinical characteristics.

Compared to placebo, treatment with cyclobenzaprine produced a significantly greater degree of improvement in the patients' experience of musculoskeletal stiffness and aching and in the quality of sleep. Moreover, the global ratings made by both patients and physicians indicated significantly greater proportions of patients with moderate or marked improvement at the end of the six-week course of treatment with cyclobenzaprine. Improvement was predicted by a few baseline characteristics, e.g., patients with the worst depressive symptomatology showed the most substantial improvement in the quality of sleep, while those with best pretrial tolerance of pain recorded more improvement in the level of fatigue and quality of sleep. On the other hand, changes in the perceived intensity of myalgias and severity of fatigue did not differ between cyclobenzaprine and placebo. Furthermore, the interpretation of the findings requires caution, because in a majority of cases both patients (67 percent) and physicians (77 percent) guessed correctly whether the treatment used was cyclobenzaprine or placebo. This level of discernment was substantially greater than that expected by chance alone, correlated strongly with the presence of cyclobenzaprine-induced dryness of the mouth, and had the potential to unblind the study.

These favorable results were contradicted by a carefully designed crossover study conducted at the Western Division of the Toronto Hospital, Toronto, Ontario, with help from the drug's manufacturer

(Reynolds et al., 1991). The study had the dual goals of attempting to confirm the efficacy of cyclobenzaprine on the symptoms of fibromyalgia and of trying to understand the agent's mechanism of action, particularly its effect on the nonrestorative sleep pattern considered characteristic for this disorder. The study cohort comprised 12 patients selected from recent referrals to the hospital's rheumatology clinic who met the authors' criteria for fibromyalgia, i.e., had complained of diffuse aching, nonrestorative sleep and fatigue, and had been found to have point tenderness at seven or more of 16 specified musculoskeletal sites. Patients with clinical or laboratory evidence of other disorders were not eligible for the trial.

The trial started with a two-week washout period, after which patients were assigned to receive either cyclobenzaprine or placebo for four weeks. This was followed by another two-week washout interval and then a four-week period of treatment with the alternate regimen. The starting dose of cyclobenzaprine was 10 mg three times daily, which was increased to 10 mg four times every day or decreased to 10 mg twice a day as determined by side effects and perceived effectiveness. Baseline and posttreatment assessments included patients' ratings of the severity of muscle pain, morning stiffness, sleep disturbance and fatigue, overnight polysomnographic evaluations, and dolorimetric measurements at five predesignated locations.

Of the 12 patients enrolled, nine completed the study. The three withdrawals were due to a diagnosis of nocturnal myoclonus, inconsistent use of the study medication (placebo) during the first treatment period, and excessive sleepiness developing after three weeks of treatment with placebo. Side effects were infrequent; dry mouth, nausea, and weakness serious enough to require reduction in dose developed in only one patient (11 percent).

Only two of the nine patients (22 percent) who completed the study reported clinically meaningful improvement of their fibromyalgia syndrome after treatment with cyclobenzaprine, and even they chose not to continue due to lack of persistent improvement. Of all symptoms recorded, cyclobenzaprine improved only the severity of fatigue felt in the evening; the data for pain, sleepiness, tender point count, and dolorimetry scores showed no difference between placebo and cyclobenzaprine and between washout and treatment intervals. Similarly, with the sole exception of a slight, and clinically insignificant, prolongation of the average total sleep time, treatment with cyclobenzaprine did not have a measurable effect on sleep architecture, sleep efficiency, and severity of alpha intrusions during nonrapid-eye-movement sleep.

The fourth attempt to define the effectiveness of cyclobenzaprine in fibromyalgia was described in a Canadian multicenter study performed with support from the drug's manufacturer (Carette et al., 1994). It is, however, the only research effort that employed the American College of Rheumatology criteria (Wolfe et al., 1990) to diagnose fibromyalgia among the patients, who were receiving outpatient rheumatological care at nine university clinics and two private practices. Patients fulfilling these diagnostic criteria were not included if they had evidence of inflammatory joint disease or other untreated bone, neurologic, or endocrine diseases or history of myocardial infarction, arrhythmias, congestive heart failure, glaucoma, or urinary retention.

The design of the study required random assignment to a 24-week course of treatment with placebo or cyclobenzaprine, which was administered at a daily dose of 10 mg at bedtime in the first week, 20 mg at bedtime from the second through the twelfth weeks of the trial, and 10 mg in the morning and 20 mg at bedtime for the remaining 12 weeks of the study period. The dose was reduced to the previous level or discontinued in case of adverse reaction or lack of tolerance. Baseline and monthly follow-up assessments measured patients' ratings of pain, fatigue, quality of sleep, feeling refreshed or exhausted upon awakening, morning stiffness, and global description of the burden of illness. Patients also provided data on standardized instruments with regard to functional disability, anxiety and depression, and completed a personality inventory. Participating physicians measured tenderness at ten (five pairs) specified musculoskeletal sites and recorded their global impression of the progress made by each patient.

Eighty-two patients were treated with cyclobenzaprine and 42 received placebo. The mean age (43 years in the cyclobenzaprine group versus 47 years in the placebo group), female preponderance (95 percent versus 93 percent), education level, marital status, and employment status were similar in the two groups. Median duration of fibromyalgia was shorter in the cyclobenzaprine group (median three years) than in the placebo group (median five years), but the difference was not statistically significant. The fibromyalgia symptoms, number of tender points, and the functional and psychological characteristics were also similar in the two study groups.

A total of 24 patients (29 percent) in the cyclobenzaprine group and 14 patients (33 percent) from the placebo group withdrew before the completion of the trial. Lack of response constituted the reason for stopping the study medication for six (7 percent) of the cyclobenzaprine-treated patients and seven (17 percent) of those treated with placebo. Adverse reactions led to the withdrawal of 13 patients (16 percent) on cyclobenzaprine and of two (5 percent) of those treated with placebo. Intolerable dizziness (five patients), abdominal pain (three patients), and somnolence (three patients) were the most common serious side effects recorded in the cyclobenzaprine-treated group.

Statistically, cyclobenzaprine was superior to placebo after one month of treatment, but the clinical significance of the finding is questionable given the fact that it reflects the difference between an improvement rate of 12 percent in the cyclobenzaprine group and 0 percent in the placebo group. After three months of treatment, improvement was reported by 19 percent of patients treated with cyclobenzaprine and 13 percent of those treated with placebo, a statistically insignificant difference. At the completion of the six-month trial the proportion of patients whose condition had improved rose to 33 percent in the cyclobenzaprine group and 19 percent in the placebo group; again, the difference was not statistically significant. Although the investigators assessed the global change produced by cyclobenzaprine as superior to placebo, most of the individual measures used to determine the outcome of the therapeutic intervention were similar in the two groups. The baseline variables that predicted initial favorable response to cyclobenzaprine were a normal personality profile and a higher education level.

SELECTIVE SEROTONIN REUPTAKE INHIBITORS

Three studies have evaluated the effect of serotonin reuptake inhibitors in fibromyalgia, an attempt justified by the authors' impression that the condition is associated with a serotonergic deficient state and a substantial overlap with depressive disorders (Wolfe, Cathey, and Hawley, 1994; Norregaard, Wolkmann, and Danneskiold-Samsoe, 1995; Goldenberg et al., 1996). However, the review of the literature demonstrates that the validity of these assumptions was not entirely supported by the available evidence. First, although initial data from Harvard Medical School indicating that the frequency of depressive symptomatology and prevalence of depressive disorders were significantly higher in fibromyalgia patients as compared with patients with rheumatoid arthritis (Hudson et al., 1985) was confirmed by studies done in Israel (Alfici, Sigal, and Landau, 1989) and Denmark (Krag et al., 1994), it was contradicted firmly by the results of work performed in Canada (Kirmayer, Robbins, and Kapusta, 1988) and at Dartmouth Medical School (Ahles et al., 1991). Second, serum serotonin levels were found to be lower than those of healthy control subjects in one study (Russell, Michalek, et al., 1992), but similar to those of patients with rheumatoid arthritis, a disorder not considered to have a pathophysiologic link with mood disorders (Stratz et al., 1993). Moreover, although a large population survey showed lower serum serotonin levels in patients with fibromyalgia, the range of values was wide and no meaningful association was found between serum serotonin levels and the clinical manifestations of fibromyalgia, such as number of tender points or severity of pain (Wolfe et al., 1997). Third, in studies measuring 3H-imipramine binding, a biochemical indicator of serotonin uptake by platelet receptors, patients with fibromyalgia had similarly contradictory findings, i.e., serotonin deficiency in a group of 22 patients evaluated in San Antonio, Texas (Russell, Michalek, et al., 1992), but not among ten nondepressed women with fibromyalgia evaluated in Chicago, Illinois (Kravitz et al., 1992). Nevertheless, the research is justified because the link between depression and fibromyalgia is supported by the confirmed excess in the prevalence of depression among first-degree relatives of patients with fibromyalgia (Hudson et al., 1985; Katz and Kravitz, 1996), and the serotonergic deficiency supported by studies that have found lower levels of serotonin and its metabolites in the cerebrospinal fluid of fibromyalgia sufferers (Houvenagel et al., 1990; Russell, Vaeroy, et al., 1992).

Fluoxetine

The first clinical trial of fluoxetine in fibromyalgia was conducted at the Arthritis Research and Clinical Centers by investigators affiliated with the University of Kansas School of Medicine and Wichita State University in Wichita, Kansas, with support from the drug's manufacturer (Wolfe, Cathey, and Hawley, 1994). The investigators enrolled 42 female patients with fibromyalgia followed in a single outpatient rheumatology clinic. The diagnosis was based on the presence of widespread pain and point tenderness at a minimum of seven of 14 musculoskeletal locations. Screening ensured that none of the subjects had other rheumatic diseases or previous treatment with fluoxetine. The participants were randomly assigned to receive fluoxetine (20 mg each morning) or placebo for six weeks. Measurements were carried out at baseline and after each week of treatment and included tender point evaluations by physicians and patients' ratings of global severity of illness, pain, quality of asleep, fatigue, depression, anxiety, and side effects and adverse reactions of treatment. Outcome analyses were carried out by comparing baseline data with those recorded after three and six weeks of treatment.

The fluoxetine and placebo groups were similar with regard to age (48 versus 53 years) and proportion of ethnic whites (100 percent versus 95 percent). Subjects assigned to the fluoxetine group were significantly more likely to have completed high school (90 percent versus 62 percent) and to have a longer duration of illness at entry in the study (16 versus 10 years). Pain, sleep disturbance, functional disability, global severity, and tender point counts were similar for the two groups. Patients assigned to receive fluoxetine had higher scores on two measures of depression, but the magnitude of the difference between the groups was statistically insignificant. Of the 21 patients entered in each arm of the study, six dropped out during the first three weeks of the trial. None of the patients receiving fluoxetine, but six of those treated with placebo withdrew in the last three weeks of the study. Of the six patients from the fluoxetine group who dropped out, one listed gastrointestinal side effects as the reason for withdrawal, one was noncompliant with the trial's requirements, and four stopped taking the drug because of perceived lack of efficacy. Of the 12 withdrawals from the placebo group, lack of efficacy was cited by eight subjects, one was lost to follow-up, and three discontinued the placebo because of adverse reactions consisting of gastrointestinal symptoms in one case and rash in two cases.

Treatment with fluoxetine was not better than placebo and produced no measurable improvement compared with baseline for any of the clinical descriptors of the pain syndrome, i.e., patients' ratings of pain, morning stiffness, and global severity of illness and physicians' ratings of tender point count and dolorimetry score. After six weeks of treatment, fluoxetine appeared to decrease the severity of depression and fatigue compared with baseline, but there was no statistical evidence that the fluoxetine group was more vigorous or less depressed than the placebo-treated group. An analysis by intention to treat (i.e., a model retaining the patients who withdrew during the first three week of the trial) confirmed the absence of a therapeutic effect of fluoxetine on any of the study's variables. Of interest is the fact that fluoxetine did not seem to improve the depressive symptoms of any subgroup of patients, including those whose condition fulfilled diagnostic criteria for major depression.

The second attempt to measure the therapeutic effect of fluoxetine was included in a trial comparing fluoxetine, amitriptyline, and the combination fluoxetine-amitriptyline with placebo in a crossover double-blind study. The methodology for patient selection and main measurements has already been described earlier in this section (Goldenberg et al., 1996). The fluoxetine treatment phase consisted of a six-week period during which one 20 mg tablet was administered each morning. Of the 31 patients entered in the study, 19 completed the trial; four patients withdrew during the fluoxetine phase because of an increase in fibromyalgia symptoms (three patients) or adverse drug effect (one patient). Compared with placebo, patients' ratings indicated that fluoxetine was better than placebo with regard to severity of pain, quality of sleep, global well-being, and impact of illness. The fluoxetine-induced benefit was similar to the change produced by low-dose amitriptyline treatment. As mentioned, the therapeutic effect of the combination amitriptyline-fluoxetine was superior to that of either drug used alone.

Citolapram

Citolapram is a selective serotonin reuptake inhibitor that has been recently approved for use as an antidepressant agent in the United States. The drug's efficacy for the treatment of fibromyalgia was tested in a carefully designed controlled trial carried out by investigators from Frederiksberg Hospital in Copenhagen, Denmark, with support from the drug's local manufacturer (Norregaard et al., 1995). A total of 43 individuals were selected from among 150 patients given the diagnosis of fibromyalgia according to standard criteria (Wolfe et al., 1990). None of the subjects had inflammatory rheumatic disorders or evidence of other physical diseases and none carried a diagnosis of endogenous depression or had been treated in the past with antidepressant drugs. Random assignment created a placebo group (21 patients) and a citolapram group (22 patients). During the first four weeks of the trial the subjects took one tablet of either placebo or 20 mg of citolapram daily, after which they were instructed to increase the dose to two tablets daily if they did not report a substantial improvement in their perception of pain. Measurements included objective identification of tender points and isokinetic muscle strength at the start and the completion of the trial. Patients contributed weekly self-reports of symptoms, the impact of illness, and the presence and severity of depression, pain, and sleep disturbance.

The citolapram and placebo groups were similar in age (48 versus 50 years), duration of illness (ten years in both groups), and number of patients requiring acetaminophen, other nonsteroidal anti-inflammatory medications, or codeine for pain control during the trial (11 versus 9 patients). One patient developed vertigo after one day of treatment with citolapram and was excluded from further treatment; all other patients completed at least three weeks of treatment. Moderate or severe side effects were relatively common in both groups and included headache (24 percent of both the citolapram and the placebo groups), dry mouth (5 percent versus 10 percent), and nausea or vomiting (5 percent in both groups). Eight subjects did not complete the entire study protocol, but the specific reasons for their withdrawal were not provided.

Seventeen of 19 patients in the citolapram group and all 19 patients from the placebo group failed to demonstrate significant improvement after four weeks of treatment and doubled the daily dose of medication for the balance of the trial. Despite this adjustment, by the end of the trial, the patients' ratings of pain, fatigue, and global status of condition did not improve compared with baseline in either group. Treatment with citolapram had no advantage over placebo with regard to physical function, isometric muscle strength, pain, fatigue, morning stiffness, anxiety, and depression. The clinicians' global assessment indicated that only two of the 19 patients treated with citolapram for eight weeks could be classified as markedly improved and one patient was considered to show minimal improvement. On the other hand, three patients from the citolapram group and one patient treated with placebo worsened during the study period.

S-ADENOSYLMETHIONINE

S-Adenosylmethionine (SAMe) is a methyl donor that has been evaluated for the treatment of fibromyalgia by investigators from Italy (Tavoni et al., 1987) and Denmark (Jacobsen et al., 1991; Volkman et al., 1997). Although the agent's mechanism of action has not been defined, its use on a trial basis in fibromyalgia appeared justified by its demonstrated effectiveness and safety as an antidepressant (Kagan et al., 1990; Salmaggi et al., 1993) and analgetic agent (Caruso and Pietrogrande, 1987).

The first controlled trial of SAMe was performed by researchers associated with the Rheumatic Diseases Unit at the University of Pisa, Pisa, Italy, with limited technical support from the drug's manufacturer (Tavoni et al., 1987). The authors recruited 25 patients who had been given a diagnosis of fibromyalgia according to the following criteria: pain or stiffness at three anatomic locations for at least three months; a specified number of tender points; and a specified number of minor criteria. At least three tender points and five minor criteria or five tender points and three minor criteria were required in each case. The minor criteria included modulation of symptoms by stress, physical activity, or weather; fatigue; sleep disturbance; persistent headache; irritable bowel syndrome; subjective swelling; paresthesias; and anxiety.

Using a crossover design, the investigators randomly assigned the subjects to receive intramuscular injections of SAMe (200 mg) or placebo daily for three weeks. The placebo was not characterized in the methods section of the study and no data were offered with regard to the osmolality of the two injectable treatments. Following this first phase of the trial the patients completed a two-week washout period, after which they were given the alternate treatment for a three-week period. Baseline, interim (day 21 and day 35) and end-of-study measurements included the number of objectively identified tender points as well as the number and severity of depressive symptoms assessed by self-report and structured interview.

Six of the 25 patients (24 percent) dropped out without explanation and the possibility of adverse drug effects was not investigated. Two patients were withdrawn from the trial after developing abscesses at the intramuscular injection site. In the remaining 17 patients, treatment with SAMe produced significant improvement in the number of painful sites and depression scores as compared with the pretreatment status while the administration of placebo did not lead to a change in the parameters studied. However, data generated by a direct comparison of changes induced by SAMe and placebo were not reported. The authors' conclusion that intramuscular administration of SAMe is effective and safe in fibromyalgia is not supported by the facts presented in their report.

The second attempt to evaluate the effectiveness of SAMe in fibromyalgia was designed by investigators from Frederiksberg Hospital and Hvidovre Hospital, Copenhagen, Denmark (Jacobsen et al., 1991). The 44 patients included in the trial were randomly selected from a countrywide registry maintained by the authors. Diagnostic criteria were similar to those used by Tavoni et al. (1987), i.e., a chief complaint of pain and stiffness at a minimum of three anatomic sites for at least three months; at least three other symptoms from a list that included sleep disturbance, fatigue, chronic headaches, subjective swelling, and modulation of symptoms by weather, anxiety, stress, and physical activity; and the presence of at least four tender points on the physical examination of 14 specified locations. None of the participants had any other established diagnosis for their symptoms and all had normal results on comprehensive laboratory evaluations.

One patient dropped out because of a dental infection before the start of the trial. The remaining 44 subjects were randomly assigned to receive identical-looking enteric-coated tablets of placebo or SAMe (400 mg) twice daily for a period of six weeks. The use of analgetic drugs was restricted to one 500 mg tablet of acetamino-phen every four hours. Other concomitant medications were held at the same dosage throughout. Measurements carried out at baseline and after 21 and 42 days of treatment included tender point ex-amination; assessment of muscle strength by isokinetic dynamome-try of both quadriceps muscles; self-scoring on visual analog scales of overall well-being, pain at rest and on movement, quality of sleep, and fatigue; mood parameters; duration of morning stiffness; and physicians' impression of changes in the severity of the disease.

The SAMe and placebo treatment groups were well-matched with regard to gender distribution (more than 75 percent females in each group), and mean age (49 years) and duration of chronic pain (4.5 years). In both groups, patients had on average greater than 10 tender points and more than 90 percent endorsed the symptoms of fatigue, sleep disturbance, and modulation of symptoms by physical activity. A majority of patients in each group had been previously treated with analgesics or nonsteroidal anti-inflammatory drugs. In contrast, prior treatment with antidepressant agents was infrequent (two of the 22 patients assigned to receive SAMe and three of the 22 subjects entered in the placebo arm of the trial).

Eight patients treated with SAMe (36 percent) developed side effects, which led to the discontinuation of the treatment in four of them. In three of the patients who stopped taking SAMe, the ad-verse effects were related to the gastrointestinal tract; the remaining patient withdrew after experiencing severe dizziness. Among the patients taking placebo, seven (32 percent) reported adverse effects and one of them dropped out because of headache.

After six weeks of treatment, the assessments made by patients indicated that SAMe was superior to placebo with regard to the severity of fatigue and nonexertional pain. The patients also felt that the severity of pain experienced during physical activity, the quality of sleep, and the overall well-being were not changed by either treatment. The physicians' assessments identified a positive effect of SAMe on the degree of discomfort produced by the examination of tender points and on the duration of morning stiffness. Isokinetic muscle strength was not significantly changed. Psychometric evaluations gave contradictory results; one instrument indicated substantial SAMe-related improvement in mood, while another measure failed to identify any difference between SAMe and placebo. A similar number of acetaminophen tablets was used by each of the two groups. The physicians felt that the condition had improved after six weeks of treatment in 47 percent of patients who had received SAMe but only in 14 percent of patients enrolled in the placebo arm of the trial.

Researchers from Frederiksberg Hospital in Copenhagen, Denmark, in collaboration with investigators employed by the German manufacturer of the drug, have also completed work evaluating the efficacy of intravenous treatment with SAMe in fibromyalgia (Volkman et al., 1997). The inception cohort was assembled from the medical records maintained by the hospital's rheumatology unit. Of the 179 potential enrollees, 54 agreed to participate and 34 of them qualified for inclusion in the trial. The participants met the American College of Rheumatology diagnostic criteria for fibromyalgia (Wolfe et al., 1990) and in addition had at least three of the following: generalized fatigue, sleep disturbance, chronic headache, symptoms compatible with irritable bowel syndrome, subjective swelling, paresthesias, and modulation of symptoms by physical activity, stress, anxiety, and weather conditions. The subjects agreed to forgo all other analgesics other than acetaminophen for the duration of the trial.

The 34 fibromyalgia patients were randomly assigned to receive intravenous SAMe or placebo and then crossed over to the alternate treatment after an eleven-day washout period. The intravenous injection delivered 600 mg of SAMe diluted in 15 ml or a similar volume of placebo over five minutes in the antecubital vein. Patients, physicians, and medical technicians were unaware of the substances administered, which were available as similar-looking powders in blinded vials. Although some suspensions had a slight yellow color, the patients did not indicate awareness of this fact. After the first two injections in each treatment phase the patients were carefully observed for immediate reactions to the intravenous treatment. Baseline and outcome measurements included assessments of tender point sensitivity; isokinetic muscle strength; self-scored questionnaires for pain at rest; assessment of mood and impact of illness; and a global impression regarding the change in condition at the end of the study.

Side effects of SAMe led to the withdrawal of four subjects (12 percent): three of these patients developed intolerable nausea, vomiting, and diarrhea, and one had an anaphylactic reaction after the first injection. Nonspecific paresthesias, dizziness, headache, and mild gastrointestinal symptoms were some of the other side effects of SAMe, but specific data regarding their prevalence were not provided. In addition to the four patients withdrawn as a consequence of SAMe-induced adverse reactions, one patient dropped out for nonmedical reasons.

The 29 patients who completed the trial had the demographic characteristics expected of a population with fibromyalgia, i.e., female preponderance (91 percent women) and middle age (mean 49 years), and had been experiencing the pain syndrome for an average of 8.5 years. Subjective assessments indicated that SAMe was better than placebo only with regard to the decrease in the severity of pain experienced at rest. The pain associated with movement, severity of fatigue, quality of sleep, and overall well-being were similarly influenced by the intravenous administration of SAMe and by that of the placebo solution. Treatment with SAMe was no better than placebo with regard to the number of tender points and the magnitude of their pain response to pressure, which were the main objective measurements of the study. No differences were noted in isokinetic muscle strength or in measures of the severity of depression. The physicians' global assessment of efficacy indicated improvement in 30 percent of patients after treatment with SAMe and 20 percent after administration of placebo, a statistically insignificant difference.

Chapter 9

Ineffective Drugs

NONSTEROIDAL ANTI-INFLAMMATORY AGENTS

Nonsteroidal anti-inflammatory drugs (NSAIDs) are almost universally part of the empirical pharmacologic treatment of fibromyalgia (Cathey, Wolfe, and Kleinheksel, 1986)) despite the fact that an inflammatory process has not been identified as the biological cause or consequence of this functional somatic syndrome.

Ibuprofen

Ibuprofen is a widely prescribed and inexpensive NSAID, available in the United States as an over-the-counter analgesic remedy. The drug is the *p*-isobutylhydratropic acid, a substance thought to exert its anti-inflammatory effect by inhibiting the synthesis or release of prostaglandins; the analgesic action of the drug is peripheral rather than central, but its mechanism has not been elucidated (American Hospital Formulary Service, 1997, p. 1499). The therapeutic efficacy of ibuprofen in fibromyalgia was first studied by investigators from the University of Illinois College of Medicine at Peoria with financial support from the drug's manufacturer (Yunus, Masi, and Aldag, 1989). The subjects were 46 patients with "primary" fibromyalgia, i.e., widespread, chronic musculoskeletal pain and multiple tender points in the absence of history of other rheumatologic disorder, systemic disorder, or trauma known to produce similar symptoms. Appropriate laboratory investigations were carried out and gave negative results in all of these patients. The great majority of these patients (83 percent) had been treated with at least one NSAID in the past.

The study started with the discontinuation of all anti-inflammatory and pain medications and a one-week washout period, after which the patients were randomly assigned to receive either 600 mg of ibuprofen (22 patients) or placebo tablets (24 patients) four times daily for three weeks in a double-blind mode. Following this, all patients received ibuprofen 600 mg four times daily for three weeks in an open manner. Measurements carried out at baseline and after the second and third weeks of the double-blind and open trials included self-assessments of symptoms and examination of specified tender points.

The treatment was well tolerated; gastrointestinal symptoms such as nausea, constipation, diarrhea, and abdominal pain were reported by five of the patients (23 percent) treated with ibuprofen and four of the patients (15 percent) receiving placebo during the double-blind phase of the trial. Three patients dropped out of the study; one patient developed severe headaches within one week of treatment with ibuprofen, one patient assigned to receive placebo withdrew because of gastrointestinal symptoms and nervousness, and one developed an unrelated illness.

The ibuprofen and placebo groups were similar with regard to demographic and clinical characteristics. The mean age in both groups was 39 years, the duration of the pain syndrome averaged seven years, and 95 percent of participants were women. Five patients in the ibuprofen group and six in the placebo group were taking amitryptiline and continued to receive stable doses of the tricyclic antidepressant agent throughout the trial. Treatment with ibuprofen was not better than placebo for pain, sleep disturbance, duration of stiffness and fatigue, and subjective swelling and paresthesias. The total number of pain sites and total tender points decreased compared with baseline data but were similar after three weeks of treatment with placebo or ibuprofen. Ibuprofen administration was followed by significant pain relief in 26 percent of patients after three weeks of treatment; 29 percent of patients treated with placebo also reported marked decrease in their pain symptoms. The open-label phase of the trial was followed by significant pain relief in 44 percent of patients originally started on ibuprofen and in 55 percent of the patients who had received placebo in the double-blind phase of the trial. The concomitant administration of amitriptyline did not change the response to ibuprofen. These findings were correctly interpreted to indicate a "study effect" or the result of increased patient-physician interaction, rather than a specific effect of the ibuprofen. The authors established the important corollary that the lack of analgesic effect, which in the case of NSAIDs is obtained peripherally through decreased prostaglandin synthesis, suggests that the pain in fibromyalgia is likely to be of central origin.

The second study to evaluate the effectiveness of ibuprofen as a therapeutic agent for fibromyalgia was designed and executed by investigators from the University of Texas Health Science Center, San Antonio, Texas, in collaboration with the Epidemiological Research Division, Brooks Air Force Base, Texas, and with support from the drug's manufacturer (Russell et al., 1991). The authors recruited 102 consecutive patients given the diagnosis of primary fibromyalgia on the basis of persistent musculoskeletal pain for at least three months and pain response to the palpation of at least five of 16 specified tender points. None of the patients had other rheumatic disorders, chronic infections, psychiatric disorders, or evidence of peptic ulcer. Of the initial cohort, 78 patients agreed to discontinue all medications previously prescribed for pain and sleep disturbance and were entered in a placebo-controlled clinical trial comparing the efficacy of ibuprofen with that of a combination of ibuprofen and alprazolam, a high-potency benzodiazepine. Sixty-eight of the 78 patients (87 percent) met the standard criteria for the diagnosis of fibromyalgia as defined by the American College of Rheumatology (Wolfe et al., 1990). The participants were randomly assigned to receive identical-looking oral medications for treatment with placebo, ibuprofen (600 mg four times daily), and ibuprofen (600 mg four times daily) plus alprazolam (initial dosage 0.5 mg at bedtime, followed after the second week of treatment by increments of 0.5 mg up to a daily maximum of 3.0 mg administered in divided doses). The trial was preceded by a two-week washout period during which only acetaminophen was allowed for pain relief. At the end of the trial, the treatment was tapered off over a one-week period. Measurements were carried out at time zero (just before the beginning of the trial) and two weeks after the end of the full-dose treatment and included assessments of the severity of tenderness at

16 specified soft tissue sites by dolorimetry and digital palpation, patients' perception of pain, physicians' ratings of global severity of fibromyalgia, and questionnaires evaluating functional and psychological status.

As a group, the 78 participants had the usual characteristics of fibromyalgia research populations, i.e., middle age (mean 47 years), female predominance (88 percent) and non-Hispanic white (80 percent). In addition to pain, most patients complained of generalized fatigue (87 percent), subjective swelling (68 percent), dysesthesias (64 percent), and anxiety (60 percent). Fifteen patients (19 percent) had elevated erythrocyte sedimentation rates and two patients had abnormal titers of antinuclear antibodies of uncertain etiology and clinical significance. Fifteen patients withdrew before the end of the clinical trial: six failed to report for follow-up, five (7 percent) developed adverse side effects, and four took unauthorized medications. Of the patients who dropped out because of adverse side effects, only one had been assigned to treatment with ibuprofen; he was a 78-year-old patient whose pain worsened and who developed rash, adenopathy, headaches, and swelling.

Treatment with ibuprofen was not better than placebo in this six-week clinical trial. Analysis of variance indicated that all treatments produced significant improvement compared with baseline; however, neither of the two treatment modalities, i.e., ibuprofen alone or the combination of ibuprofen with alprazolam, produced a measurably superior outcome when compared to placebo treatment with regard to any of the clinical, functional, and psychometric variables.

Naproxen

A placebo-controlled trial of naproxen, a propionic acid derivative structurally and pharmacologically related to ibuprofen (American Hospital Formulary Service, 1997, p. 1536), was reported by investigators from Boston University School of Medicine (Goldenberg et al., 1986). The authors compared the therapeutic effect of naproxen to that of amitriptyline and the combination of the two drugs in a six-week trial involving 62 patients with fibromyalgia diagnosed according to criteria already described in the analysis of this work contained in the amitriptyline subsection. The findings reported with regard to the patients who received naproxen 500 mg twice daily or the same amount of naproxen plus amitriptyline 25 mg at bedtime, or placebo. The prevalence and severity of fibro-myalgic symptoms were similar in the three treatment groups. Naproxen had no significant effect on any of the main outcome parameters (pain, tender point score, fatigue, sleep disturbance, and global severity of the condition). No significant synergy was found between naproxen and amitriptyline, i.e., the combination did not outperform its components.

Tenoxicam

The effectiveness of tenoxicam (a long-acting anti-inflammatory agent not available in the United States) for the treatment of fibro-myalgia was tested in a well-designed clinical trial performed at the Hospital Universitario Virgen del Rocio, Seville, Spain, with limited technical support from the drug's manufacturer (Quijada-Carrera et al., 1996). The authors invited the participation of 285 patients diagnosed in the hospital's rheumatology clinic with fibromyalgia according to standard criteria (Wolfe et al., 1990). Patients were not eligible if they had a history of peptic ulcer disease or other gastro-pathies (17 patients), liver disease (6 patients), hypersensitivity to NSAIDs (5 patients), or if they were pregnant (3 patients). Participation in the study required discontinuation of all psychotropic and analgesic drugs. A total of 164 patients (mean age 43 years; 93 percent women) were enrolled in the study and assigned to receive tenoxicam (20 mg each morning), bromazepan (3 mg at bedtime), tenoxicam and bromazepan, or placebo. The four treatment groups were well matched with regard to the study's main baseline measurements, which were severity of pain, presence of sleep disturbance, number of tender points, and duration of morning stiffness. The group treated with tenoxicam had a somewhat shorter average duration of illness (7.7 years) than the three other treatment groups. The main outcome variable was the patients' assessment of fibro-myalgia after the eight-week trial as worse, unchanged or minimally improved, markedly improved, or asymptomatic.

Side effects were experienced by 52 patients (32 percent) and were severe enough to induce nine patients (5 percent) to withdraw from the trial. Stomach pain, heartburn, or nausea were reported by

17 patients (21 percent) taking tenoxicam (with or without the addition of bromazepan) and by eight patients (10 percent) treated only with bromazepan or placebo. Dizziness and headache were experienced by seven patients from the two groups receiving tenoxicam and six patients in the other two treatment groups. Six of the nine patients withdrawn from the trial had developed significant stomach pain; four of these six cases had been treated with tenoxicam.

The trial was completed by 110 of the 164 eligible subjects; in addition to the nine patients withdrawn because of adverse drug reactions, 12 patients dropped out because of insufficient therapeutic response and 33 subjects did not report for follow-up examinations. The proportions of patients reporting improvement were 22 percent in the placebo group, 12 percent in the tenoxicam group and 32 percent in the tenoxicam plus bromazepan group. The intergroup differences did not reach statistical significance, indicating that treatment with tenoxicam has no clinical utility in the management of fibromyalgia.

BENZODIAZEPINES

The therapeutic effectiveness of benzodiazepines in fibromyalgia has been tested by two independent research groups (Russell et al., 1991; Quijada-Carrera et al., 1996) in similarly designed trials that compared benzodiazepines with placebo, nonsteroidal anti-inflammatory drugs (NSAIDs), and a combination of the two nonplacebo treatments. From the outset, it is important to note that the theoretical basis of these two trials has been the perceived association between fibromyalgia and symptoms of depression and anxiety, rather than a benzodiazepine-specific central or peripheral pathophysiologic mechanism at work in the causation and maintenance of fibromyalgia.

Alprazolam

Alprazolam, a high-potency triazolobenzodiazepine widely used in the United States as an anxiolytic agent, was tested in patients with fibromyalgia at the University of Texas Health Science Center, San Antonio, and Brooks Air Force Base, Texas (Russell et al., 1991). The drug is considered an inhibitor of the neurotransmitter γ-aminobutyric acid in the hypothalamus, thalamus, and limbic structures of the central nervous system and is known to possess sedative, hypnotic, and skeletal muscle relaxing properties (American Hospital Formulary Service, 1997, p. 1799). The trial described here required a sample of 17 randomly assigned patients to take 0.5 mg alprazolam at bedtime for two weeks, after which the dose was increased by 0.5 mg increments to a tolerated daily total of up to 3 mg administered in divided doses. The outcome after six weeks of treatment was compared with the effect of placebo and to that of the combination of alprazolam and ibuprofen (600 mg four times daily). The treatment was tolerated well, as reflected by the fact that only one of 17 patients treated with alprazolam withdrew from the study because of an adverse drug effect (blurred vision). Among the 15 patients treated with the combination of alprazolam and ibuprofen, one patient withdrew because of increased pain, rash, adenopathy, and swelling. Treatment with placebo produced adverse health effects that led to the withdrawal of three out of 14 patients.

Alprazolam and placebo substantially improved the symptoms of fibromyalgia in this study; the effect of alprazolam was statistically identical to that of placebo with regard to the patients' assessment of pain, dolorimetric scores, physicians' assessments of disease severity, and the number and severity of symptoms of depression and anxiety. The combination of alprazolam and ibuprofen was only marginally better than alprazolam alone or placebo. A dose-dependent favorable effect of alprazolam was noted for the tender point sensitivity to digital palpation, but the clinical significance of this finding is questionable given the fact that after six weeks of treatment the patients treated with alprazolam felt that their pain was worse than those in the placebo-treated group.

Bromazepan

Bromazepan, a benzodiazepine not marketed in the United States, was used for the treatment of fibromyalgia in a study conducted at the Hospital Universitario Virgen del Rocio, Seville, Spain (Quijada-Carrera et al., 1996). Patients were randomly assigned to receive fixed doses of bromazepan (3 mg at bedtime), bromazepan and the NSAID tenoxicam (20 mg each morning), or placebo. Treatment with this benzodiazepine was accompanied by adverse drug reactions in 14 of the 33 subjects (42 percent); four patients (12 percent) taking bromazepan were unable to complete the trial because of intolerable gastralgia (two patients) and rash (two patients). The addition of tenoxicam did not change the side effects profile and only one of the 37 patients receiving this therapeutic combination discontinued participation because of adverse drug effects.

Treatment with bromazepan for at least three weeks was considered successful in 15 percent of patients, an improvement rate lower than that observed among patients treated with placebo (22 percent). The analysis by intent to treat did not change this reality; improvement was apparent in 12 percent of patients treated with bromazepan and 17 percent of those assigned to receive placebo.

NONBENZODIAZEPINE HYPNOTICS

The use of nonbenzodiazepine hypnotics zopiclone and zolpidem in fibromyalgia is based on a conceptual framework postulating that the condition is, at least in part, due to a reduction in the delta type of electrical activity (7-11 Hz), which normally constitutes most of the non-rapid eye movement of the third and fourth sleep stages (Moldofsky et al., 1975). In contrast with traditional benzodiazepines, which have the potential to worsen the delta sleep deficit, both agents induce an increase in the delta sleep duration (Mouret et al., 1990; Patat et al., 1994; Yamadera et al., 1997).

Zopiclone

The therapeutic efficacy of the cyclopyrrolone hypnotic zopiclone, a drug not available for sale in the United States, was first tested in fibromyalgia by investigators affiliated with Viborg County Hospital, Viborg, Denmark, with support from the drug's manufacturer (Drewes et al., 1991). The 45 subjects recruited for the study had been diagnosed with fibromyalgia according to a set of criteria validated in a controlled investigation (Yunus et al., 1981). Using a double-blind, parallel group design, the patients were randomly assigned to receive zopiclone (7.5 mg) or placebo at bedtime for 12 consecutive weeks. No other sleep-modifying drugs were allowed during the trial. Data collected included patients' self-scoring of the severity of pain, stiffness, muscle fatigue, pain produced by pressure on a specified tender point, and global status of illness, and daily assessments of sleep characteristics using structured instruments. Investigators assessed tender point sites using calibrated dolorimeters and conducted interviews to determine the severity of the main symptoms at baseline, midpoint, and end of the trial period. Polysomnographic evaluations were performed at baseline and at the end of the trial on 11 patients assigned to receive zopiclone and on ten patients from the placebo group and data analyzed blindly after the treatment was completed. Precautions were taken to exclude the "first night in the sleep laboratory" effect.

Four of the 45 patients (9 percent) dropped out of the study because of inability to comply with the study's investigational requirements. None of the dropouts had adverse reactions to zopiclone or placebo. Among the 41 patients completing the trial, zopiclone produced side effects in four of 20 subjects (20 percent); three patients reported dysgeusia (taste alteration), and one had episodic sleepwalking. Among the 21 placebo-treated patients, side effects were reported by two (10 percent) patients, who complained of nightmares and taste alteration.

All patients who completed the trial were women whose age ranged from 36 to 59, with a median of 50 years. The zopiclone and placebo groups were well matched with respect to the number of tender points present at the initial examination. The groups differed with regard to the duration of illness, which averaged ten years for the zopiclone group but only four years in the placebo group.

Compared with placebo, treatment with zopiclone improved consistently and significantly patients' perception of the quality of sleep and sleep onset latency. Self-scores of the feeling on awakening gave inconsistent results. These subjective assessments were not supported by the objective polysomnographic evaluations, which indicated no quantitative change in any of the sleep stages during treatment. Alpha intrusions during slow-wave sleep were found in 56 percent of the timed epochs at baseline and 51 percent during treatment with the nonbenzodiazepine hypnotic. The number of recorded awakenings were likewise statistically similar for the two treatment groups. An attempt to correlate subjective improvement with recorded sleep characteristics revealed no significant associations. With the exception of an improvement in daytime tiredness, the main clinical features of the fibromyalgia syndrome, i.e., widespread pain, morning stiffness, and headache were not changed by treatment with zopiclone. The tender point evaluation at the end of the trial indicated no detectable effect of zopiclone therapy.

Support for these findings has been provided by a group of Finnish investigators who utilized the clinical resources of the University Central Hospital, Helsinki, and Kivela City Hospital, Helsinki, Finland, with support from the drug's manufacturer (Gronblad et al., 1993). Employing the same set of diagnostic criteria (Yunus et al., 1981) as their colleagues from Denmark (Drewes et al., 1991), the authors recruited 49 patients with fibromyalgia who were randomly assigned to receive zopiclone (7.5 mg in the evening) or placebo for eight consecutive weeks. Physical, laboratory, and radiologic evaluations excluded other causes for the patients' musculoskeletal pain complaints. No other medications were allowed during the trial. Main measurements were based on symptom scores provided by patients and obtained by investigators at baseline and after four and eight weeks of treatment; neither patients nor clinicians were aware of the treatment group assignment. Dolorimetric evaluations of specified anatomic sites were carried out only in a minority of patients and objective evaluations of sleep were not performed.

Three of the 24 patients assigned to receive zopiclone dropped out for personal reasons. Seven of the remaining 21 patients (33 percent) experienced symptoms attributed by them to zopiclone and withdrew. The adverse effects consisted of diarrhea (two patients), bitter taste (two patients), nightmares and headache (one patient), nausea (one patient), and fatigue, constipation, and paresthesias (one patient). None of these adverse effects were considered severe by the investigators. The placebo group (n = 25) had three dropouts caused by lack of compliance with the research protocol. Three of the remaining 22 patients (14 percent) developed adverse effects attributed to treatment and withdrew before the end of the trial. These adverse effects of placebo therapy consisted of nausea, arrhythmia and symptoms suggestive of thrombophlebitis.

The trial was completed by 14 patients from the zopiclone group and 19 treated with placebo. Data generated by five patients assigned to take placebo were discarded as part of a planned effort to ensure an adequate match between the two groups with respect to baseline sleep characteristics. After eight weeks of treatment, blinded investigators concluded that the fibromyalgia syndrome had improved in 50 percent of patients treated with zopiclone and 50 percent of those who had received placebo. Patients' assessments indicated improvement in 43 percent of the zopiclone group and 29 percent of the placebo group, a difference with statistical significance. Zopiclone was no better than placebo with regard to self-scored quality of sleep, sensitivity of tender points, and severity of morning stiffness and generalized pain.

Zolpidem

Zolpidem is an imidazopyridine derivative which has selective affinity for the BZ1 benzodiazepine receptor in the central nervous system and thus has sedative effects but lacks noticeable anxiolytic or muscle-relaxing properties (American Hospital Formulary Serice, 1997, p. 1849). The agent is commonly used for the treatment of insomnia in North America, and has been tested for efficacy in fibromyalgia by an experienced group of investigators from the University of Toronto's Center for Sleep and Chronobiology and Toronto Hospital, Western Division, Toronto, Ontario, Canada (Moldofsky et al., 1996). The authors recruited 19 subjects (mean age 42 years) who had been diagnosed with fibromyalgia according to standard criteria (Wolfe et al., 1990). All patients had experienced nonrestorative sleep and fatigue for at least three months prior to the onset of the trial. Baseline polysomnographic evaluations had identified significant alpha intrusions during slow-wave sleep in all subjects. None of the patients had an active major physical or psychiatric disorder, including sleep apnea or nocturnal myoclonus. Patients were required to discontinue all benzodiazepines, antidepressants, and analgesics, (other than aspirin or acetaminophen) two weeks before they entered the trial. The study was conducted according to a modified crossover design for a total of 20 days of treatment divided into five four-day units, one of which was a placebo period. During the other four units patients received increasing doses of zolpidem (5, 10, 15 mg) and placebo at bedtime. The night selected for placebo administration varied during each sequence. The effect of treatment was assessed by comparing the self-scored severity of symptoms and the results of tender point evaluations at baseline and those obtained after each treatment sequence.

Three of the 19 patients studied failed to complete the trial. One patient was dropped out because of lack of compliance with the research requirements. The other two (10 percent) withdrew after developing adverse effects of medication, which consisted of migraine occurring on the day of treatment with 10 mg of zolpidem and lightheadedness and nausea following intake of placebo. The zolpidem dose of 15 mg led to significant arterial hypotension in one patient (5 percent). Anxiety, hallucination, and depersonalization were reported by four patients (20 percent), two each after zolpidem and placebo. Minor side effects (headache, flu-like symptoms, diarrhea, and abnormal dreaming) were common, being reported by 44 percent of patients after 5 mg of zolpidem, 40 percent after 10 mg, 54 percent after 15 mg, and 56 percent after placebo administration.

Zolpidem was no better than placebo with regard to the subjective severity of pain, ache, and stiffness experienced in the morning or afternoon. No improvement was detectable by the objective dolorimetric evaluation of tender points. Assessments of the fatigue/energy level gave conflicting results; on one hand, zolpidem and placebo treatments did not appreciably change the degree of tiredness recorded on patient-kept diaries; on the other hand, the data suggested that zolpidem did in fact increase evening energy levels. Sleep quantity improved after zolpidem therapy (10 and 15 mg at bedtime), as reflected in the decrease of the time to fall asleep and increase in the total sleep time. However, sleep quality did not change and the severity of morning sleepiness and ability to concentrate were not different at the end of the trial.

Chapter 10

Unreplicated Trials

ONDANSETRON

Ondansetron, a serotonin (5-hydroxytryptamine, 5-HT) type 3 receptor antagonist, was tested for potential efficacy in the treatment of fibromyalgia by investigators from the Karol Marcinkowski University of Medical Sciences, Poznan, Poland, and Hochrhein Institute for Rehabilitation Research, Bad Sackingen, Germany, and Rheinfelden, Switzerland (Hrycaj et al., 1996). The 21 patients offered participation were recent referrals to a rheumatology clinic who fulfilled standard criteria for the diagnosis of fibromyalgia (Wolfe et al., 1990); had not been treated with antidepressant drugs for at least two months prior to the trial; and agreed to discontinue all pain and sleep medications upon entering the study. After a one-week washout period, patients were randomly assigned to receive ondansetron (8 mg orally twice daily) or the over-the-counter analgesic paracetamol (500 mg twice daily) for five consecutive days. Next followed a three-day washout period, after which the patients were treated for five days with the alternate regimen. During the study subjects were not allowed to take other medications for symptomatic relief of the syndrome and received a regularly scheduled physical therapy regimen. Main measurements included self-scoring of pain intensity in 24 anatomical areas and severity of 14 other clinical variables (e.g., cold feet or hands, sicca syndrome, diaphoresis, dizziness, sleep disturbance, and headache); dolorimetric evaluation of 24 potentially tender point and eight control anatomical sites; and determination of serum serotonin concentrations using a specific immunoassay.

One of the 21 patients (5 percent) enrolled in the trial had a serious adverse effect (allergic rash) and discontinued the study medication. The 20 participants (19 women) who completed the trial had a mean age of 44 years and average duration of fibromyalgic symptoms of six years. Other than the hypersensitivity reaction described, side effects of ondansetron were constipation (20 percent) and dry mouth (15 percent). The administration of paracetamol was not associated with any notable adverse reactions.

In this short-term crossover trial, ondansetron was superior to control therapy with the over-the-counter analgesic paracetamol with regard to subjective reports of pain intensity and objective findings of tenderness at specified musculoskeletal sites. The tender point examination indicated mild worsening after treatment with paracetamol. Overall, significant improvement in condition, defined as a 40 percent or more decrease in pain intensity, was noted in 11 patients (55 percent) at the end of the five-day course of treatment with ondansetron but only one patient (5 percent) in response to therapy with paracetamol. A global increase in the serum serotonin levels was produced by ondansetron, but no correlation was seen between this change and response to therapy in individual cases.

RITANSERIN

The effectiveness of ritanserin in fibromyalgia was tested by investigators affiliated at the time of writing with Huddinge Hospital, Karolinska Institute, Stockholm, Sweden, and University of Tübingen, Tübingen, Germany, in collaboration with the Swedish manufacturer of ritanserin (Olin, Klein, and Berg, 1998). An unusual dimension of this trial was the effort to correlate changes in clinical condition with the presence of autoantibodies to 5-hydroxytryptamine, which have been previously described among fibromyalgia patients by the same group of investigators (Klein, Bansch, and Berg, 1992).

The study group included 54 women referred for evaluation and treatment at the National Social Insurance Hospital in Tranas, Sweden, a facility receiving patients from all regions of the country. Most of the patients admitted had long-term illnesses, which in about 10 percent of cases were diagnosed as fibromyalgia. The cohort entered in the trial fulfilled the American College of Rheumatology standard diagnostic criteria (Wolfe at al., 1990) and had no evidence of major physical or psychiatric disorder, took no psy-chotropic medications, were not pregnant and were not breast-feeding. The subjects were randomly assigned to receive ritanserin (10 mg daily) or placebo for 16 weeks, the first four of which were in the hospital. Data recorded at baseline and after four and 16 weeks of treatment included self-reports of the severity of pain, fatigue, sleep disturbance, and morning stiffness; psychometric scales; and tender point evaluations. Antibodies to serotonin were detected by en-zyme-linked immunosorbent assays.

Three of the 54 patients (6 percent) withdrew before the end of the trial. All had been assigned to receive ritanserin; one of these patients developed pulmonary embolism, another discontinued the study medication because of flu-like symptoms, and the third was noncompliant with the trial's requirements. No adverse effects were reported by the patients treated with placebo.

Ritanserin was no better than placebo in treating the symptoms of pain, fatigue, sleep disturbance, morning stiffness, and anxiety ex-perienced by this group of fibromyalgia patients. Correspondingly, there was no significant difference in physical performance and in the amount of analgesic drugs taken during the trial by the patients assigned to the ritanserin or placebo groups. Objective measure-ments of sensitivity of the fibromyalgic tender points did not indi-cate improvement after ritanserin therapy. Positive effects of ritan-serin were noted for only two clinical variables, i.e., headache and feeling refreshed in the morning. Antiserotonin antibody activity was detected in 47 percent of participants at levels that were not significantly influenced by treatment with ritanserin or placebo.

PREDNISONE

The only controlled trial of corticosteroids in fibromyalgia was designed and executed by researchers from the Oregon Health Sciences University (Clark, Tindall, and Bennett, 1985). The authors recruited 20 rheumatology clinic patients who had been given the diagnosis of fibrositis based on their symptoms, the presence of pain at a minimum of seven out of 14 defined anatomic sites, and the absence of clinical and roentgenographic evidence of collagen vascular disease, axial or peripheral degenerative joint disease, hypothyroidism, hypercalcemia, and diabetes mellitus. The design required a blinded 28-day crossover trial during which the patients took either 15 mg of the synthetic glucocorticoid prednisone (deltacortisone) or an identical-looking placebo capsule each morning for 14 consecutive days and then were switched to the alternate treatment modality. Baseline and outcome measurements included assessments of pain severity, quality of sleep, morning stiffness, fatigue, and dolorimetry scores of the pain response of 14 potentially tender points. A prospective decision was made to use a 50 percent or more improvement in any one score as the only criterion for beneficial response to treatment.

The 20 subjects enrolled in the trial had a mean age of 45 years and an average duration of illness of seven years. One patient had been previously diagnosed with hypothyroidism and had this condition corrected with appropriate treatment. One patient each had mildly abnormal titers of rheumatoid factor and antinuclear antibody, but without evidence of collagen vascular disease over the 12-month period preceding the trial. Five patients were found at baseline to have slight increases in their serum level of creatin-phosphokinase, but without evidence of primary or secondary myopathy. All patients completed the trial without notable adverse effects.

Treatment with prednisone did not produce improvement in any of the clinical variables measured. The administration of placebo was likewise insignificant when outcome data after 14 days and 28 days of treatment were compared with baseline findings. Compared with placebo, only two of the 20 patients (10 percent) could be considered improved by treatment with prednisone. One patient reported significant improvement in morning stiffness and fatigue after the two-week course of prednisone; however, pain severity, dolorimetry score, and degree of sleep disturbance were not affected by corticosteroid therapy. In another patient, prednisone therapy produced a favorable decrease in the dolorimetry scores but only minimal positive changes in the overall pain experience, morning stiffness and fatigue, and a clear-cut deterioration in the quality of sleep. The authors appear justified in their conclusion that a positive response to corticosteroid treatment in patients diagnosed with fibromyalgia is so unusual as to indicate that the patient may actually have been misdiagnosed and that the cause of the pain syndrome is a corticosteroid-responsive rheumatic condition.

CHLORMEZANONE

Chlormezanone, a skeletal muscle relaxant not available in the United States, has been tried for the treatment of fibromyalgia by a group of investigators from City Hospital, Nottingham, United Kingdom, who believed that the drug combines properties attractive for the improvement of this condition, i.e., a peripheral muscle relaxing effect by decreasing efferent discharges to the motor fibers of the muscle spindle and a benzodiazepine-like effect on sleep architecture (Pattrick, Swanell, and Doherty, 1993). The authors received limited technical support from the drug's manufacturer. The 42 subjects were recruited from among patients newly referred to a specialized unit for evaluation; all met diagnostic criteria, which included the presence of typical symptoms and pain at ten or more specified musculoskeletal sites. Clinical and laboratory evaluation excluded other significant physical disorders. None of the patients were currently treated with psychotropic or hypnotic therapy. Participants were randomly assigned to receive chlormezanone (400 mg daily at bedtime) or placebo for six consecutive weeks. Main measurements included self-scored assessments of morning pain, morning alertness, morning stiffness, and sleep quality; objective determination of the number of tender points; and the patient's and physician's global assessment of the severity of illness.

Of the 42 patients recruited for the study, two were excluded because they did not have the required number of tender points at the onset of the trial. One patient (5 percent) treated with chlormezanone developed nausea that was severe enough to lead to discontinuation of medication and withdrawal from the trial. Adverse effects were reported by ten patients (50 percent) treated with chlormezanone and by seven patients (33 percent) from the placebo group and consisted mostly of headache and nausea.

Chlormezanone had no therapeutic effect on any of the symptoms and objective findings of patients with fibromyalgia included in this trial. In fact, after six weeks, placebo-treated patients had significantly fewer tender points than patients treated with the muscle relaxant. Placebo also improved sleep quality and morning alertness as compared with baseline, an effect not observed in the chlormezanone-treated group. Morning aching and stiffness improved with placebo but not with chlormezanone at the three-week evaluation. At the end of the trial 44 percent of the patients treated with chlormezanone and 50 percent of the subjects in the placebo group considered themselves improved; the corresponding frequencies as judged by the physician-investigator were 38 percent for the chlormezanone group and 47 percent for the placebo group. The amount of medication (paracetamol) needed for rescue analgesia was similar in the two groups.

GROWTH HORMONE

The effectiveness of growth hormone therapy in fibromyalgia was recently studied by investigators from the Oregon Health Sciences University, Portland, Oregon, in a trial supported in part by a grant from the drug's manufacturer (Bennett, Clark, and Walczyk, 1998). A role for growth hormone in the pathophysiology of fibromyalgia was postulated by the authors based on evidence indicating that patients with fibromyalgia have a disturbance that reduces the amount of time spent in stages 3 and 4 of the non-rapid-eye-movement sleep (Moldofsky et al., 1975). Since growth hormone is secreted predominantly during these sleep stages, a deficiency state may ensue and has in fact been confirmed by decreased levels of a surrogate marker for growth hormone (insulin-like growth factor 1), which have been identified by the Oregon investigators in a subset of close to one-third of patients with fibromyalgia (Bennett et al., 1992).

The study group included only subjects from this subset, i.e., women with fibromyalgia who had an IGF-1 level of less than 160 ng/ml at baseline. The diagnosis of fibromyalgia was made in accordance with standard criteria (Wolfe et al., 1990). In all cases the fibromyalgia had its onset more than five years prior to the trial and the absence of pituitary and other endocrinologic disorders was carefully established. In addition, the participants did not carry diagnoses of depression or any past or present malignancy. The 50 eligible subjects were randomly assigned to receive daily subcutaneous injections of growth hormone or an identical placebo for a nine-month period. The growth hormone was a recombinant protein with an amino acid sequence reproducing the naturally occurring pituitary hormone. The initial dose was 0.0125 mg/kg, which was administered daily for one month, after which the dose was adjusted at monthly intervals to maintain an IGF-1 level of around 250 ng/ml. The dose was decreased to the initial level whenever side effects such as arthralgia, edema, or carpal tunnel syndrome occurred and was kept unchanged at that dose until the resolution of the adverse reaction. Dose adjustments were made by an investigator aware of the type of treatment and serum IGF-1 level who did not interact with patients. Every dosage change in a patient receiving growth hormone was matched by a similar adjustment in the amount of injectable material received by a patient assigned to treatment with placebo.

Main measurements were made by an investigator blinded to the treatment group to which patients belonged, and consisted of a questionnaire assessing pain, fatigue, morning stiffness and tiredness, anxiety, depression, physical functioning, job difficulty, work record, and overall well-being as well as the objective evaluation of 18 specified anatomical locations to detect fibromyalgia tender points.

Of the 50 patients enrolled in the study, five withdrew before the end of the trial. Three of these patients had been receiving growth hormone and dropped out because of medical reasons independent of the effect of medication (sciatic nerve tumor and cardiomyopathy, respectively) and one for reasons of noncompliance. Of the two patients assigned to receive placebo who dropped out, one had been noncompliant with the trial protocol and the other had an undefined medical reason. Carpal tunnel syndrome developed in seven of the 22 completers (32 percent) treated with growth hormone and in one of the 23 subjects (4 percent) treated with placebo. The authors indicate that this adverse effect occurred during the early stages of the trial and was treated with nighttime wrist splints and instructions to lower the amount of medication self-administered by subcutaneous injection. As required by the protocol, each time a patient treated with growth hormone developed symptoms of carpal tunnel syndrome, a presumably asymptomatic patient from the placebo group was also instructed to lower her dose of medication. The sum effect may have been the unblinding of the assignment to growth hormone or placebo for at least 13 of the 45 patients (29 percent) who completed the trial, a potential pitfall not commented upon by the authors of this report. The substantial frequency of this major complication is not surprising; in a study of elderly men with low IGF-1 concentrations treated with growth hormone, carpal tunnel syndrome was the most common side effect, occurring in ten of 47 patients (21 percent) (Cohn et al., 1993). Moreover, there is evidence that the carpal tunnel syndrome produced by growth hormone may be the result of irreversible narrowing of the carpal tunnel rather than transient soft tissue edema (Kameyama et al., 1993). The frequency and type of other adverse reactions in this group of patients with fibromyalgia were not described; instead, a statement indicated that "no unexpected adverse reactions that could be attributed to the growth hormone were encountered" (Bennett, Clark, and Walczyk, 1998, p. 230).

The groups treated with growth hormone and placebo were considered similar with regard to age (mean 46 versus 48 years), initial IGF-1 level, and number of patients concomitantly treated with NSAIDs (55 percent versus 35 percent), tricyclic agents (50 percent versus 39 percent), and estrogens (55 percent versus 83 percent). Treatment with growth hormone was found to be superior to placebo on the basis of questionnaire data and reduction in the number of tender points. However, the clinical significance of the difference appears doubtful, given the fact that no patient had a complete remission of symptoms and that the average number of tender points at the end of the trial, although decreased from 18 to 13, was still amply sufficient for an unequivocal diagnosis of fibromyalgia. Given the authors' indication that a nine-month course of treatment with growth hormone at the dose used in this trial will cost each patient $13,500 and the possibility that the extent of the modest improvement was influenced by the potential unblinding effect of carpal tunnel syndrome in almost one-third of the patients, this therapeutic modality appears unconvincing and cost-ineffective.

CALCITONIN

Calcitonin, a hormone that participates in calcium homeostasis and is used in the treatment of hypercalcemia and osteoporosis, has been tried in a group of patients with fibromyalgia in a study designed by investigators from Centre Hospitalier Universitaire de

Quebec, Sainte-Foy, Quebec, Canada, and Brigham and Women's Hospital, Harvard Medical School, Boston, Massachusetts (Bessette et al., 1998). The authors postulated that calcitonin will reduce the symptoms of this pain syndrome through a mechanism involving the brain serotonin mechanism. The 11 patients enrolled in the trial fulfilled standard diagnostic criteria (Wolfe et al., 1990) and had baseline evaluations indicating substantial severity of both the pain and the other clinical manifestations of the syndrome. Ten of the 11 patients were women, the mean age of the group was 44 years, and the average duration of fibromyalgia was nine years. All antidepressant or anti-inflammatory drugs were discontinued at least one week prior to the trial and care was taken to make sure that none of these subjects had active bony disorders or endocrine or infectious conditions. Subcutaneous injections of salmon calcitonin (100 IU suspended in 1 ml) or placebo (1 ml of isotonic saline) were administered daily for four weeks, after which the patients entered a four-week washout period followed by four weeks of treatment with the alternate regimen. All patients and investigators were stringently blinded to treatment assignment for the entire duration of the trial. Baseline and monthly follow-up examinations recorded the self-assessed severity of pain, fatigue, sleep disturbance, morning stiffness, the refreshed feeling on awakening, and the degree to which subjects were troubled by their illness. The physician-investigators measured tenderness at five pairs of musculoskeletal sites included in the definition of fibromyalgia and scored the general progress of the condition. A standardized questionnaire was used to measure functional disability and the psychosocial impairment produced by the syndrome.

Ten of the 11 patients completed the trial in full compliance with the assigned treatment and follow-up evaluation. The direction of the crossover was from calcitonin to placebo in five cases and from placebo to calcitonin in six. One patient developed severe nausea and vomiting after two weeks of treatment with calcitonin and discontinued this phase of the trial but completed the placebo phase without incident. Side effects of calcitonin were extremely common, and included nausea (91 percent of patients), facial flushing (45 percent), palmar or plantar erythema (36 percent), and pruritus

(27 percent). The side effects recorded during the placebo phase were not listed in the published report.

Calcitonin was no better than placebo for the treatment of fibromyalgia patients included in this trial. Favorable response, defined by a 50 percent or greater decrease in pain and in the global severity of illness was observed in only one patient (9 percent) after four weeks of injectable calcitonin therapy. Two patients were considered partial responders, i.e., had a 25 percent improvement in the same parameters. After treatment with placebo, two patients obtained partial response. None of the individual variables assessed indicated a statistical difference between calcitonin and placebo. For the majority of outcome measures (nine out of 11), therapy with calcitonin did not produce any meaningful change from baseline.

MALIC ACID AND MAGNESIUM

Malic acid, a dicarboxylic acid that occurs naturally and is a component of apple juice (4-8 g/l) and other fruits and vegetables, has been tried for the treatment of fibromyalgia in a study performed at the University of Texas Health Science Center, San Antonio, Texas, with financial support from the manufacturer of a proprietary tablet containing 200 mg of malic acid and 50 mg of magnesium hydrochloride (Russell et al., 1995). The rationale for the study invoked the reduced high-energy phosphate (ATP) levels in the painful muscles of patients with fibromyalgia (Bengtsson, Henriksson, and Larson, 1986) and postulated that treatment with malic acid and magnesium may increase the mitochondrial synthesis of ATP.

The authors recruited 29 sequential patients who fulfilled the diagnostic criteria for fibromyalgia in accordance with the standard established by the American College of Rheumatology (Wolfe et al., 1990) and who agreed to discontinue all other medications prescribed for the treatment of this condition. However, five patients were unable to comply with this requirement, so that only 24 patients entered the controlled, crossover trial and were randomized to start treatment with three tablets twice daily for four weeks of either the combination malic acid and magnesium or a similar number of placebo tablets, which were similar in appearance and taste.

This first four-week treatment period was followed by a two-week washout interval, after which the patients received the alternate form of therapy for the last four weeks of the study. The patients were allowed to take only acetaminophen at a maximum dosage of 650 mg once daily as needed for severe headache. Baseline and outcome measures consisted primarily of subjective assessments of pain and objective determination of the severity of tenderness at the nine pairs of musculoskeletal sites specified by the standard definition of fibromyalgia (Wolfe et al., 1990).

The study group had a mean age of 49 years and the expected female predominance (87.5 percent). Of the 24 patients who started the trial, four (17 percent) dropped out for reasons not described in the published report. Adverse effects were reported by three subjects during treatment with the malic acid and magnesium combination and consisted of nausea, dyspepsia, and diarrhea in one case each. Two patients developed diarrhea and one complained of dyspepsia while taking placebo.

The combination malic acid and magnesium was no better than placebo in this double-blinded crossover study. Compared with baseline, the treatment did not provide any measurable decrease in the subjective experience of pain (pain score on analog scale 7.3 at the outset and 6.8 after four weeks of treatment) or dolorimetric response of the fibromyalgic tender points. Separate analyses taking into account the use of acetaminophen for rescue analgesia did not change the completely negative findings of the trial.

Chapter 11

Evidence-Based Therapy of Fibromyalgia

The results of the numerous controlled clinical trials of drug therapy in fibromyalgia indicate that only the tricyclic antidepressant
amitriptyline has shown the ability to improve the main characteristics of this condition in a manner clinically distinguishable from that
of placebo. With the important caveat created by the fact that only a
minority of patients will show consistent and substantial amelioration of their symptoms (Abeles, 1998), and the sobering lack of data
regarding the outcome of long-term therapy, the evidence indicates
that amitriptyline is the only reasonable first-line treatment for fibromyalgia. If not contraindicated, the treatment must be initiated in all
patients regardless of the presence and severity of depressive symptoms. Standard instructions should be carefully consulted and the
drug should not be used when its anticholinergic potential can wors-
en preexisting conditions such as urinary retention, benign prostatic
hypertrophy and other types of bladder outlet dysfunction, angle-
closure glaucoma, hyperthyroidism, or treatment with synthetic or natural thyroid hormones. The drug is contraindicated in patients recover-
ing from a myocardial infarction and in subjects with a history of
hypersensitivity reactions to any tricyclic agent (American Hospital
Formulary Service, 1997, p. 1677). The drug should not be prescribed
to women who are or plan to become pregnant, or are lactating or
planning to breast-feed. Extreme caution is called for whenever the
treatment with amitriptyline is contemplated in patients with preexisting cardiovascular disease, seizure disorder of any etiology, broncho-
pulmonary disorders, and alcohol or sedative-hypnotic abuse or dependence. The potential for drug-drug interactions must be carefully
explored before the first prescription, with great attention paid to
patients treated by multiple physicians and direct inquiry as to

whether the patient is, or has recently been, taking monoamine oxidase inhibitors, hypotensive agents, sedative or hypnotic agents, adrenergic agents, drugs with anticholinergic effect, and cimetidine (American Hospital Formulary Service, 1997, p. 1678).

The treatment can be started with a dose as low as 10 mg daily, and increments of 10 mg made every week with careful monitoring of symptom response and adverse drug reactions. Although the controlled trials of amitriptyline have tested only doses on the low side of the accepted range, we see no pharmacological reason not to continue to increase the amount until at least the moderate dose of 100 mg daily is reached. At this or greater dosages, periodic electrocardiograms are needed for early detection of cardiac toxicity, which leads to increase in the QRS duration and the prolongation of the Q-T interval. Compliance and efficiency of gastrointestinal absorption can be assessed by measuring plasma levels of amitriptyline, a laboratory test that is both available and affordable in this country.

Among the nonpharmacological approaches tested in controlled trials, an impressive body of work has reported the results of aerobic exercise on the manifestations of fibromyalgia. In the first trial, investigators from University of Western Ontario, London, Canada, compared the effect of cardiovascular fitness training with that of simple flexibility exercises (McCain et al., 1988). After 20 weeks of treatment, the patients' self-assessment indicated no significant change in the severity of pain, extent of body area affected by fibromyalgic symptoms, and sleep disturbance. Similarly negative results were reported after a 20-week trial of physical fitness training performed at the Sanitetsforening Rheumatism Hospital, Oslo, Norway (Mengshoel, Komnaes, and Forre, 1992); there were no differences in the severity of pain and fatigue or in ability to cope with pain. A common denominator of these two trials is the fact that the exercise programs were effective with regard to their specific target, i.e., they produced the expected increases in cardiovascular fitness, muscle strength, and endurance. In contrast, a six-week trial of physical training and self-management education involving patients followed at Sahlgren University Hospital, Gothenburg, Sweden (Burckhardt et al., 1994), showed significant positive changes. In another six-week trial of aerobic exercise, researchers from the University of Calgary, Alberta, Canada (Martin et al., 1996) reported a decrease in the total myalgic score and the number of tender points, which reached significance in comparison with the posttreatment status of a control group treated with relaxation therapy. Finally, recent controlled work performed at the Missouri Arthritis Rehabilitation Research and Training Center, University of Missouri, Columbia, Missouri (Buckelew et al., 1998), has indicated some improvement in physical activity after an exercise intervention. Of some concern is the fact that fibromyalgia patients undergoing aerobic exercise treatments may experience substantial exercise-related pain, develop significant postexercise pain and fatigue (Mengshoel, Vollestad, and Forre, 1995), and notice a worsening in their functional ability (Nichols and Glenn, 1994). Therefore, given its mostly negative results and potential for adverse effects, a prescription for exercise does not appear justified for most patients with fibromyalgia.

Controlled trials of cognitive therapy have also produced discouraging results. A large-scale randomized trial planned and executed at the Institute for Rehabilitation Research, Hoensbroek, Netherlands (Vlaeyen et al., 1996), compared the cognitive/educational intervention with an education/discussion approach and a separate "waiting list" control. Both interventions improved the ability to cope with pain, but the cognitive therapy did not change the severity of pain, a failure attributed to poor compliance, difficulty of homework assignments, and lack of individual support. Support for these findings was provided by a controlled study of a 10-week comprehensive behavioral intervention performed by researchers from the California School of Professional Psychology, San Diego, California (Nicassio et al., 1997), which produced no surplus value with regard to myalgia scores and self-reported pain behaviors despite improved coping and reduced helplessness. Somewhat more encouraging data were recently reported by academic investigators from Basel, Switzerland (Keel et al., 1998), which have shown that early use of integrated group therapy (cognitive-behavioral strategies, relaxation, and physical exercise) was better than nonspecific training on measures of pain and activities of daily living, but the clinical significance of the findings is limited by the small number of patients included in the trial and the fact that four-month follow-up data indicated persistent improvement only in a negligible minority.

SECTION III:
IRRITABLE BOWEL SYNDROME

Chapter 12

Definition and Methodological Issues

The standard for the diagnosis of irritable bowel syndrome is a set of criteria generated by what is known as the Rome group, a multinational working committee of gastroenterologic investigators (Thompson et al., 1989). The first criterion is the presence of at least three months of recurrent or continuous abdominal pain or discomfort that is either relieved with defecation or associated with a change in frequency or consistency of stool. Care must be taken to determine that the pain symptom is not part of a different functional gastrointestinal disorder, such as functional dyspepsia or functional constipation. The second criterion requires the presence of at least two of the following five symptoms: altered stool frequency, altered stool consistency, altered stool passage, passage of mucus, and feeling of abdominal distention. Altered stool frequency is generally understood to mean fewer than three bowel movements each week or more than three bowel movements each day. Altered stool consistency refers to feces that are loose and watery or hard and lumpy. Altered stool passage is indicated by the report of symptoms such as a feeling of incomplete evacuation, or straining or urgency to defecate. Based on the type of stool frequency and consistency, patients with irritable bowel may be classified as having the constipation-predominant or diarrhea-predominant variant of the syndrome. Physical examination, endoscopic investigation of the large bowel (sigmoidoscopy or colonoscopy), contrast radiologic studies, and stool analysis for blood, microorganisms, or evidence of malabsorption are useful only to exclude organic pathology (Longstreth, 1998).

The methodologic issues raised by controlled treatment trials in irritable bowel syndrome were defined more than a decade ago

(Klein, 1988). The main issue was considered the difficulty of measuring efficacy in the absence of objective markers of a favorable change. The solution has been a dizzying array of arbitrary rating scales that have attempted to quantify the effect of treatment on as many as 15 dimensions of the illness or as few as a single global score. A related problem is the continuing need to ensure that the main objectives of the trial are assessed with specific instruments, i.e., one should not assume that the drug tested has been efficacious based on decreased frequency of bowel movements if the severity of abdominal pain has not diminished. Thus, an overall measure carefully weighing the contribution of the changes induced by therapy in the major manifestations of the syndrome is advisable, but difficult to construct and validate and prone to recording only the subjective sense of heightened well-being, which may be due to the correction of fundamental abnormalities but may also reflect only a change in the patients' sick role and illness behavior. Data generated by asking the patients to indicate a preference between placebo and the drug treatment are also fraught with uncertainties, to the extent that placebo may be chosen on the basis of its lack of side effects or the active drug selected for having improved the mood state rather than the gastrointestinal features of the syndrome. Furthermore, given a placebo response rate that can exceed 50 percent of the study group, investigators must ensure a sufficient sample size and either utilize a crossover design or establish a high degree of baseline similarity between placebo and active treatment groups as prerequisites to obtaining precision in the assessment of efficacy. The intrinsic variability of the condition implies that only trials of sufficient duration will be able to offer meaningful information and Klein recommended a minimum of eight to 12 weeks for both the placebo and active treatment phase of the trial.

Chapter 13

Effective Therapies

TRICYCLIC ANTIDEPRESSANTS

Amitriptyline

The therapeutic usefulness of the tricyclic antidepressant amitriptyline in patients with irritable bowel syndrome was first tested in a well-designed crossover double-blind trial executed by an interdisciplinary team from the Departments of Psychiatry and Medicine at Albany Medical College, Albany, New York, with technical assistance from the drug's manufacturer (Steinhart, Wong, and Zarr, 1981). The cohort studied comprised 14 subjects (11 females) with "spastic colon syndrome" of at least six months' duration. The mean age of the cohort was 41 and the average duration of illness 5.1 years. All subjects had adequate open-label trials of a smooth muscle relaxant (dicyclomine hydrochloride) and a periphery-acting antimuscarinic agent (propantheline bromide) without significant improvement. The most common symptoms were abdominal pain (75 percent), diarrhea (71 percent), flatulence (50 percent), and nausea or vomiting (50 percent). Mental status examination identified eight patients (57 percent) as depressed and 11 patients (79 percent) as anxious. The majority of the patients (8 of 14) had abdominal pain, diarrhea, and/or constipation occurring at least three times daily or lasting more than 15 minutes each day; the severity of the symptoms was not substantially disabling, i.e., the symptoms did not interfere with more than eight hours of work each week. Three of the 14 patients had severe symptoms, which led to the loss of at least five days of work each month. The remaining three patients described abdominal pain and abnormal bowel habits that occurred only once or twice daily for a total daily duration of less than 15 minutes. All patients had normal findings on physical examination, stool testing for blood and enteric pathogens, lactose tolerance testing, and sigmoidoscopy. All female patients younger than 50 years of age had normal pelvic examinations just prior to enrolling in the trial.

The experimental conditions required that amitriptyline (50 mg orally at bedtime) and placebo be administered daily for a four-week period each. The study started with a one-week drug-free period. A two-week washout followed the first four-week medication trial. Patients were instructed to keep diaries of their symptoms and were given a total of five follow-up evaluations during the study.

Amitriptyline improved the symptoms of 11 of the 14 patients studied (79 percent). The improvement reached a highly significant level when baseline symptoms were compared to the status immediately following the administration of the tricyclic drug. The direct comparison of the effects of amitriptyiline and placebo indicated that the difference was close to the level of statistical significance. Compared with baseline, placebo treatment had no effect on the number and severity of symptoms. Amitriptyline-induced improvement was more frequently observed among patients whose irritable bowel syndrome was of moderate severity and among those whose baseline evaluation indicated high depression and anxiety scores. The authors noted that the positive effect of amitriptyline was clinically manifest within one to two days of treatment.

Trimipramine

Trimipramine, a dibenzazepine-derivative tricyclic compound with antidepressant and antisecretory properties (American Hospital Formulary Service, 1997, p. 1687), was tried in patients with irritable bowel syndrome in a multicenter Norwegian study coordinated by investigators from the Laboratory of Gastroenterology, Ulleval Hospital, Oslo, Norway (Myren et al., 1982). A total of 61 patients (33 women, average age 39 years) whose symptoms had been present for at least several months were recruited for the study. In all cases, the diagnosis of irritable bowel syndrome was established after organic disease was excluded on the basis of clinical and laboratory evaluations that included radiologic or endoscopic examinations of the upper and lower gastrointestinal tract.

The design of the study required that patients be randomly assigned to receive either trimipramine (50 mg before bedtime) or identical-looking placebo tablets for four weeks. The trial was preceded by a one-week washout period of all previous medications. The placebo and trimipramine groups were similar with respect to age, gender distribution, duration of symptoms, and basic laboratory values. The target symptoms of the investigation were abdominal pain, nausea, vomiting, belching, headache, sleeplessness, tiredness, anxiety, and depression, and were recorded by physicians on visual analog scales before and after treatment. The presence of mucus in stool was graded by patients on a semiquantitative scale.

At baseline, the frequency and severity of symptoms were similar among the two groups, with the exception of vomiting, which was more bothersome to patients assigned to receive placebo. Compared with placebo, treatment with imipramine significantly reduced the severity of vomiting, sleeplessness, and depression, as well as the presence of mucus in stool. However, for the other six target symptoms, including the cardinal complaint of abdominal pain, the frequency and severity was reduced to a similar degree in both the placebo and trimipramine groups. Tiredness decreased more in the placebo group than in the trimipramine-treated group, a difference noted by the authors but not substantiated by statistical analysis.

Several years later, the Norwegian investigators reported the results of a much larger trial of trimipramine efficacy in irritable bowel syndrome (Myren et al., 1984). This time, the multicenter study was expanded to include 88 general practitioners and 14 gastroenterologists who enrolled a total of 428 patients (216 women; median age 36.5 years). Patient selection and analysis of therapeutic effect was based on clinical criteria identical to those employed in the authors' previous effort (Myren et al., 1982). After a two-week washout, the patients were randomly assigned to receive 50 mg of trimipramine at bedtime (92 subjects), 10 mg of trimipramine in the morning and 40 mg in the evening (93 subjects), 35 mg of trimipramine at bedtime (71 subjects), 10 mg of trimipramine three times daily (77 subjects), or placebo (75 patients) for six consecutive weeks. The groups were similar with regard to all demographic and clinical variables.

Compared with placebo, treatment with 50 mg of trimipramine daily (given either as a single bedtime dose, or 10 mg in the morning and 40 mg in the evening) produced a statistically significant improvement in abdominal pain, nausea, and depression. On the other hand, with the exception of depression, treatment with lower doses of trimipramine was not superior to placebo for any of the target symptoms. Tiredness and morning drowsiness increased during the first two weeks of treatment with trimipramine, but by the end of the six-week trial their severity was similar to that reported by the patients treated with placebo.

Desipramine

Closely related to trimipramine, the dibenzazepine-derivative desipramine (American Hospital Formulary Service, 1997, p. 1681) has been the focus of a very well designed crossover study in which its action was compared with atropine and placebo on a patient sample assembled by investigators from the Departments of Medicine and Psychiatry at the College of Human Medicine, Michigan State University, East Lansing, Michigan (Greenbaum et al., 1987). The initial cohort comprised 41 patients (27 women) who were given the diagnosis of irritable bowel syndrome according to the following criteria: at least three months of abdominal pain with constipation and/or diarrhea and the absence of an organic diagnosis for these symptoms. The symptoms had to occur at least twice each week and patients were classified into diarrhea- or constipation-predominant irritable bowel syndrome. Baseline evaluations included routine thorough history and physical examination; routine hematologic and biochemical testing; examination of stools for blood, ova, parasites, and enteric bacterial pathogens; proctosigmoidoscopy; and barium enema. In addition, all patients completed a standard comprehensive personality inventory, a brief psychiatric rating scale, and a depression questionnaire.

The study design required a four-week period of observation, followed by three six-week treatment periods, during which the patients received 50 mg of desipramine and placebo, 0.4 mg of atropine and placebo, or only placebo. One tablet of each (active medication and placebo, or two placebo tablets) was administered at bedtime during the first week of treatment, two the second week, and three tablets of each from the third through the sixth week of each treatment period. Data were collected by patients in a diary that recorded the frequency and intensity of abdominal pain and distress, stool frequency and consistency, and mood changes. Assessments were also made by using structured questionnaires administered at biweekly clinic visits, repeated psychometric tests, rectosigmoid manometry, and desipramine blood levels. Data analysis was restricted to the last four weeks of each treatment period to avoid drug overlap and washout effects.

Of the 41 patients entered in the study, five were found to be noncompliant with the medication regimen, and five patients dropped out for a variety of reasons not related to treatment. A total of nine (22 percent) patients developed adverse effects while treated with desipramine, consisting mainly of anxiety, tremulousness, xerostomia, sweating, palpitations, and constipation; the severity of these symptoms was sufficiently severe to require discontinuation of desipramine and termination of the participation in the trial. Xerostomia, palpitations, and constipation developed also among seven patients during treatment with atropine, but the symptoms were relatively mild. The incidence of adverse effects during placebo administration was lower; three patients complained of tremors, xerostomia, nausea, or urticaria requiring discontinuation of the agent after four or more weeks of treatment. Therefore, the trial was completed by 28 patients, 19 of whom had diarrhea-predominant and 9 constipation-predominant irritable bowel syndrome.

Of these 28 patients, 26 reported improvement during at least one of the three phases of the trial: 15 (54 percent) were shown to improve during treatment with desipramine, six (21 percent) felt better while taking atropine, and five (18 percent) responded favorably to placebo. The diarrhea-predominant cases were more likely to respond to desipramine (68 percent) than the constipation-predominant subgroup (22 percent). Compared with placebo and atropine, desipramine proved superior in alleviating the abdominal pain of patients suffering from diarrhea-predominant irritable bowel syndrome. In the same subgroup, as compared with placebo therapy, treatment with desipramine significantly reduced the number of stools and the frequency of episodes of diarrhea. In the constipation-predominant subgroup, desipramine insignificantly increased the severity of constipation. These data correlated well with desipramine-induced changes in rectosigmoid manometry, which consisted of a substantial decrease in the number, force, and total duration of contractions. At steady state the serum concentrations of desipramine ranged from 12 to 560 ng/ml; the levels did not correlate with or predict the therapeutic response. As expected, desipramine therapy led to a decrease in the depression scores when compared with atropine treatment, but the trend was not confirmed by subgroup analyses, suggesting that mood changes played only a minor role in the improvement noted in the majority of patients with diarrhea-predominant irritable bowel syndrome. These clinical findings are supported by recent experimental work assessing the effect of two tricyclic agents, imipramine and desipramine, on the magnitude of the response of mechanosensitive pelvic nerve afferent fibers to colorectal distention in rats (Su and Gebhart, 1998). Tricyclic agents reduced the mean afferent fiber response to 20 percent of the values recorded for untreated control preparations. The action appeared specific to this group of agents, as it was clearly superior to the effect of the serotonin reuptake inhibitor clomipramine.

Chapter 14

Controversial Therapies

BULKING AGENTS

Ispaghula

Ispaghula husk, a bulking agent sold in many countries as an over-the-counter remedy for irritable bowel syndrome, was tested for efficiency in controlled trials performed in the United Kingdom (Prior and Whorwell, 1987) and India (Jalihal and Kurian, 1990).

In the first of these studies, investigators based at the University Hospital of South Manchester, Manchester, England, enrolled 80 consecutive outpatients diagnosed with irritable bowel syndrome (Prior and Whorwell, 1987). The diagnosis required the presence of abdominal discomfort and distention associated with an abnormal bowel habit of frequent bowel movements, constipation, or alternating constipation and frequent movements. The absence of organic gastrointestinal disease was confirmed by sigmoidoscopy in patients younger than 40 years of age, and by colonoscopy or air contrast barium enema in those older than 40. Hematologic and biochemical tests gave normal results in all patients. The members of the cohort were randomly assigned to receive a brand name of flavored ispaghula husk or placebo three times daily for 12 weeks. The starting dose consisted of 6.4 g of coarsely ground material containing exipient and 3.6 g of mucilloid ispaghula; the placebo doses contained only the exipient. Patients were allowed to decrease the dose in case of "unacceptable loosening" of the stools. Upward adjustment of the dosage was permitted if the bowel habit improved but did not normalize. Measurements included daily self-scoring of the severity of abdominal pain and characteristics of the bowel habit and assessments of the overall change in condition and whole gut transit time using a carmine dye marker.

Only 53 (66 percent) of the 80 participants completed the trial. Eight subjects assigned to take ispaghula and 15 subjects from the placebo group withdrew from the study. Serious adverse affects were uncommon. One patient treated with ispaghula withdrew because of flatulence and one patient taking placebo dropped out after developing persistent nausea. Most of the withdrawals (four in the ispaghula group and ten in the placebo group) were due to the patients' perception that the treatment was ineffective. The remainder of withdrawals were caused by noncompliance with the study's requirements or need for unrelated medical interventions.

Treatment with ispaghula was no better than placebo with regard to the principal symptoms of abdominal pain, abdominal distention, and the presence of frequent bowel movements. The bulking agent performed better than placebo by improving habitual constipation, an effect confirmed by the substantial reduction in the whole gut transit time from an average of 36 hours to 22 hours. At the end of the study, overall assessments of the change in condition indicated that treatment was considered a success by 53 percent of patients treated with placebo and 82 percent of those who had completed therapy with ispaghula, a statistically significant difference. The discrepancy between the lack of effectiveness on specific symptoms and the improved sense of well-being produced by treatment with ispaghula remained unexplained. However, unblinding may have contributed to this result, as the mucilaginous consistency of the ispaghula may have been detected by some of the patients.

The second important clinical trial of ispaghula in patients with irritable bowel syndrome was conducted at the Christian Medical College and Hospital in Vellore, India (Jalihal and Kurian, 1990). The authors recruited 23 patients with at least a two-year history of irritable bowel syndrome. The diagnosis was established by the presence of recurrent abdominal pain and/or flatulence and alteration in bowel habit. The search for organic disorders included standard hematologic and biochemical screening tests, stool examination for blood and parasites, and visual examination of the large bowel with colonoscopy or barium enema. None of the pa-

tients had a history of abdominal surgery and none had been previously treated with ispaghula-containing remedies.

The crossover design assigned patients randomly to treatment
with ispaghula husk (30 g administered once daily) or placebo (a
mixture of wheat flour and powdered rice, visually identical to the
ispaghula powder) for four weeks. This phase of the trial was followed by a seven- to ten-day washout period, after which the patients took the alternate treatment for four weeks. To avoid the
potential for unblinding created by the mucilaginous consistency of
the moistened ispaghula powder, patients were instructed to empty
the packets of powder in the back of the mouth and wash it down
immediately with water. No dietary changes were suggested and no
other medications were permitted during the trial. The main measurements relied on structured interviews and daily ratings regarding severity of pain and flatulence, number and consistency of
bowel movements, degree of satisfaction with bowel movements,
and assessment of global improvement. Baseline and posttreatment
whole-gut transit time was measured using radiopaque markers.

Twenty (15 women and five men, median age 38 years) of the 23
patients completed the trial. One patient declined participation and
two dropped out after enrollment, but the specific reasons for withdrawal were not disclosed. No adverse effects were described. Of
the 20 patients studied, 15 had diarrhea-predominant and five had a
constipation-predominant syndrome.

The abdominal pain improved in five (25 percent) patients after
ispaghula therapy and six (30 percent) after treatment with placebo.
A similar observation was made for flatulence (abdominal distention), which improved in five patients given ispaghula and two
subjects treated with placebo. Ispaghula seemed more effective with
regard to the subjective feeling of "satisfaction with one's bowel
activity," which improved in 17 patients (85 percent) as compared
with only five patients (25 percent) reporting a similar degree of
satisfaction after treatment with placebo. Overall, 85 percent of
patients felt that their condition had improved after treatment with
ispaghula, while treatment with placebo led to improvement in 40
percent of cases, a difference that reached marginal statistical significance. The magnitude of the improvement was higher after ispaghula (mean 35 percent) than after placebo (mean 11 percent)

therapy. Improvement correlated only with the evidently subjective satisfaction with bowel movements, but not with the severity of abdominal pain or number of bowel movements.

Psyllium

Psyllium, a hydrophilic mucilloid, has been studied in a well-designed trial conducted by a group of investigators from the Southern California Permanente Medical Center, San Diego (Longstreth et al., 1981). The authors recruited 77 patients with a history of abdominal pain improved after defecation and abnormal bowel habits (constipation, diarrhea, or both) for at least three months. Exclusion criteria were the presence of other gastrointestinal disorders (except for uncomplicated colon diverticulosis), pregnancy, and clinical evidence of lactose intolerance. Patients with a history of previous psyllium use were not included in the study group.

The patients recorded and graded daily their pain symptoms, "gas" symptoms (flatulence, bloating, rumbling, and belching), number of bowel movements and consistency of stools, and the extent to which these symptoms interfered with their usual activities. Diaries were kept for a two-week period prior to the study and throughout the eight-week trial. At the completion of the treatment period the patients provided a global rating of their status as compared to baseline. Before starting the trial, all patients had psychometric testing with an abbreviated version of the Minnesota Multiphasic Personality Inventory validated for medical patients (Newmark and Raft, 1976). The subjects were randomized to receive either psyllium or placebo. The psyllium was administered in the form of 6.4 g of an effervescent preparation containing 56 percent psyllium mucilloid taken three times daily in water. The placebo was presented in an identical packet and had a similar taste. The placebo contained cornstarch, dextrose, and polyvinylpyrrolidone. All patients were instructed to continue their usual diet and to take no other medications.

Seventeen patients failed to complete the study, including seven on psyllium and three on placebo who opted out because they noticed no improvement or because they disliked the treatment. Of the 60 patients completing the trial, 34 had been assigned to placebo and 26 to the psyllium group. The groups were well matched with respect to age, gender distribution, educational achievement, symptom duration and current severity, and psychometric abnormalities on the hypochondriasis, hysteria, and depression scales.

After eight weeks of treatment, the severity of abdominal pain and the number of normal stools improved in both treatment groups as compared with baseline. A significant improvement in the frequency of episodes of pain and the severity of "gas" symptoms was recorded by the subjects on placebo, but not by those on psyllium. There was no difference between placebo and psyllium in the proportion of patients who considered themselves "much better" (30 percent on psyllium and 40 percent on placebo) after treatment. The "much better" category was best predicted by results of the baseline psychometric testing indicating fewer abnormalities in the depression, psychastenia, and schizophrenia domains. A discriminant formula based on these three scores correctly identified 19 of the 21 patients who felt "much improved." Improvement was not predicted by any other demographic, clinical, or social variable, or by any other group of variables examined.

Calcium Polycarbophil

Calcium polycarbophil is another agent recommended for use in patients with irritable bowel syndrome on the basis of its ability to increase the bulk of the stool. The agent is not metabolized and exerts its hydrophilic activity predominantly in the alkaline environment of the bowel. Its effect has been studied in a randomized, double-blind crossover study by investigators from the University of Florida College of Medicine, Gainesville, in close collaboration with the product's manufacturer (Toskes, Connery, and Ritchey, 1993). A group of 28 patients were enrolled sequentially in the trial. None of the subjects had a past history of gastrointestinal surgery, gastrointestinal malignancy, lactose intolerance, diabetes mellitus, and nephrolithiasis and none were taking laxatives, antidepressants, anticholinergics, antibiotics, or supplemental calcium. The patients fulfilled the authors' criteria for irritable bowel syndrome, which required the presence of any one of the following combination of symptoms at least twice each week for at least three months: abdominal pain and alternating constipation and diarrhea; abdominal pain and diarrhea; and constipation associated with abdominal distention or pain. The patients recorded their symptoms on a daily basis and each month rated the overall effect of the treatment.

Patients were randomized to receive either 12 tablets of calcium polycarbophil daily (total dose six g) or identical placebo tablets containing dicalcium phopshate for a period of 12 weeks, after which they crossed over to receive the alternate treatment for 12 weeks. The amount of calcium was similar in the two types of tablets.

Twenty-three of the 28 patients completed the trial and submitted the interim and final data. The group included 16 women and seven men, with a mean age of 48 years. At the end of the trial, there were no statistically significant differences between the two treatments as measured by global scores, by the specific symptom scores for abdominal pain, abdominal distention, nausea, and stool consistency, and by the proportion of patients who favored one of the treatments over the other. Ease of stool passage was the only variable for which the treatment with calcium polycarbophil appeared superior to placebo.

SMOOTH MUSCLE RELAXANTS

Dicyclomine Hydrochloride

Dicyclomine hydrochloride is a selective muscarinic antagonist that has a high affinity for the neuronal M1-receptor of the gastrointestinal tract (Kilbinger and Stein, 1988) but only low affinity for the cardiac and glandular receptors (Giachetti et al., 1986). This selectivity is the basis of its pharmacologic use as a smooth muscle relaxant, and more specifically as a spasmolytic agent not encumbered by a full, atropine-like, anticholinergic spectrum of activity. Its effect on patients with irritable bowel syndrome was tested in a multi-investigator clinical trial supervised and reported by researchers employed by the drug's manufacturer in Cincinnati, Ohio (Page and Dirnberger, 1981). The diagnostic formulation required at least one of the following symptoms: abdominal pain, most severe after breakfast; persistent abdominal pain accompanied by the desire to move one's bowels; cramplike, i.e., sharp lower quadrant pain relieved by passing gas; and straining at stool. Alteration in bowel habit was not a requirement, but the clinician-investigators were encouraged to enroll patients complaining of constipation and subjects whose irritable bowel syndrome had been present for at least five years. The participants had to have negative results on sigmoidoscopy and barium enema performed within one year of the trial, no blood or parasites in stool, and no other significant physical or laboratory abnormalities.

After confirmation of eligibility, the participants started the trial with a week of single-blind placebo therapy. Patients were instructed to avoid foods known from previous experience to be related to their symptoms and to eat a "bulk" diet. The subjects whose symptoms improved at the end of this interval were considered placebo responders and were dropped out of the study. The 97 participants who did not respond to the single-blind placebo trial were randomly assigned to a two-week treatment with dicyclomine hydrochloride (40 mg in two tablets four times daily) or placebo. During the double-blind phase subjects were not allowed laxatives, antacids, or anticholinergic or antispasmodic agents. Measurements were based on patients' daily recordings of presence, timing, and severity of pain and on investigators' ratings of the complaints of abdominal pain, change in bowel habits, tenderness to abdominal palpation, and overall status of clinical condition.

Efficacy analyses were carried out on data provided by 71 of the 97 participants (73 percent). Criteria for excluding more than one-quarter of the study cohort were not disclosed, except to indicate that most of the dropouts had no episodes of pain during the single-blind placebo phase of the trial. Of the 71 patients whose data were used to assess the outcome of the trial, 34 had taken dicyclomine and 37 had been treated with placebo. The two treatment groups were well matched with regard to age, gender distribution, overall duration of illness, and duration of the current episode.

Adverse effects were reported by 69 percent of the 48 patients who started treatment with dicyclomine but only 16 percent of the 49 patients assigned to treatment with placebo. As expected, most of the dicyclomine-related symptoms were a direct consequence of the agent's anticholinergic activity, which produced dry mouth, blurring of vision, and dizziness. Seven patients (14 percent) from the dicyclomine group felt that the adverse effects were intolerable and stopped their participation in the trial. In 12 cases (24 percent) patients were able to continue the treatment only after the dicyclomine dose was reduced from 160 mg/day to an average of 90 mg/day.

The physicians assessed the posttreatment abdominal pain symptom as absent in 44 percent of patients treated with dicyclomine and 11 percent of those treated with placebo. The physician-investigators appreciated that abdominal tenderness had improved in 94 percent of dicyclomine-treated patients and 62 percent of the participants treated with placebo, and that bowel habits were better in 85 percent of cases after dicyclomine and 54 percent of patients who took placebo. The overall assessments indicated that 94 percent of dicyclomine-treated patients and 54 percent of those who took placebo had improved. These ratings are consistent with those made by patients, the corresponding proportions being 84 percent and 54 percent. Only 3 percent of the patients who completed the two-week course of dicyclomine felt worse, compared with five patients (17 percent) who had just finished placebo therapy. Treatment with dicyclomine exacerbated the abdominal pain in two patients (6 percent); in contrast, 13 patients (35 percent) treated with placebo reported increased abdominal discomfort during the second week of the double-blind phase of the trial.

Mebeverine

Mebeverine is widely used for the treatment of irritable bowel syndrome in the United Kingdom (Washington et al., 1998) and Australia (Evans, Bak, and Kellow, 1996). The agent has a prokinetic action on the small bowel (Evans, Bak, and Kellow, 1996; Washington et al., 1998) but decreases the motility of the large bowel, as evidenced by decreased mass movements in the ascending colon (Washington et al., 1998). Despite its apparent popularity, our extensive literature search indicates that the drug's effectiveness has been tested correctly only once in the past two decades, by investigators from Klinikum Grosshadern, University of Munich, Munich, Germany (Kruis et al., 1986). For their placebo-controlled trial of mebeverine, the researchers recruited 80 outpatients diagnosed with irritable bowel syndrome on the basis of abdominal pain, irregular bowel habits, and severe abdominal distention by gas (flatulence). The diagnosis required the absence of food intolerance and normal findings on physical examination, upper gastrointestinal endoscopy, and colonoscopy (or on contrast radiologic studies of the entire gastrointestinal tract when endoscopy was not performed) and ultrasound examination of the abdomen. In patients complaining of diarrhea, additional investigations included thyroid function tests, determination of lactase activity in biopsies of small bowel mucosa and lactose tolerance tests, and a search for parasites and pathogenic bacteria in stool. After the initial diagnostic workup the patients were randomly assigned to receive mebeverine (100 mg orally four times daily) or placebo for 16 weeks. Instructions were given to avoid taking any other medications, to continue usual diet, and to maintain a daily fluid intake of at least 1500 ml. The patients were instructed to rate the severity of their symptoms and to report side effects every four weeks throughout the trial.

The mebeverine and placebo groups were well matched with regard to median age (43 versus 41 years) and gender distribution (proportion of women 58 percent versus 55 percent). The clinical characteristics of the syndrome were similar in the mebeverine and placebo groups, as reflected by almost identical frequencies of abdominal pain (93 percent versus 100 percent), irregular bowel habits (78 percent versus 73 percent), and severe abdominal distention (75 percent versus 78 percent).

Eight patients (20 percent) treated with mebeverine and ten patients (25 percent) assigned to the placebo group dropped out before the end of the 16-week trial. The reason for discontinuation was perceived lack of efficacy of the study medication, which was invoked by four patients from the mebeverine group and seven from the placebo group. Adverse effects included abdominal pain, nausea, constipation, dry mouth, and malaise and were not considered clinically significant; no data were provided with regard to group-specific prevalence of these iatrogenic symptoms. Compliance with the study medications deteriorated over time, and at the 16-week end point only 40 percent of patients from the mebeverine group and 50 percent of the patients assigned to the placebo group were still following the therapeutic protocol.

Mebeverine was no better than placebo for symptom relief in irritable bowel syndrome. With regard to abdominal pain, only 23 percent of patients treated with mebeverine and 28 percent of patients taking placebo reported partial or complete improvement. The rate of improvement was even smaller for irregular bowel habits (13 percent with mebeverine and 25 percent with placebo) and negligible for abdominal distention (3 percent with mebeverine and 8 percent with placebo).

Trimebutine

A clinical trial of trimebutine published in 1979 has indicated that this agent reduces the stool transit time in patients with the "spastic form of irritable colon" and improved their symptoms of abdominal pain and constipation after eight weeks of therapy (Moshal and Herron, 1979). Later pharmacologic research indicated that the drug has a number of distinct, and sometimes contradictory, effects on the gastrointestinal tract, including selective inhibition of the propulsive activity of the proximal two-thirds of the colon in patients with irritable bowel syndrome (Frexinos, Fioramonti, and Bueno, 1985); stimulation of motor activity of the small intestine and colon in healthy subjects, an action suppressed by naloxone and therefore considered mediated by opiate receptors (Valori et al., 1987); increased myoelectric propagating bursts in patients with chronic constipation (Schang, Devroede, and Pilote, 1993); and reduction in the pain produced by rectal distention in animals with experimentally induced rectocolitis and stress (Lacheze et al., 1998). Yet despite the intense research activity, the literature of the past 20 years contains only one satisfactorily blinded and controlled trial of trimebutine for the treatment of irritable bowel syndrome (Luttecke, 1980), but the study is hampered by the very short duration of the treatment period and the limited outcome data obtained.

The trial was conducted in Mainz, Germany, with technical support from the drug's manufacturer. The group comprised 45 outpatients (mean age 47 years) who had symptoms compatible with irritable bowel syndrome for an average of 16 months. Organic disorders were excluded by what is described only as a "full investigation," which included radiographic examination. All patients were symptomatic at the time of the trial, with moderate or severe abdominal pain (95 percent of patients), abdominal distention (91 percent), constipation (48 percent), and diarrhea (23 percent). Thirty-nine patients were enrolled in a double-blind crossover trial of trimebutine (200 mg three times daily) or placebo, each given for three consecutive days. The two treatments were separated by a one-day washout interval. Twenty-six subjects participated in a trial similar to the one just described except that the dose of trimebutine was 100 mg three times a day. Outcome was judged only on the basis of the patients' preference after the second three-day treatment period.

One (3 percent) of the 39 patients enrolled in the first trial dropped out because of vomiting, which developed on the second day of treatment with 200 mg of trimebutine three times daily. The other reported side effects did not lead to withdrawal from the trial and consisted of fatigue (16 percent of the entire study group) and "hot and cold" sensations (14 percent). Treatment with 200 mg of trimebutine three times daily was considered superior to placebo because 69 percent of patients expressed preference for the drug as compared to 5 percent who felt better after treatment with placebo. In the trial using the lower dose of trimebutine, 42 percent preferred trimebutine and 19 percent placebo, a difference that did not reach statistical significance.

Octylonium

Octylonium bromide is a quaternary ammonium spasmolytic agent manufactured in Italy that has demonstrated, in experiments performed on rats, a combination of anticholinergic (antimuscarinic) and calcium channel blocking properties (Evangelista et al., 1998). Recent work in healthy human volunteers has shown little anticholinergic effect as measured by visual accommodation and stimulated salivary flow and no change in the orocecal transit time; the whole-gut transit time increased compared with placebo, indicating greater affinity for receptor sites in the colon than in the more proximal segments of the gastrointestinal tract (Sutton, Kilminster, and Mould, 1997).

The efficacy of octylonium was tested for the first time in a large clinical trial conducted in Italy by investigators from eight gastroenterology units, with support from the drug's manufacturer and direct involvement of its employees in at least the preparation of the published report (Baldi et al., 1992). The study cohort included patients with a chief complaint of chronic and at least moderately severe abdominal pain (three days each week for a minimum of six months) relieved by bowel movements. The diagnostic evaluation relied on endoscopic or radiologic evaluation of the colon and upper gastrointestinal tract; oral cholecystogram or abdominal ultrason-ography; tests for lactose intolerance; and examination of stools for parasites. Extensive exclusion criteria included pregnancy and lacta-tion; previous major surgical interventions on the abdomen or gas-trointestinal system; and current treatment with drugs interfering with intestinal motility, bacterial flora, or central nervous system function. Eligible subjects entered a two-week single-blind placebo interval during which baseline data were collected and then were randomly assigned to receive octylonium (40 mg three times daily before meals) or placebo for four weeks. The study concluded with another two-week single-blind placebo interval, which enabled collection of outcome data regarding the presence and severity of abdominal pain, abdominal distention, alteration in bowel habit; type and frequency of side effects of therapy; and manometric evaluation of the distal sigmoid coupled with determination of the sensitivity threshold to gradual distention of the bowel.

Seventy-one of the 72 patients completed the trial; the lone drop-out did not comply with the study protocol. The octylonium and placebo groups were well matched with regard to age and gender. Adverse effects were extremely rare, the only report being that of mild nausea in one patient. Compared with placebo, treatment with octylonium led to a decrease in the severity of abdominal pain, but had only limited effect on the frequency of abdominal pain, did not influence the discomfort produced by abdominal distention, and did not change the altered bowel habits characteristic of the syndrome. Objective data indicated that sensitivity thresholds to sigmoid dis-tention changed significantly after both placebo and octylonium therapy. The sigmoid motility response to distention, and pain was decreased only by octylonium, but the clinical significance of the finding is questionable given the fact that there was no correlation between the volume of gas eliciting pain and the sigmoid motility response.

A second group of Italian researchers sponsored by the drug's manufacturer has recently published the results of an even larger study of octylonium's effect in patients with irritable bowel syndrome (Battaglia et al., 1998). The authors organized the trial at 23 clinical sites throughout Italy. A total of 378 subjects were recruited; all fulfilled diagnostic criteria that required the presence on a continuous or recurrent basis of abdominal pain (or discomfort) relieved by defecation or associated with changes in the consistency or frequency of stools, and an irregular pattern of defecation at least 25 percent of the time. Not included were individuals with previous gastrointestinal surgery, confirmed pregnancy, food intolerance, malignancies, and treatment with agents known to modify gut motility or pain threshold. Organic disorders were excluded by normal findings on colonoscopy or barium enema, hydrogen breath test, liver and thyroid function tests, and stool examination for bacterial pathogens and ova and parasites. Subjects then entered a two-week run-in period of single-blinded placebo therapy, and patients who were still symptomatic and had demonstrated compliance with treatment and daily data collection were randomly assigned to treatment with octylonium (40 mg three times daily before meals) or placebo for 15 consecutive weeks.

Of the 378 subjects recruited for the study, 53 (14 percent) failed to qualify for the double-blind phase of the protocol. The eligible patients were assigned to receive octylonium (n = 160) or placebo (n = 165); the two groups were well matched with respect to gender distribution (2.3:1 female:male ratio), mean age (47 years), proportion of smokers and alcohol users, and severity of the main symptoms, stool characteristics, sigmoid colon tenderness, and overall well-being. Twenty-two patients (14 percent) treated with octylonium withdrew before the end of the trial; unnamed adverse effects were the reason for withdrawal in two cases and six patients dropped out because of perceived lack of therapeutic effectiveness. Losses were essentially similar in the placebo group; 32 patients (19 percent) failed to complete the trial, one of them because of adverse effects and five due to lack of efficacy.

Compared with baseline, treatment with octylonium or placebo decreased the frequency and severity of abdominal pain episodes. Intergroup comparisons showed no statistical difference in terms of pain severity, as assessed by patients, at any point during the trial. In contrast, investigators rated the effectiveness of therapy with regard to this symptom as excellent in 55 percent of patients treated with octylonium and 40 percent of the placebo-treated patients, a significant variance. The same discrepancy in judging the outcome is apparent with regard to abdominal distention, for which patients indicated no difference between octylonium and placebo; in contrast, investigators judged octylonium to be effective in 42 percent of patients as compared with a 30 percent effect of placebo, a difference reaching (but only barely) the statistical level of significance. Placebo and octylonium were equally effective in improving the frequency of bowel movements, feeling of incomplete evacuation, and the presence of mucus in stools. Marginal statistical significance in this study with multiple comparisons was also reached in favor of octylonium with regard to the rate of disappearance of sigmoid colon tenderness (48 percent versus 33 percent in the placebo group). The global assessment made by the investigators at the end of the study indicated that treatment was efficacious in 65 percent of patients treated with octylonium as compared to 50 percent in the placebo group; although the difference reaches statistical significance because of the large sample size, it is not impressive from a clinical standpoint.

CALCIUM CHANNEL BLOCKING AGENTS

The calcium channel blockers nifedipine (Narducci et al., 1985), pinaverium bromide (Fioramonti et al., 1988, Malysz et al., 1997, Awad et al., 1997), and diltiazem (Malysz et al., 1997) reduce gastrointestinal motility in animal experiments and in patients with irritable bowel syndrome. Two of these agents, diltiazem (Perez-Mateo et al., 1986) and pinaverium bromide (Awad et al., 1995), have also been the object of controlled clinical trials that have produced contradictory results.

Diltiazem

The clinical efficacy of diltiazem was tested by investigators from the Hospital de Insalud de Elche and the University of Alicante, Alicante, Spain (Perez-Mateo et al., 1986). The drug is a benzothiazepine derivative that decreases the transmembrane influx of extracellular calcium ions, an action leading to the inhibition of the smooth muscle contractile process (American Hospital Formulary Service, 1997, p. 1226). The study group comprised nine men and 11 women with irritable bowel syndrome who were symptomatic at the time of entry in the trial, were off medications used to treat the manifestations of the irritable bowel, had no significant hepatic or renal impairment, and were not bradycardic. The nine-week trial had a crossover design, that is, the patients received the sequence diltiazem-placebo-diltiazem or placebo-diltiazem-placebo. Each phase lasted three weeks. Identical-looking capsules of diltiazem (60 mg) or placebo were administered before meals three times a day. Data collected at entry and every three weeks thereafter included patients' assessments of the severity of abdominal pain, flatulence, diarrhea, gastric heaviness, headache, and palpitations. In addition, the investigators recorded the overall response to treatment and the presence, severity, and type of adverse reactions.

Two of the 20 patients enrolled in the trial failed to report for follow-up without giving an explanation and were dropped out. No adverse effects were recorded. Compared with baseline, the symptoms of abdominal pain and diarrhea became less severe during the trial, but the effect of placebo was similar to that of diltiazem. Diltiazem appeared to be slightly more effective than placebo when it was the first treatment used in the crossover sequence of the trial, but, again, the overall outcome after nine weeks indicated no meaningful advantage. None of the other symptoms scored during the trial showed any significant difference compared with baseline data. Altogether, the effect of the treatment with diltiazem was judged as imperceptible by this group of patients with irritable bowel syndrome.

Pinaverium

Pinaverium bromide, a calcium channel blocker without cardiac electrophysiologic effects (Guerot et al., 1988), which is not marketed in the United States, was used in controlled conditions for the treatment of irritable bowel syndrome by a group of investigators from the Unidad de Medicina Experimental, Hospital General de Mexico in Mexico City (Awad, Dibildox, and Ortiz, 1995). The researchers screened 315 outpatients referred for evaluation of disorders of gastrointestinal motility and identified 53 patients who had at least seven of the following ten symptoms: abdominal pain relieved by moving bowels; more frequent stools at the onset of pain; softer stools at the onset of pain; abdominal distention; passage of mucus per rectum; feeling of incomplete evacuation after defecation; altered stool frequency; altered stool shape; straining with defecation; and fecal urgency. Forty of these 53 patients agreed to undergo a complete clinical evaluation including rectosigmoidoscopy and air contrast barium enema, which failed to discover an organic cause for the multisymptomatic illness in all cases. The patients (all females) were then randomly assigned to receive pinaverium (50 mg) or placebo three times daily for three weeks. Data recorded at the beginning and the end of the three-week treatment period consisted of the patient's assessment of characteristics of their pain symptoms (frequency, severity, and duration), severity of abdominal distention, frequency of bowel movements, changes in the consistency of stool, and the other manifestations of irritable bowel.

The placebo and pinaverium groups were similar with regard to age (33 versus 30 years), education, occupation, and duration of symptoms, which averaged five years. More patients had the constipation-predominant variant of the syndrome in the pinaverium group (45 percent versus 20 percent); the rate of the diarrhea-predominant variant was identical at 20 percent in the two groups. Both groups lost one participant each before the end of the trial; one patient from the pinaverium group developed a salmonella infection and a patient receiving placebo withdrew for personal reasons. Side effects were uncommon, and consisted of mild headache in one patient taking pinaverium.

The severity of abdominal pain and the frequency of painful episodes, as well as the severity of abdominal distention, decreased significantly after treatment with both pinaverium and placebo, and intergroup comparisons did not reveal a difference between these treatments. Pinaverium was superior to placebo with regard to the decreased pain duration, normalization of stool frequency and consistency, presence of mucus in stool, and improvement in the feeling of incomplete evacuation. The total symptom score improved significantly after both treatments, but pinaverium was clearly superior to placebo from this vantage point.

Of the two calcium channel blocking agents tested in clinical trials, pinaverium but not diltiazem appears to offer short-term benefit. The explanation of this discrepancy has been suggested by animal studies using canine colonic circular smooth muscle (Malysz et al., 1997). Both diltiazem and pinaverium reduced spontaneous contractile activity and response to cholinergic stimuli, but the effect of pinaverium was much more pronounced.

CISAPRIDE

Cisapride is a synthetic piperidinyl benzamide which enhances gastrointestinal motility by stimulating the acetylcholine release from the postganglionic neurons of the myenteric plexus, either directly or through a serotonergic mechanism involving 5-HT4 receptors (American Hospital Formulary Service, 1997, p. 2269). Experimental data recording motility changes after oral administration of the drug has shown no significant effect in patients with constipation-dominant irritable bowel syndrome and had produced the undesired increase of clustered contractions in patients with the diarrhea-predominant variant of the illness (Evans, Bak, and Kellow, 1997). Cisapride's efficacy in irritable bowel syndrome was in the past decade the focus of four European-controlled trials (Van Outryve et al., 1991; Schutze et al., 1997; Farup et al., 1998; Noor et al., 1998), which produced strikingly conflicting results.

The first attempt to establish the therapeutic effect of cisapride was planned and conducted by clinical investigators affiliated with the University Hospital of Antwerp, Edegem; St. Elizabeth Hospital, Aalst; and Onze Lieve Vrouw Hospital, Kortrijk, Belgium (Van

Outryve et al., 1991). After an open study during which four of 46 subjects (9 percent) experienced adverse drug reactions (diarrhea, headache, nausea, and vertigo), the authors recruited patients with constipation-predominant irritable bowel syndrome for the double-blind trial. The diagnosis required only the presence of constipation and nonmenstrual abdominal pain for at least six months and the absence of an organic or overtly psychogenic explanation for these symptoms. The diagnostic threshold for constipation was reached in cases in which the bowel movements occurred less than three times each week or the stools were hard. The abdominal pain had to occur at least three times each week and interfere with normal activities. Patients with diverticulosis or laxative abuse as well as those with evidence of abnormal colonic motility or tone were not included in the study group. After confirmation of eligibility, a total of 72 subjects were randomly assigned to treatment with cisapride or placebo for 12 weeks. The initial dose was one tablet (placebo or 5 mg cisapride) three times daily shortly before the main meals. After four weeks, the dose was doubled if the symptoms had not already improved or was reduced to one-half tablet if abdominal pain had worsened. Efficacy was determined by analysis of the change in the severity of symptoms and the overall condition at four-week intervals throughout the trial.

The trial was completed by 60 (83 percent) of the 72 initial participants. Four patients treated with cisapride dropped out on account of loose stools (one patient), absence of all symptoms (one patient), and lack of improvement (two patients). Among the patients assigned to receive placebo, five patients discontinued their participation because of lack of improvement (four patients) and personal reasons (one patient). Two other patients were withdrawn after developing evidence of nondigestive pathology, and one was lost to follow-up. There were no other cisapride-related adverse effects. The cisapride and placebo groups were well matched with regard to median age (48 years in both groups), female predominance, duration of complaints, frequency and clinical characteristics of the main symptoms, and previous drug and dietary treatments of their irritable bowel syndrome.

During the 12-week trial, 31 percent of patients from the cisapride group and 46 percent of patients assigned to treatment with placebo doubled the dose of their daily regimen. The dose was halved by two cisapride and four placebo-treated patients. Treatment with cisapride improved constipation, as shown by the fact that 52 percent of patients passed stools every day, as compared with 15 percent of the patients treated with placebo. After eight and 12 weeks of treatment, data generated by patients indicated that the frequency of pain relief was statistically similar in the two groups. In contrast, clinicians felt that the symptoms of abdominal pain and flatulence responded well to treatment in 73 percent of cisapride patients and 36 percent of patients treated with placebo, a difference that reached statistical significance. Cisapride was not superior to placebo with regard to any of the other gastrointestinal symptoms (abdominal distention, feeling of incomplete evacuation, postprandial fullness, defecation urge, eructation, heartburn, and postprandial nausea). At the end of the trial, the overall score for response to treatment indicated improvement in 80 percent of patients treated with cisapride and 55 percent of those receiving placebo, a difference for which our calculation finds only marginal statistical significance.

The effect of cisapride on the symptoms of abdominal discomfort and constipation experienced by 96 patients with irritable bowel syndrome was studied by a group of investigators from Hanusch Hospital and Regional Public Medical Insurance Outpatient Clinic, Vienna; General Hospital, Graz; and University of Innsbruck, Innsbruck, Austria (Schutze et al., 1997). The sample size was based on the prediction that cisapride and placebo treatments will produce response rates of 65 percent and 35 percent, respectively. The subjects were recruited at nine specialized Austrian clinical sites and were carefully evaluated to ensure that they had the constipation-predominant variant of the syndrome, as defined by the accepted standard (Thompson et al., 1989). Pregnant or lactating women and patients with blood in stool, evidence of organic disorders, history of alcoholism or heavy cigarette smoking, or recent weight loss were not eligible for the trial. The study participants were randomly assigned to receive either placebo or cisapride (5 mg) tablets three times daily for four weeks, after which the dose was doubled if the therapy was judged to be ineffective on a self-scored instrument. No other dosage changes were permitted for the remainder of the

12-week trial. Concomitant treatment with medications known to influence gastrointestinal motility were not permitted, except for "rescue" laxatives given when no stools were passed after three consecutive days. Patients were instructed to keep a symptom diary and were followed up at four-week intervals throughout the trial. The primary outcome measures were the scores assigned by patients and investigators for the severity of symptoms; in addition, the investigators rated the global therapeutic effect.

The cisapride and placebo groups were well matched to median age (44 versus 45 years) and median age at the time the irritable bowel syndrome had been diagnosed (33 versus 35 years), as well as female predominance, weight, aggregate severity of symptoms, and previous therapies. The daily dose was increased in about a quarter of the patients in both groups. Side effects were infrequent; four patients (8 percent) treated with cisapride developed abdominal pain and diarrhea, and treatment had to be discontinued in one of these cases. Diarrhea was reported by only one patient from the placebo group. Two patients were withdrawn from treatment with placebo because of vomiting.

The investigators' double-blinded observations indicated that cisapride was not better than placebo with regard to the main symptoms of the irritable bowel syndrome. Abdominal pain improved in 36 percent of patients treated with cisapride and 32 percent of those receiving placebo. Similarly, abdominal distention disappeared in 31 percent of patients given cisapride and 21 percent of the placebo group. Cisapride improved the constipation of 64 percent, but 59 percent of patients treated with placebo also reported a significant favorable change in their bowel habits. Cisapride and placebo were equally efficacious in treating the symptoms of depression (67 percent versus 86 percent), anxiety (76 percent versus 86 percent), tenseness (86 percent versus 86 percent), and nervousness (62 percent versus 66 percent). The global assessments of the severity of illness made by patients indicated no significant differences between cisapride and placebo. Of the symptoms rated by patients, only the ease of passage of stool was significantly better in the cisapride group, while the general well-being, frequency and consistency of stools, feeling of incomplete evacuation, abdominal pain, and bloating were not.

Disappointing results were also reported by a group of Norwegian researchers who studied the effect of 12 weeks of therapy with cisapride or placebo on 70 patients recruited through nine gastroenterological practices (Farup et al., 1998). The investigators received financial and administrative support from the drug's manufacturer. Only patients with the constipation-predominant variant of the syndrome were included in the study cohort, and care was taken to exclude subjects who had been recently started on a fiber-rich diet and those treated with drugs known to affect gastrointestinal motility. The design of the trial was essentially identical to that employed by Schutze et al. (1997), including the option of doubling the dose of placebo or cisapride (5 mg three times daily) in patients without noticeable improvement after four weeks of therapy.

The cisapride (n = 33) and placebo (n = 37) groups were well matched with regard to age and gender distribution but differed with respect to the age at which the diagnosis of irritable bowel had been made (26 versus 35 years). Three of the patients (9 percent) assigned to the cisapride arm of the trial were withdrawn after developing adverse drug reactions, which were not further described in the published report. One patient in each group dropped out because of lack of improvement.

After 12 weeks of therapy, the investigators found the response to be good or excellent in 59 percent of patients treated with placebo and 39 percent of those who had received cisapride. The self-scored assessments made by patients reflected no significant difference between cisapride and placebo with regard to changes in any of the clinical manifestations of irritable bowel syndrome and no therapeutic effect on the global severity of the illness.

The latest attempt to confirm a therapeutic role for cisapride in irritable bowel syndrome was made by a team of surgeons and epidemiologists from Ninewells Hospital and Medical School, Dundee, Scotland (Noor et al., 1998). The investigators had access to a cohort of 79 patients and selected 50 women and 10 men to participate in a placebo-controlled study of oral treatment with cisapride (5 mg) administered three times daily for 12 weeks. The diagnosis of irritable bowel syndrome was established in each case in accordance with standard criteria (Thompson et al., 1989). Of the 60 patients entered in the study, 21 had the constipation-predominant variant of the syndrome, i.e., had histories indicating at least two of the following symptoms: a maximum of three stools each week; passage of hard stool; feeling of incomplete evacuation, urgency, or straining; and passage of mucus. The diarrhea-predominant variant was diagnosed in 17 patients who had "excessive" mucus in stool or at least two loose stools each day. Therapeutic effectiveness was measured by comparing the pre- and posttreatment severity of symptoms and performance on the 24-hour ambulatory jejunal manometry.

Technical problems and lack of patients' compliance reduced the study group to 38 patients, which were equally divided between the cisapride and placebo treatments. The distribution of the diarrhea-predominant and constipation-predominant cases was balanced across the two groups. The treatment appears to have been tolerated well, given that no adverse reactions to cisapride or placebo were included in the report.

The most important effect of treatment was an increase in the abdominal pain experienced by patients with diarrhea-predominant irritable bowel syndrome treated with cisapride. Among patients with the constipation-predominant variant of the syndrome, cisapride therapy was better than placebo with regard to the number of bowel movements, but did not influence stool consistency or the straining, urgency, and feeling of incomplete evacuation. Significant, and undesired, enhancement of jejunal motility was observed only among patients with diarrhea-predominant irritable bowel.

Chapter 15

Ineffective Therapies

DIETARY FIBER

The treatment of irritable bowel syndrome with dietary fiber is extremely popular among patients and clinicians (Drossman, 1995). Trials performed in the 1970s gave conflicting results; while Danish researchers observed subjective improvement in 52 percent of patients treated with bran supplements for six weeks and in 65 percent of subjects taking a wheat placebo (Soltoft et al., 1976), investigators from the United Kingdom reported a significant improvement in symptoms that correlated with objective changes in colonic motor activity, but their study was incompletely blinded (Manning, Heaton, and Harvey, 1977). Our evidence-based analysis will demonstrate that research performed in the past two decades has established with a high degree of certainty that the administration of dietary fiber is not useful for this syndrome.

The first trial that employed an unyielding double-blind, crossover design was performed by investigators from the Hvidovre Hospital, University of Copenhagen, Copenhagen, Denmark (Arffmann et al., 1985). They recruited 20 patients followed in their outpatient clinic who were given the diagnosis of irritable bowel syndrome as an explanation for symptoms of abdominal pain, abdominal distention, abnormal bowel habit, and abdominal rumbling. The symptoms had persisted for at least six months and could not be attributed to abdominal surgery or other organic causes after proctoscopy, barium enema, cholecystography, upper gastrointestinal endoscopy or barium radiographs of the stomach and duodenum, lactose tolerance test, and a standard battery of hematologic and biochemical tests. Clinical examinations ruled out other medical or psychiatric disorders. After the baseline evaluation, the participants were randomly assigned to start treatment with either dietary fiber (coarse wheat bran with a water-binding capacity of 4.5 ml/g of bran) or placebo (bread crumbs with a water-binding capacity of 1.3 ml/g, prepared to look and taste like the bran product). Patients ingested 15 g of the assigned substance twice daily. Other than being advised to drink 1500 ml water daily and to avoid caffeine-containing liquids, the patients had no dietary restrictions. The first treatment phase lasted six weeks and then patients crossed over to the alternate treatment without any treatment-free washout interval. The only medication allowed during the trial was, surprisingly, the prokinetic agent metoclopramide, to be used as analgesic, a practice referred to the report of work (Kjaerulff and Tojner, 1977) performed in the same country and unfortunately not available for evaluation. Outcome data were generated by symptom diaries kept by patients and by their recording of the frequency of bowel movements and number of tablets of metoclopramide used. A brief hospital stay at the end of the trial was used to measure the weight and fat content of the stools and to determine the intestinal transit time and rectosigmoid intraluminal pressures.

The use of metoclopramide was described as slight, and similar during the placebo and bran phases of the trial. Among the 18 subjects who finished the trial, the scores for the severity of abdominal pain, bloating, abdominal rumbling, the number of bowel movements, and the fat content of stools were no different after fiber supplementation with bran as compared to treatment with placebo.

The effect of increasing oral intake of fiber in irritable bowel syndrome was carefully assessed in a well-designed, placebo-controlled crossover trial involving 44 patients newly referred to the outpatient clinics of St. Bartholomew's Hospital, London (Lucey et al., 1987). All patients fulfilled the authors' stringent diagnostic criteria, which required the absence of an underlying gastroenterological disease and the presence of at least three of the following six symptoms: abdominal pain relieved by defecation, increased frequency of bowel movements at the onset of abdominal pain, decreased stool consistency at the onset of pain, abdominal distention, passage of mucus, and the sensation of incomplete stool evacuation. For all patients, the diagnostic workup included physical examination, screening hematological and biochemical tests, and a sigmoidosco- py. Other tests, such as stool cultures, fecal fat measurement, bari- um enema, and jejunal biopsy were performed if deemed necessary in individual cases. Of the 44 initial cases, 28 (19 women and nine men with a median age of 32 years and a median duration of symptoms of five years) completed the trial. The group was demo- graphically and clinically similar to the 16 patients who withdrew from the study.

The study design required the patients to add 12 biscuits to their diet. One type of biscuit contained 1.3 g of dietary fiber; the placebo biscuit contained 0.23 g of fiber. The source of fiber was wheat bran. Each type of biscuit was used daily for three consecutive months. Baseline and monthly measurements included an inventory of symptoms and dietary questionnaires. At the end of each three- month treatment period, a three-day stool sample was collected and brought to the clinic for weighing. The symptoms recorded ad- dressed frequency and severity of abdominal pain, stool frequency and characteristics of defecation, and the presence of nausea, vomit- ing, abdominal distention, and severe flatus.

After three months there was significant improvement in 71 per- cent of the placebo and 74 percent of the bran-treated patients. No additional improvement was noted after the second three-month period with the alternative treatment. There was no significant dif- ference in symptom scores between placebo and bran treatments when compared before and after crossover. The mean 24-hour stool weight was 123 g while on placebo and 148 g while on bran, an insignificant difference. There was no correlation between symp- tomatic improvement and stool weight; in fact, of the 15 patients whose stool weight increased during the bran therapy period, eight reported worsened symptoms compared to the placebo treatment period.

A small but well-planned long-term crossover trial compared the effect of dietary fiber with placebo in a group of 14 patients receiv- ing care in the gastroenterology clinic at McMaster University Medical Centre, Hamilton, Ontario, Canada (Cook et al., 1990). All patients had normal findings on lactose tolerance testing, stool cul- ture, rigid sigmoidoscopy, and either barium enema or colonoscopy.

The irritable bowel syndrome was defined as the presence of at least three of the following six symptoms: abdominal pain relieved by defecation, increased frequency of stools with the onset of abdominal pain, looser stools with the onset of pain, abdominal distention, a feeling of incomplete evacuation after defecation, and the presence of mucus in stool. The symptoms were quantified at entry and at four-week intervals on a standardized questionnaire. The trial was conducted in a double-blind manner and required the patients to ingest either placebo or 20 g of corn fiber daily. Treatments were administered as identical cookies twice every day. Fiber and placebo treatments lasted 12 weeks each and were separated by a four-week washout period. Rectosigmoid pressures were carefully recorded at entry and after each phase of the trial.

Nine patients completed the study. Their mean age was 26 years and eight were female. Their pretrial dietary fiber intake at entry in the study did not correlate with their symptoms of abdominal pain and altered bowel habits. Treatment with placebo and fiber improved most symptoms within the first four weeks, but there were no significant differences between the two types of treatment. Severity of abdominal pain and the total number of symptoms were the variables that changed the most with placebo and fiber. Fasting and postprandial motility at both proximal and distal rectosigmoid recording sites decreased to a similar extent following both placebo and fiber, and paralleled the favorable change observed with regard to the severity of abdominal pain.

Dietary supplementation with bran had no effect on the symptoms of irritable bowel syndrome in another well-designed double-blind, placebo-controlled, crossover study conducted at the Royal Hampshire County Hospital, Winchester, United Kingdom (Snook and Shepherd, 1994). All patients received the diagnosis of irritable bowel syndrome according to standard criteria (Thompson et al., 1989) and had no evidence of organic bowel disease (other than uncomplicated colonic diverticulosis). The group included 67 women and 13 men with a median age of 40 years. Abdominal pain was considered the worst manifestation of the syndrome by 60 percent of the patients. The group's estimated baseline dietary fiber intake ranged from 16 to 29 g daily; the median daily amount was 24 g. Five patients had been consuming a high-bran cereal on a regular basis.

This type of cereal and all other medications taken for irritable bowel syndrome were stopped prior to the start of the trial.

The study started with a two-week observation period, followed by a seven-week treatment period, a two-week washout period and then the crossover to the second seven-week treatment period. The patients were provided individual daily boxes of placebo or the fiber preparation. The placebo consisted of wheat and rice flour without measurable fiber content. The fiber preparation included 40 g of wheat bran, corresponding to 12 g of fiber. The placebo and the fiber preparation were similar in appearance, texture, and taste. The content of the boxes was presented to the group as two different fiber breakfast supplements in order to compare their effect on the irritable bowel syndrome. No other dietary advice was provided. The patients were instructed to score their symptoms daily; upon the completion of each treatment phase, the patients were interviewed by a blinded investigator to provide an overall assessment score.

Of the 80 patients making up the inception cohort, 71 completed the study and 65 provided complete symptom diaries. The overall assessment scores indicated symptomatic improvement with placebo in 54 percent of patients; bran supplementation improved 52 percent of patients. The proportion of patients feeling "much better with treatment" was identical (17 percent) for the placebo and bran supplementation. The proportion of patients feeling "much worse with treatment" was 14 percent after bran supplementation and 7 percent after placebo. Treatment with placebo was statistically superior to that with bran supplementation for the 22 patients with pretrial alternating diarrhea and constipation and in the 29 patients whose main symptom was abdominal distention, excessive flatulence, or disturbance in bowel habit. Patients whose main symptom was abdominal pain and those whose bowel habit disturbance consisted of either diarrhea alone or constipation alone noted no difference between bran and placebo. The analysis of the daily symptom records indicated significantly worse flatulence during the bran supplementation period; the severity of all the other symptoms was similar throughout the trial.

Additional support for the finding of lack of effect of dietary fiber in irritable bowel syndrome was provided by investigators from the Western General Hospital, Edinburgh, in a study that has also advanced our understanding of the placebo response observed in these trials (Fowlie, Eastwood, and Prescott, 1992). The cohort comprised 49 patients receiving care in an outpatient gastroenterology unit. All patients had normal findings on physical examination and sigmoidoscopy, as well as on extensive laboratory testing that included liver and thyroid function tests. Double contrast barium enema was performed in 48 patients and showed no significant abnormalities. To fulfill the criteria for the diagnosis of irritable bowel syndrome, all patients had, for at least six months, frequent episodes of abdominal pain relieved by defecation, abdominal distention, and abnormal bowel habits.

The subjects were randomized to receive either placebo tablets (24 patients) or fiber tablets (25 patients) every day for a total of three months. The placebo was a mixture of starch, lactose, and calcium phosphate with a fiber content of 0.4 g daily. The fiber tablets contained cereal and fruit fiber; the total daily supplement of fiber was 4.1 g. During the week prior to the onset of the trial the patients completed a diary recording the occurrence of the abdominal pain, type of stool, and frequency of bowel movements. A 14-item questionnaire and visual analog scales measuring depression and anxiety were also obtained at baseline. The placebo and fiber-supplemented groups were similar in all measured dimensions and also with regard to age, gender distribution, and pretrial daily fiber intake. Symptom measurements were repeated after four weeks of treatment and again at the end of the trial.

Five patients taking placebo and two patients assigned to the fiber supplementation group withdrew from the study. Among the remaining patients, 70 percent of those assigned to placebo therapy and 59 percent of the fiber-treated group reported feeling "generally better" after the three-month trial period. The global symptom score and the severity scores for each of the gastrointestinal symptoms improved during the trial in the placebo group, but the direct comparison with the fiber-treated group showed no significant difference. The patients who were the most constipated at baseline recorded the smallest degree of change in their gastrointestinal symptoms after both placebo and fiber therapy. The outcome of the treatment was best predicted by the baseline severity of the depressive symptomatology, i.e., the patients who improved had been significantly less depressed at the initial assessment. A correlation was also noted between the severity of pain and depression at baseline, but the initial pain score did not predict well those subjects who improved with these treatments, suggesting that the severity of depression is the independent variable most useful to selecting irritable bowel syndrome patients for a therapeutic trial with placebo.

LACTASE

Lactose maldigestion can be identified in close to one-third of patients diagnosed with irritable bowel syndrome, and the characteristics of abdominal pain, abdominal distention, altered bowel habits, mucus content of stool, and relief with defecation do not allow the clinical identification of this subgroup (Tolliver et al., 1996). Therefore, correction of lactose intolerance and maldigestion with exogenous lactase appears a reasonable way for reducing these symptoms and has been attempted in controlled trials by investigators from the United States (Newcomer et al., 1983) and Central America (Lisker et al., 1989).

The first of these two double-blind randomized studies was performed at the Mayo Clinic and the Mayo Foundation in Rochester, Minnesota, with partial support from the National Dairy Council (Newcomer et al., 1983). The therapeutic agent was unfermented acidophilus milk, which is obtained by supplementing cooled pasteurized milk with cultured *Lactobacillus acidophilus*. The product is commercially available and, when maintained at the usual household refrigeration temperature of less than 40°F, is similar in taste to nonsupplemented milk. *L. acidophilus* multiplies rapidly in warm milk, survives the bile-containing environment of the small bowel, and has substantial lactase (beta-D-galactosidase) activity demonstrated both in vitro (Rao and Dutta, 1978) and in vivo (McDonough et al., 1987). To test the clinical effectiveness of this enzymatic activity, the Mayo Clinic group recruited 67 patients with irritable bowel syndrome and proven lactase sufficiency, 18 patients with lactase deficiency, and ten healthy subjects. The diagnosis of irritable bowel syndrome was based on a "typical history" and the absence of organic pathology on proctosigmoidoscopy and radiologic examinations of the upper and lower gastrointestinal tract. Lactase deficiency was carefully ruled out in all subjects with irritable bowel syndrome with the standard hydrogen breath test. In contrast, the hydrogen breath test confirmed lactase deficiency in the 18 control subjects who reported milk intolerance; five of these individuals also had symptoms compatible with irritable bowel syndrome. The ten-week trial was divided into five consecutive two-week periods. For the second period, the patients with irritable bowel syndrome and the healthy control subjects were randomly assigned to receive either unaltered milk (240 ml three times daily with meals) or an equal amount of unheated acidophilus milk (three billion *L. acidophilus* organisms daily). The alternate product was ingested during the fourth period. The first, third, and fifth two-week periods were treatment-free observation intervals. No other milk products were allowed for the entire ten-week trial period, and careful dietary instructions were given so that patients would avoid gas-producing foods. All anticholinergic, laxative, and antidiarrheal drugs were stopped. The design was modified for the lactase-deficient subjects, who received unadulterated milk or acidophilus milk during the first and fourth week in a double-blind manner; the amount of milk was individualized according to previously established tolerance. Data were collected daily by the patients and by weekly telephone interviews.

Six of the 67 patients (9 percent) dropped out during the trial because their symptoms did not improve with treatment. The remaining 61 patients (age range 20 to 82 years) had symptoms compatible with irritable bowel syndrome for at least one year. The predominant symptom at baseline was abdominal pain (constant or cramping) in 19 patients, abdominal distention in 16, and diarrhea (at least two loose stools daily at least five days each week) or constipation (no more than three bowel movements each week, all with hard stool) in 13 patients each. Treatment with acidophilus milk did not change the frequency and severity of abdominal pain, bloating, constipation, and diarrhea. Among the 18 patients with lactase deficiency, improvement was noted only during the milk-free periods, as both the unadulterated and acidophilus milk consumption was associated with a significant symptomatic worsening. The subjects from the healthy control group remained asymptomatic throughout the trial. These data indicate that acidophilus milk has no therapeutic value in irritable bowel syndrome. However, given the lack of effect in patients with well-documented lactase deficiency, the product may have had insufficient enzymatic activity for a meaningful pharmacologic role.

The second attempt to test the clinical effectiveness of lactase in the management of irritable bowel syndrome took place at the Instituto Nacional de la Nutricion "Salvador Zubiran" in Mexico City, Mexico (Lisker et al., 1989). The authors enrolled 18 subjects who had received the diagnosis of irritable bowel syndrome in the outpatient gastroenterology clinic on the basis of chronic symptoms of abdominal pain and altered bowel habits. All subjects were milk drinkers, i.e., their regular diet included at least 240 ml of milk or an equivalent lactose intake each day. During the first month of the trial, the presence and severity of symptoms was established by self-report questionnaires completed daily. For the following three months, patients were randomly assigned to either lactase-placebo-lactase or placebo-lactase-placebo treatment sequences, with each component lasting one month. The microbial lactase used in the trial was obtained from cultures of *Kluyveromyces lactis* available as a liquid suspension. The placebo liquid was identical in color and viscosity and contained polydextrose. Vials containing these suspensions were provided for the dairy products consumed at home and for use with lactose-containing meals eaten away from home. The enzymatic activity of the lactase product was tested in each subject with a bioassay measuring the postprandial concentration of hydrogen in the expired air after an oral load of 12.5 g of lactose. Outcome data relied on daily assessments of symptoms.

Of the 18 patients entered in the trial, three patients declined participation and three were dropped out after one month because they were unable to comply with the research protocol. The 12 patients (nine women and three men) who completed the trial had an age range of 29 to 72 years and had had the symptoms of irritable bowel syndrome for a minimum of three years. The daily milk intake averaged 250 ml in four patients, 500 ml in four, 750 ml in one, and 1000 ml in the remaining three patients. Eight of the 12 subjects were shown to be lactose maldigesters.

The gastrointestinal symptoms of this group of patients with irritable bowel syndrome were not changed by treatment with lactase. Five of the eight lactose maldigesters felt improved after both lactase and placebo therapy. The other lactose-maldigesters reported that their symptoms remained the same (one patient), got steadily worse during the three-month crossover trial (one patient), or got worse during the first month of treatment with lactase but better during the second lactase period. Among the four lactose digesters, one improved and the other three saw essentially no change in their symptomatology. The hypothesized pattern of improvement after lactase therapy but not after placebo was observed in only one patient, a lactose digester. Although the lactase suspension had a slightly sweeter taste than the placebo preparation, patients interviews indicated no recognition of this difference and therefore there was no reason to suspect that the study's "blind" design had failed.

In a more recent report, *Lactobacillus acidophilus* was tested in patients with irritable bowel syndrome by researchers from the School of Medicine, University of California, Davis, California, with support from the manufacturer of a drug containing the heat-stabilized LB strain of this microorganism (Halpern et al., 1996). The authors enrolled 30 patients whose condition was diagnosed after clinical examination and exclusion of organic pathology to conform to the current diagnostic standard (Thompson et al., 1989). The treatment consisted of two capsules twice daily; each capsule contained five billion *L. acidophilus* organisms and a total of 85 mg of lactose. The placebo capsule contained 235 mg of lactose each, an amount described in the report as being well below the symptomatic threshold of patients with lactose intolerance. The trial required random assignment to one of the two treatments, which was continued for six weeks. After a two-week washout period the subjects switched to the alternate therapy for a second six-week period. Baseline and follow-up assessments were based on structured questionnaires recording the severity of the main symptoms and the general physical state.

Only 18 of the 30 patients fulfilled all the requirements of the trial. No adverse effects were reported. Compared with baseline, treatment with *L. acidophilus* improved the condition of 17 of the

18 patients (94 percent), while treatment with placebo was effective in 13 subjects (72 percent), for which our calculation indicates statistical insignificance.

ONDANSETRON

The role of serotonin (5-hydroxytryptamine or 5-HT) in the functioning of the enteric nervous system has stimulated work on its gut-specific receptors and the contribution to the motility and pain responses of compounds such as ondansetron, granisetron, tropisetron, and zacopride that block, with various degrees of specificity, the 5-HT^3 receptors widespread in the gastrointestinal tract (Talley, 1992). In the rat visceral hypersensitivity model, some of these agents (granisetron and zacopride) but not others (ondansetron and tropisetron) were shown to inhibit the abdominal contractions that were the result of irritating the colon with acidic solutions (Langlois et al., 1996). In patients with irritable bowel syndrome, the intravenous administration of granisetron after instrumental rectal distention significantly reduced the rectal sensitivity, i.e., the discomfort, desire to defecate, urgency, and sensation of excessive gas without changes in motor activity, rectal compliance, or anal pressures; dose-dependent decrease in the postprandial motility was also observed (Prior and Read, 1993). Other data have confirmed the heterogeneity of this class of agents, demonstrating that single doses of intravenous ondansetron given to patients with irritable bowel syndrome did not influence visceral perception, but did induce increased rectal compliance and promoted rectal relaxation (Zighelboim et al., 1995). Although granisetron has been considered to have more therapeutic potential than ondansetron (Langlois et al., 1996), by the end of 1998 only the latter had been the subject of clinical trials employing placebo-controlled designs (Steadman et al., 1992; Goldberg et al., 1996; Maxton, Morris, and Whorwell, 1996).

The first clinical trial of ondansetron was performed by investigators from the Gastroenterology Research Unit, Mayo Clinic, Rochester, Minnesota, with financial support from the drug's manufacturer (Steadman et al., 1992). Because the research hypothesis postulated that ondansetron will slow colonic transit and reduce visceral hypersensitivity, the study's major goals were to document the effect of the drug on the frequency and consistency of stools and on pain symptoms experienced by patients with diarrhea-predominant irritable bowel syndrome.

The candidates for the study were identified by medical record review, contacted by mail, and invited to participate if they had abdominal pain and at least three stools per day. Inclusion in the study group also required the presence of at least three of the following six symptoms: abdominal distention, feeling of incomplete evacuation, pain relieved by passing stool, more frequent stools at the onset of pain, looser stools at the onset of pain, and passage of mucus. Patients with a history of any gastrointestinal surgery and any major medical condition or psychiatric disorder were not considered eligible for enrollment. The study group comprised 14 patients (six women and eight men) whose age ranged from 28 to 61 years. Ondansetron (16 mg three times daily) or placebo were administered for 28 consecutive days, after which the patients entered a washout period sufficiently long to enable the return of the symptoms present at baseline. After washout, the patients completed the second 28-day therapeutic phase with the alternate agent. Throughout the drug trial, the patients were advised to attempt to maintain a diet with 20 to 25 g of indigestible fiber each day. Before entering the study, and every two weeks thereafter, the patients provided self-scored recordings of their main symptoms, were interviewed to uncover adverse effects of therapy, and had a brief physical examination. Stool weights (24-hour collections) were obtained at the end of each treatment period. Physiologic studies of gastrointestinal function were also performed at the completion of each phase of therapy and consisted of measurements of orocecal and colonic transit time and of the levels of gastrointestinal hormonal peptides.

Eleven of the 14 initial participants completed the trial. Among the three patients withdrawn from the study, one developed intolerable symptoms (headache, tiredness, dry mouth) while taking placebo, another had to be operated on for a mechanical intestinal obstruction occurring during the placebo phase of the trial, and the third because she became pregnant during the ondansetron phase of the trial.

Treatment with ondansetron did not decrease significantly the severity of abdominal pain or the total number of symptoms experienced during the trial. Stool consistency increased after ondansetron therapy, so that only one of the 11 patients was still complaining of loose or watery stools. In contrast, this degree of diarrhea was reported by eight of the 11 patients at the end of the placebo phase of the trial. The improvement in the consistency of stool was not accompanied by a significant change in the amount (weight) of the stool. The orocecal and colonic transit time were not substantially changed by ondansetron, and the circulating levels of gastrointestinal hormonal peptides (human pancreatic polypeptide, neurotensin, and peptide YY) were similar during the ondansetron and placebo phases of the trial.

The effect of ondansetron on the abdominal pain experienced by patients with irritable bowel syndrome and its relation to modification of visceral sensitivity was also studied in a small but well-designed study conducted at St. Mark's Hospital, London, with limited technical support from the drug's manufacturer (Goldberg et al., 1996). The investigators recruited nine patients with irritable bowel syndrome whose chronic symptoms included abdominal pain and distention and either constipation with bowel movements at more than three-day intervals and/or diarrhea occurring at least four times daily. Appropriate steps were taken to exclude organic gastrointestinal disorders and ingestion of drugs known to alter bowel motility and digestive function. A control group included 12 healthy volunteers who were on no medications and had no gastrointestinal symptoms.

The randomized two-way crossover trial started with a two-week baseline observation period during which the participants knowingly received placebo tablets. During the following two-week period, the subjects were randomly assigned to ingest either ondansetron 16 mg or placebo three times daily. This was followed by a two-week washout requiring the open-label administration of placebo tablets and a final two-week interval during which the subjects double-blindly crossed over to the alternate treatment they had not previously received. Outcome data included daily assessments of symptoms, frequency of bowel movements, and stool consistency. In addition, objective measurements of anal sphincter pressures, rectal compliance, rectal sensitivity to distention, and anal and rectal sensitivity to electrical stimulation were carried out at the end of each treatment period.

Three of the nine patients and two of the 12 control subjects dropped out of the study. Only one of these participants withdrew due to adverse effects (nausea and vomiting) that developed during the active phase of the trial, and the event resolved four days after ondansetron was discontinued. Treatment with ondansetron was not better than administration of placebo with regard to pain severity, abdominal distention, straining, number of loose bowel movements, and general well-being. However, ondansetron decreased the number of episodes of abdominal pain, a change not correlated with modification of rectal sensitivity threshold to distention and electrical stimulation.

A larger clinical trial of ondansetron in irritable bowel syndrome was conducted at the University Hospital of South Manchester, Didsbury, Manchester, United Kingdom, with financial support from the drug's manufacturer (Maxton, Morris, and Whorwell, 1996). The stated goal of the study was to assess not only changes in the defining colonic symptoms, but to evaluate the effect of ondansetron on the non-colonic manifestations of the syndrome.

The 50 patients (39 women and 11 men) recruited for the study met standard symptom criteria for the diagnosis of irritable bowel syndrome (Thompson et al., 1989). Twenty-eight patients had a diarrhea-predominant illness and 20 patients were found to have the constipation-predominant presentation of the syndrome. The patients' ages ranged from 22 to 65 years and the diagnosis of irritable bowel syndrome had been established an average of four years prior to entering the trial. Laboratory investigations were normal and evaluation of the large bowel with barium enema or colonoscopy confirmed the absence of structural abnormalities.

The trial used a randomized, placebo-controlled, crossover design to test the efficacy of ondansetron at a dose of 4 mg orally three times each day, an amount four times smaller than that used by Steadman et al. (1992) at the Mayo Clinic. Following a two-week observation period, ondansetron or placebo were given for 28 days. After a two-week washout, the subjects were given the alternate therapy. Baseline and outcome measurements (performed at biweekly intervals throughout the trial) included assessments of the severity of abdominal pain, abdominal distention, nausea, belching, heartburn, postprandial discomfort, lethargy, backache, urinary frequency, urgency, urge incontinence, depression and anxiety, stool consistency, and frequency of bowel movements. Care was taken to ensure that the subjects took no other medications, did not alter their diet during the study period, and did not change the amount of dietary fiber, which was kept at approximately 20 g each day. Therapy with ondansetron or placebo was well tolerated and the trial was completed by 49 of the 50 patients.

Ondansetron was similar to placebo with regard to its effect on abdominal pain, abdominal distention, backache, urinary symptoms, and depression and anxiety. The only symptoms improved by ondansetron in this population of patients with irritable bowel syndrome were postprandial discomfort, belching, and heartburn. This pattern of limited and selective symptomatic improvement was similar among patients with diarrhea-predominant and those with constipation-predominant illness. In the diarrhea-predominant group, therapy with ondansetron increased the stool consistency and decreased the frequency of bowel movements.

Chapter 16

Unreplicated Trials

STREPTOCOCCUS FAECIUM

Freeze-dried cultures of *Streptococcus faecium* were tried in a group of 58 patients with irritable bowel syndrome assembled by investigators employed by the manufacturer of this preparation from among patients receiving care for this condition through 13 general practices in Jutland, Denmark (Gade and Thorn, 1989). A mechanism of action was not hypothesized, but the authors indicated that the bacteria may colonize the intestinal tract and change bowel patterns by increasing the intraluminal concentration of lactic acid. Our review of the literature indicates only partial support for these assumptions because while the oral administration of *Streptococcus (Enterococcus) faecium* affects the distal intestinal microflora (Nielsen et al., 1994), it has no antidiarrheal properties in infectious enteritis (Mitra and Rabbani, 1990). In the study presented here, the authors included patients with complaints of constipation and/or diarrhea, abdominal pain, abdominal distention, and flatulence who were not concomitantly treated with antibiotics, spasmolytics, laxatives, or antidiarrheal agents. Eligible patients were assigned to receive identical-looking tablets of placebo or freeze-dried cultures of *S. faecium* for four weeks, and compliance and side effects were monitored at regularly scheduled visits. A visual analog scale was used by patients to rate the global severity of their illness prior to the start of the trial. Evaluation of efficacy relied on the clinicians' overall assessment of the change in condition at the midpoint and endpoint of the four-week course of treatment.

No adverse effects were recorded, and 54 of the 58 participants completed all the requirements of the trial. The groups treated with *S. faecium* (n = 32) and placebo (n = 22) were well matched with regard to the frequency of baseline symptoms. After four weeks of treatment, *S. faecium* was not substantially better than placebo for any of the symptoms evaluated. Clinicians' assessments indicated that 81 percent of patients treated with *S. faecium* and 41 percent of those who had received placebo had a favorable change in their condition, a statistically significant difference. Although all of the patients not improved by *S. faecium* were female, response to treatment was not correlated with gender.

FEDOTOZINE

Fedotozine (phenyl-trymethoxy-dimethyl-propylamine), a peripheral agonist of the opioid kappa receptors that has been shown to block colonic pain response in animal (Langlois et al., 1997) and human experiments (Delvaux, 1999), was tested for efficacy in patients with irritable bowel syndrome in a multicenter trial organized by investigators from Hotel Dieu, Clermont-Ferrand, France, and the drug's manufacturer (Dapoigny, Abitbol, and Fraitag, 1995). The authors obtained the collaboration of 64 gastroenterologists from France, Belgium, and Tunisia to recruit 313 patients whose irritable bowel syndrome was characterized by moderate or severe abdominal pain and by at least two other symptoms from a list that included diarrhea alternating with constipation, constipation, excessive flatus, feeling of incomplete evacuation after defecation, and abdominal pain relieved by defecation. Patients were enrolled only if these symptoms had been present for at least one year and at least during three days each week. In all cases, the absence of organic gastrointestinal pathology was demonstrated by clinical, laboratory, and endoscopic evaluations. Patients treated with anticonvulsants, neuroleptics, hormones, barbiturates, and corticosteroids were ineligible for the study.

After a single-blind placebo phase designed to document the presence and severity of symptoms and compliance with treatment and data recording, the 238 eligible patients were randomly assigned to a six-week treatment phase with fedotozine or placebo. The drugs were administered in a parallel-group, dose-response fashion, i.e., patients received either 3.5, 15, or 30 mg of fedotozine three times daily before meals. Concomitant therapy with analgesic and antidepressant agents was allowed if it had been continued at the same dose for more than three months prior to the start of the study medication. The primary self-scored and clinician-rated outcome measure was the intensity of pain; other variables recorded were the severity of abdominal distention and alteration in bowel habits. Patients and clinicians also assessed the global change in condition at the end of the trial.

Adverse drug reactions led to the withdrawal of 14 of the 238 participating subjects (6 percent), but no details were provided regarding the clinical presentation of these complications or how many of them were due to fedotozine. A total of 265 side effects were reported by the 238 participants, the most common being headache (22 percent), vertigo (14 percent), fatigue (13 percent), nausea (13 percent), faintness (8 percent), and diarrhea (6 percent). There were no significant differences between the frequency of these complications as recorded in the fedotozine and placebo groups. Laboratory and electrocardiographic follow-up data showed no significant abnormalities.

The study was completed by 182 patients. Fourteen patients withdrew because of adverse drug reactions, seven patients dropped out because they felt that the treatment made no difference in their condition, and one subject discontinued the study drug because of complete cure of the symptoms. The remaining patients were not included in the analysis because they or the referring physicians did not comply with the research protocol. Analysis of efficacy was performed by intent to treat and took into account the fact that some of the clinical features were unevenly distributed among groups (i.e., there were more women in the low-dose fedotozine group and a lower proportion of patients previously treated for irritable bowel syndrome in the high-fedotozine group). Treatment with the high-dose fedotozine regimen (30 mg daily) was better than placebo with regard to the severity of abdominal pain and abdominal distention. Abnormal defecation patterns and changes in stool consistency were not significantly influenced by therapy with fedotozine.

CHINESE HERBAL MEDICINE

A well-designed and carefully executed randomized controlled trial of Chinese herbal medicine was carried out by investigators from the University of Sydney, Macquarie University, two teaching hospitals, and five private gastroenterological practices from Sydney, New South Wales, Australia (Bensoussan et al., 1998). Appropriate consent from local government authorities was obtained to use herbal substances available as over-the-counter remedies throughout Australia. A total of 116 patients with a diagnosis of irritable bowel syndrome made in accordance with the standard criteria (Thompson et al., 1989) were recruited at the seven clinical sites participating in the trial. Eligibility for the trial required that the subject be free of detectable liver disease, not pregnant, not currently using drugs or alcohol, and not having an organic gastrointestinal disorder or a current psychiatric diagnosis.

After a two-week observation period designed to detect changes in condition due to mere enrollment in the clinical trial, the subjects were randomly assigned to treatment with placebo (n = 35), standard (n = 43), or individualized (n = 38) preparations of Chinese herbs. The standard preparation contained parts of 20 different plants. The individualized preparation was formulated by a practitioner of Chinese medicine after direct contact with the patient; the decision rules leading to the selection of herbs and their proportions were not disclosed. All patients received their treatment as five capsules three times daily. Testing on five independent volunteers indicated that the placebo capsules were indistinguishable from the capsules containing the dried, powdered Chinese herbs. The effectiveness of the therapeutic interventions was judged on the basis of visual analog scales rating the severity of each symptom at the beginning and end of the trial.

Of the 116 subjects enrolled, 19 were withdrawn before the completion of the trial; two patients developed gastrointestinal discomfort associated with the use of Chinese herbal medicine. Among the other 17 dropouts, 11 were lost to follow-up, four withdrew because they felt that the treatment was ineffective, and two broke the research protocol. Eight subjects were lost to follow-up among those assigned to receive individualized preparations of Chinese herbal medicine (21 percent), but none among those assigned to treatment with placebo.

The standard preparation of Chinese herbal medicine was more effective than placebo with regard to the severity of symptoms and the illness's interference with life activities. Patients treated with placebo showed an overall improvement in the severity of their condition of 22 percent, while those who took the preparation of Chinese herbal medicine improved by an average of 44 percent. The group treated with individualized preparations of Chinese herbal medicine improved by 42 percent. The proportions of subjects who indicated a decrease in the degree to which irritable bowel syndrome interfered with life activities were 37 percent in the placebo group but 63 percent among patients treated with the standard preparation of Chinese herbal medicine.

Although the results are encouraging, these findings need independent replication, complete disclosure of the composition of the individualized preparations, and meticulous clinical and laboratory follow-up of all participants. The latter requirement is extremely important from the standpoint of safety, because ingredients of Chinese herbal medicines have been shown to produce severe nephropathy (Vanherweghem, 1998), liver injury (Kane, Kane, and Jain, 1995), lead poisoning (Chan et al., 1977), and hormonal disruptions (DiPaola et al., 1998).

INDIAN HERBAL MEDICINE

An Ayurvedic preparation containing extracts of the Northern Indian plants locally known as *Bilva (Aegle marmelos correa)* and *Brahmi (Bacopa monniere Linn.)* was tested for its efficacy in a placebo-controlled trial organized at the Institute of Medical Sciences, Banaras Hindu University, Varanasi, India (Yadav et al., 1989). The study cohort included patients given the diagnosis of irritable bowel syndrome on the basis of chronic alteration in bowel habits accompanied by abdominal pain, abdominal distention, or a sense of incomplete evacuation. Parasitic infection and other organic gastrointestinal disorders were excluded by stool examinations, sigmoidoscopy, and barium enema. Psychiatric evaluations identified abnormalities in more than three-quarters of the sample. The subjects' illnesses were further classified as diarrhea- and pain-predominant; alternate diarrhea and constipation; abdominal distention- and pain-predominant; and painless diarrhea. These subtypes were taken into account during the random allocation of subjects to treatment with the Indian herbal medicine or placebo (corn starch), both of which were administered as identical-looking dark green granules three times daily for a total of approximately 15 g of herbal products each day for six weeks.

Fifty-seven patients were assigned to treatment with Indian herbal medicine and 52 received placebo; the groups were well matched with regard to mean age (29 versus 28 years), gender distribution (male:female ratio 7:1 versus 8:1), median duration of illness (four years in both groups), and frequency of psychiatric diagnoses (79 percent versus 81 percent). Therapy with Indian herbal medicine was well tolerated, the only adverse effect noted being drowsiness, which was reported by two patients (4 percent).

Treatment with Indian herbal medicine was no better than placebo with respect to the proportions of patients reporting improvement in the severity of abdominal pain, constipation, gaseousness, and altered bowel habits consisting of alternating diarrhea and constipation. The herbal mixture was effective in reducing the severity of diarrhea and that of symptoms of anxiety and depression. Of the five subtypes of irritable bowel syndrome, Indian herbal medicine was superior to placebo only for patients whose illness was diarrhea-predominant with or without associated abdominal pain. In light of the potential for hepatotoxicity of *Aegle marmelos,* one of the herbs used in this study (Arseculeratne, Gunatilaka, and Panabokke, 1985) and that of hematological complications (Ohnuma et al., 1982) and heavy metal poisoning possibly related to other Indian herbal products (Pontifex and Garg, 1985; Smitherman and Harber, 1991), the limited benefit identified in this trial does not support widespread use of Indian herbal medicine as a therapeutic modality for patients with irritable bowel syndrome.

Chapter 17

Evidence-Based Therapy
of Irritable Bowel Syndrome

In a recent review of the issue raised by patients with refractory functional gastrointestinal disorders, one of the most prominent U.S. writers on the topic suggests that treatment must be based on the severity and nature of the symptoms and on the degree of disability produced by the illness (Drossman, 1995). In his view, patients with mild symptoms and no significant disability can be treated with dietary and lifestyle changes, education, and reassurance. Once the functional syndrome is characterized by moderately severe symptoms, the pharmacologic treatment should focus on the most disturbing symptom. Rather than treating the syndrome, one is advised to use loperamide for diarrhea, fiber for constipation, and anticholinergic agents for pain. If the pain is severe, continuous, and not related to changes in the gastrointestinal tract's function, then tricyclic antidepressants or serotonin-reuptake inhibitors are indicated because of their "central analgesic" effect.

Support for these recommendations was not documented by evidence generated by carefully conducted double-blind trials, and practitioners have had to contend with a state of the science in which "not a single study has been published that provides compelling evidence that any therapeutic agent is efficacious in the global treatment" of irritable bowel syndrome (Klein, 1988, p. 232). However, we judge the evidence to indicate that tricyclic antidepressants are in fact effective for the totality of this illness and should constitute the first-line treatment in all cases in which the severity of the syndrome warrants intervention, provided that there are no contraindications to the use of these agents and that the potential for drug-drug interactions has been carefully explored, as indicated in the description of the evidence-based therapy of fibromyalgia.

Monotherapy with amitriptyline or desipramine should be initiated with a starting dose of 10 mg administered once a day in patients with the diarrhea-predominant variant of the syndrome. The dosage can be increased by 10 mg every week with close monitoring of adverse reactions and changes in the gastrointestinal manifestations of the syndrome. Pharmacologically, these two agents are quite similar; attention must be paid to the fact that a popular brand of desipramine contains the dye tartrazine, which may cause hypersensitivity reactions, especially in patients allergic to aspirin (American Hospital Formulary Service, 1997, p. 1682). Adjunctive therapy with a bulking agent may lead to a decrease in the overall severity of the syndrome in all patients and ameliorate the bowel habit and ease of stool passage in those with the constipation-predominant variant of the syndrome.

The limited pharmacological arsenal has stimulated controlled trials of cognitive-behavioral therapy; unfortunately, their results are contradictory and do not inspire the confidence that would justify their introduction in current clinical practice. In the first of these trials, 42 irritable bowel patients registered for care at St. Bartholomew's Hospital, London, were randomly allocated to receive either "standard" medical treatment or behavioral psychotherapy (Corney et al., 1991). After nine months, the severity of gastrointestinal symptoms had improved, but the magnitude of change was similar in the two groups. Subsequent work performed at the Center for Stress and Anxiety Disorders, State University of New York at Albany, compared the effect of a multicomponent treatment consisting of cognitive therapy, thermal biofeedback, and relaxation, first with the effect of an attention-placebo intervention and then with the changes produced by a symptom-monitoring control treatment (Blanchard et al., 1992). Symptom diaries kept by the 80 patients enrolled in the trial indicated improvement in the gastrointestinal symptoms and reduction of depression and anxiety, but the treatment that included the cognitive-behavioral intervention was not better than either of the two control therapies. A later report from the same group described the results of individualized cognitive therapy, administered during ten sessions over eight weeks to 20 patients in a controlled trial that compared the psychotherapeutic intervention with symptom monitoring (Greene and Blanchard,

1994). This time, cognitive-behavioral therapy was clearly the better of the two interventions, and the results were maintained after the three-month follow-up evaluation. Of the psychological variables influenced by cognitive-behavioral therapy, a reduction in negative automatic thoughts correlated best with the improvement in gastrointestinal symptomatology. These encouraging results were confirmed in a trial performed at the University of Nijmegen, Nijmegen, Netherlands (Van Dulmen, Fennis, and Bleijenberg, 1996) in which the long-term outcome of cognitive-behavioral therapy consisting of eight two-hour group sessions over a period of three months was compared with the natural history of disease (i.e., waiting list control). The absence of placebo therapy substantially decreases the value of the findings indicating that cognitive-behavioral therapy improved abdominal complaints and coping strategies and reduced avoidant behaviors and the fact that the favorable changes were still detectable two years later.

SECTION IV:
PREMENSTRUAL SYNDROME

Chapter 18

Definition and Methodological Issues

The current standard for the diagnosis of premenstrual syndrome was published by the U.S. experts contributing to the most recent version of the classification of psychiatric disorders (American Psychiatric Association, 1994). Presented as research criteria for "premenstrual dysphoric disorder," the diagnosis requires the evaluation of the presence and characteristics of 11 clusters of symptoms that are presented here with the original descriptive phrases:

1. *Dysphoria* (markedly depressed mood, feelings of hopelessness, or self-deprecating thoughts)
2. *Anxiety* (marked anxiety, tension, feelings of being "keyed up" or "on edge")
3. *Affective lability* (increased sensitivity to rejection, or feeling suddenly sad or tearful)
4. *Irritability* (persistent and marked irritability or anger, or increased interpersonal conflicts)
5. *Anhedonia* (decreased interest in social, occupational, or recreational activities)
6. *Difficulty with concentration*
7. *Fatigue* (lethargy, marked lack of energy, or easy fatigability)
8. *Eating disturbance* (marked change in appetite, overeating, or specific food cravings)
9. *Sleep disturbance* (hypersomnia or insomnia)
10. *Feeling overwhelmed or out of control*
11. *Other physical symptoms* (breast tenderness or swelling, headaches, joint or muscle pain, "bloating," or weight gain)

The diagnosis is confirmed if the patient indicates that symptoms from at least five of these 11 clusters (with at least one from the clusters dysphoria, anxiety, affective lability, or irritability) have been present during the premenstrual week of most of the menstrual cycles of the preceding year. To be counted toward the diagnosis, the symptoms must improve rapidly within a few days after the onset of menses; be absent in the week following the end of menstrual bleeding; produce significant deterioration in the usual occupational efficiency; and lead to avoidance or difficulties in social activities and relationships with others. The diagnostic evaluation must include careful consideration of the luteal phase exacerbation of general medical conditions (e.g., epilepsy, disorders of thyroid gland function, endometriosis, systemic lupus, or malignancies) or psychiatric disorders (e.g., major depressive disorder, dysthymic disorder, panic disorder, or personality disorder) known to manifest symptoms similar to that of premenstrual syndrome. However, because premenstrual dysphoric disorder may be superimposed on any of these medical or psychiatric disorders, the final diagnosis should be confirmed only by analysis of prospective daily ratings of the symptoms present during at least two consecutive cycles. The criteria are essentially similar to those proposed in the previous version of the *Diagnostic and Statistical Manual of Mental Disorders* (American Psychiatric Association, 1987).

The relative clarity of the American Psychiatric Association's definition must be considered as substantial progress in a research field that had been, as Halbreich and Endicott (1985) have indicated so well, plagued for decades by lack of descriptive accuracy, unreliable measurements, controversy regarding the intensity of premenstrual changes that may qualify as abnormal, variability in defining the premenstrual period, and the lack of instruments to assess and confirm the presence of premenstrual syndrome. Nonetheless, from the standpoint of the evaluator of therapeutic efficacy, some of the issues raised by Halbreich and Endicott in 1985 remain just as valid 15 years later. In the first place, these authors have questioned the comparability of studies involving populations "that happened to be available," thus creating a selection bias by age, duration of illness, parity, and health-seeking behavior. Second, they have rightly pointed out that therapeutic trials whose efficacy must be judged mostly by the subjects' self-reports are liable to the effect of expectation, social learning, and cultural beliefs. Third, other sources of bias identified by Halbreich and Endicott in the same commentary are psychosocial factors, including environmental stress or whether the trial occurs during a work period or while the subject is on vacation. Fourth, of major importance is the modulation of placebo response among patients with premenstrual syndrome, given the fact that the placebo nonresponders will show persistent dysphoria and anhedonia, as well as anxious and hostile features and tenacious impairment in social functioning.

Chapter 19

Effective Therapy

SELECTIVE SEROTONIN REUPTAKE INHIBITORS

The first experimental indication that premenstrual syndrome is caused by a functional serotonergic deficiency was provided in a study of the platelets' uptake of serotonin (Ashby et al., 1988). The research was performed at the University of Louisville and compared eight women with well-defined premenstrual syndrome with ten healthy control subjects well matched for age, marital status, and parity. Blood samples were collected in the premenstrual and postmenstrual periods, the platelets counted, and the content and uptake of serotonin measured in triplicate. The results indicated a significantly lower serotonin content and serotonin uptake during the premenstrual period in the patient group. Because the serotonergic mechanisms in platelets and serotonin-containing neurons are considered analogous, the authors interpreted their findings to indicate the probability of an alteration in serotonergic brain activities, including neuronal uptake and rate of firing.

The serotonergic deficiency hypothesis was next tested in a study measuring neuroendocrine responses to an infusion of L-tryptophan, a biological challenge that increases the availability of serotonin in the brain (Bancroft et al., 1991). The research was conducted by investigators from the Reproductive Biology Unit and Brain Metabolism Unit of the Medical Research Council, Edinburgh, on 13 women with perimenstrual mood changes, which included, in all cases, premenstrual depression. Control subjects were recruited from among the staff and were women who denied mood changes around the time of their periods. Tryptophan was administered as 1 percent solution in sodium chloride (0.72 percent) and sodium sulphite (0.05 percent) for a total dose of 5 g (500 ml) infused over 30 minutes. All participants were tested just before their menstruation and again postmenstrually at the time indicated by the subject to be "feeling at her best." Plasma levels of growth hormone and cortisol, but not prolactin, were significantly smaller in the premenstrually depressed group, an altered endocrine response interpreted by the authors to indicate a neurotransmitter abnormality that creates a vulnerability to dysphoria.

Additional support for the hypothesis attributing clinical manifestations of premenstrual syndrome to serotonin deficiency was provided by an elegant, simple, yet well-designed study of the effect of acute dietary tryptophan depletion (Menkes, Coates, and Fawcett, 1994). The procedure leads to a decrease in serotonin synthesis in the central nervous system. The experiment was conducted on a group of 16 women who had been diagnosed with premenstrual syndrome on the basis of daily self-rating of luteal phase abnormalities for at least three menstrual cycles. Subjects were tested in a randomized, double-blind, crossover manner for a total of four days during two menstrual cycles, once each during the follicular and luteal phases of these cycles. On test days, one of two amino acid mixtures disguised with chocolate flavoring was ingested. The mixtures contained 100 g of food-grade amino acids diluted to 250 ml with tap water. The mixtures were identical but for the presence of 2.3 g of L-tryptophan. During the test days the subjects were allowed to eat only tryptophan-poor food (e.g., corn flakes, canned fruit, apples, carrots, celery, and rice cakes). A strong negative correlation was noted between the severity of baseline symptoms and tryptophan levels. Tryptophan depletion produced significant worsening of irritability, restlessness, anxiety, social withdrawal, breast tenderness, and abdominal bloating.

Recent work has offered further support for the characterization of the abnormalities in serotonergic function of patients with premenstrual syndrome as detected by the serotonin response to a fenfluramine challenge, which activates serotonin neurotransmission and is followed by an increase in plasma prolactin levels (Fitz-Gerald et al., 1997). This research continued a line of inquiry that had demonstrated a favorable effect of d-fenfluramine on affective symptoms and on calorie and carbohydrate intake of patients with premenstrual syndrome (Brzezinski et al., 1990), but could not identify significant neuroendocrine responses (Bancroft and Cook, 1995). The study was conducted at the College of Physicians and Surgeons, Columbia University, New York, where the authors recruited nine clinic patients diagnosed with premenstrual dysphoric disorder and 11 healthy control subjects. Participants received 60 mg of dl-fenfluramine or placebo orally and had their prolactin levels measured at baseline and then hourly for five hours after the dose. The dose of fenfluramine was at least twice that used in previous research (Bancroft and Cook, 1995), a choice supported by a recent pharmacologic study (Goodwin, Murray, and Bancroft, 1994). All fenfluramine and placebo challenges were given in the luteal phase. The results indicated that the maximum net prolactin response to fenfluramine was significantly higher in healthy subjects than in patients with premenstrual syndrome. The statistical significance of the difference was confirmed after the data were controlled for age, body weight, and plasma levels of fenfluramine and its metabolite.

Fluoxetine

The first double-blind, randomized, placebo-controlled trial of a selective serotonin reuptake inhibitor in the treatment of premenstrual syndrome was performed by investigators from the University of Massachusetts and Brown University (Stone, Pearlstein, and Brown, 1991). The subjects were recruited from among the women who responded to a newspaper advertisement and had to fulfill standard diagnostic criteria (American Psychiatric Association, 1987) but be otherwise physically healthy. Patients with current major psychiatric disorder and those receiving antidepressants, anxiolytics, or neuroleptics were excluded. Also excluded were women with irregular menstrual cycles and those treated with hormones or diuretics.

Of the 487 women screened for the study, 71 were found to be eligible, i.e., had no active medical or psychiatric condition, took no medications, and met all diagnostic criteria indicating late luteal phase dysphoric disorder severe enough to produce at least a 30 percent increase in symptoms during the week prior to the onset of menstruation. Of this cohort, 25 patients elected to participate in the trial and were started on placebo given in a single-blinded manner.

One subject improved markedly during this first cycle of treatment; another dropped out because of intolerable side effects; a third was excluded because of alcohol and drug abuse; a fourth became pregnant; and a fifth did not return for further treatment.

The remaining 20 patients were randomly assigned to receive either 20 mg of fluoxetine or a placebo for two complete menstrual cycles. The groups were comparable in age, marital status, prevalence of past major depression (50 percent in the fluoxetine group and 40 percent in the placebo group), and severity of premenstrual symptomatology. Response to treatment was defined by significant (at least 50 percent) reduction in the mean premenstrual symptom exacerbation.

Scores generated by the daily assessment forms and global assessment scales showed a significant difference between the placebo and the fluoxetine groups. Five of the ten patients receiving fluoxetine improved to such a significant extent that they no longer met diagnostic criteria for the condition at the end of the two-month therapeutic trial. Four other patients showed a substantial decrease in their illness experience, but were sufficiently symptomatic to retain the diagnosis. Only two of the ten subjects treated with placebo showed a similar improvement, a highly significant difference from the 90 percent success rate in the fluoxetine group. All of the symptoms recorded showed a significant decrease in the fluoxetine group, the most prominent improvement being noted for depression, anxiety, loss of interest, affective lability, and irritability. Seven of the eight placebo nonresponders were offered fluoxetine at the completion of the controlled study and six of them responded favorably.

A mild side effect (insomnia, fatigue, decreased appetite, difficulty achieving orgasm) was reported by 50 percent of the patients in the fluoxetine group. With only one exception, these symptoms disappeared by the last cycle of the study. The patients enrolled in the placebo group reported more side effects, including headache, sleep disturbance, breast tenderness, nausea, anxiety, increased appetite, and decreased energy.

The pioneering work of Stone, Pearlstein, and Brown (1991) was replicated by a group of investigators representing seven Canadian university-affiliated women's health clinics (Steiner et al., 1995). The diagnosis of late luteal phase dysphoric disorder was established according to standard symptomatic criteria (American Psychiatric Association, 1987). Patients who met diagnostic criteria for any major psychiatric syndrome or had used psychoactive drugs within two months prior to the study were excluded. Patients were not included if they had used fluoxetine at any point in their lives, had a record of multiple adverse drug reactions, findings suggesting unstable medical illnesses, and if they had irregular menstrual cycles, were taking oral contraceptives, were lactating, or were considered to have anovulatory cycles. Patients taking any medications to treat premenstrual symptoms were identified and screened out.

The study began with 405 patients who entered a single-blind placebo washout period lasting two menstrual cycles. At the end of this period, 92 subjects were withdrawn: 22 did not meet diagnostic criteria, 12 responded to placebo, 15 experienced significant side effects, 20 did not report for follow-up, and 23 invoked personal reasons for discontinuation. The remaining 313 patients were randomly assigned to receive fluoxetine 20 mg daily, fluoxetine 60 mg daily, or placebo for six consecutive menstrual cycles. The mean age of the study participants was 36 years; all subjects had at least a high-school education, 55 percent were married, and 70 percent had at least one child. The placebo and treatment groups were well matched with regard to demographic and clinical characteristics. The outcome measures included reduction in premenstrual tension, irritability, dysphoria, headache, bloating, and breast tenderness scored by the patients daily on visual analog scales. A 50 percent improvement from baseline was defined as moderate improvement, while marked improvement required a 75 percent positive change compared with the pretreatment baseline.

A total of 133 patients (42 percent) failed to complete the study; most of these patients had been assigned to the placebo group (53 patients or 50 percent) or to the fluoxetine 60 mg daily group (47 patients or 44 percent). In slightly more than half of the withdrawals in the placebo group (51 percent) the reason invoked was lack of efficacy. Among those who dropped out of the fluoxetine 60 mg group, the most common reason for withdrawal was the presence of intolerable side effects, reported by 33 percent of patients. In contrast, both the total number of withdrawals (32 percent) and the number of patients dropping out because of side effects (10 percent) were smaller among those assigned to take fluoxetine 20 mg daily. There were no life-threatening events or serious medication side effects in any of the patients enrolled in the study. None of the patients had homicidal or suicidal tendencies during the study period.

The trial indicated that treatment with fluoxetine was efficacious for premenstrual syndrome; 52 percent of the patients receiving fluoxetine at either dose showed at least moderate improvement within the first cycle of treatment. The corresponding figure in the placebo group was only 22 percent improvement, a highly significant difference. The proportion of patients showing at least moderate improvement over the entire treatment period was 53 percent as compared with a 28 percent improvement rate among those receiving placebo. The proportion of cycles in which there was marked improvement was 32 percent during fluoxetine therapy, but only 14 percent for the cycles involving placebo administration. Side effects were much more likely among those receiving 60 mg fluoxetine than those receiving 20 mg fluoxetine; insomnia or disturbed sleep (26 percent versus 10 percent), nausea (24 percent versus 14 percent), tremor or shakiness (20 percent versus 5 percent), fatigue or lethargy (19 percent versus 10 percent), dizziness (14 percent versus 8 percent), anorexia or disturbed appetite (14 percent versus 5 percent), daytime somnolence or decreased ability to concentrate (14 percent versus 9 percent), sweating (11 percent versus 4 percent), visual disturbance (11 percent versus 3 percent), dry mouth (10 percent versus 4 percent), minor cardiovascular symptoms (10 percent versus 4 percent), and excessive yawning (6 percent versus 1 percent). The data were interpreted to indicate that fluoxetine at a daily dose of 20 mg significantly reduces the symptoms of premenstrual syndrome in a majority of patients and is generally well tolerated.

The second confirmation of the efficacy of fluoxetine in abolishing luteal phase symptomatology of premenstrual syndrome was obtained in a small but very well-designed study performed by researchers from the Department of Reproductive Medicine of the University of California at San Diego (Wood et al., 1992). The methodological advance consisted of a treatment crossover phase to directly assess the placebo effect in patients whose symptoms responded to fluoxetine treatment. Moreover, this study excluded all patients with a personal or family history of mood disorder or all other diagnosable psychopathology.

The patients considered for enrollment in this trial underwent a thorough and highly structured clinical evaluation to document their premenstrual syndrome and to investigate in detail the possible presence of physical and psychiatric conditions that may imitate the syndrome. The patients were instructed to use a prospective self-rating scale that scored daily 12 behavioral and 10 physical symptoms associated with premenstrual syndrome. Reliable questionnaires were used to score depression, anxiety, and psychometric abnormalities, and appropriate exclusion criteria were developed and applied. The diagnosis of premenstrual syndrome in this clinical setting was given according to the following: menstrual cycles lasting 26 to 32 days; evidence of ovulation by hormonal measurements; well-established follicular phase symptomatic improvement; symptom-associated disruption in socioeconomic activities.

The study group comprised eight women with a mean age of 38 years and a mean duration of symptoms of 14 years. Symptoms had began after a pregnancy in six of the eight patients. The randomized, double-blind study lasted six months, during which the subjects received placebo or 20 mg of fluoxetine daily for three menstrual cycles each.

As reported by seven of the eight patients, during treatment with fluoxetine both behavioral and physical symptoms of the premenstrual syndrome were significantly improved; the mean reductions were 75 percent for behavioral symptoms and 40 percent for the physical manifestations of the syndrome. The chronology of the improvement highlighted the effect of the drug on the illness experienced during the luteal phase; symptoms reported during the follicular phase were not substantially changed by fluoxetine. The administration of placebo produced insignificant symptomatic changes; this was a surprising result that was tentatively attributed by the investigators to the fact that the subjects had failed prior therapeutic attempts and had been carefully informed that the drug studied could either improve or worsen the symptoms. The frequency of recorded side effects (headache, insomnia, anxiety, nausea, and dizziness) was not significantly different between the fluoxetine and the placebo treatment periods.

Finally, the third confirmatory study available at this time is also exemplary for its use of the double-blind, randomized, crossover methodology (Menkes et al., 1993). Performed by investigators from the University of Otago Medical School, Dunedin, New Zealand, the project started with a cohort of 23 patients with a tentative diagnosis of premenstrual syndrome. After three months of baseline daily self-rating of social functioning and physical and affective symptoms, 21 of the 23 patients had the diagnosis confirmed and were randomly assigned to receive daily doses of inert placebo or 20 mg of fluoxetine. The treatment was started on the twelfth day of the menstrual cycle and continued through the end of three consecutive menstrual cycles; following a 12-day washout period, the patients were crossed over to the alternate treatment, which was administered for three additional cycles. The subjects recorded daily ratings on self-administered questionnaires identical to those used during the baseline period and completed inventories addressing the side effects of medication. Steady-state plasma levels of fluoxetine and its active metabolite, norfluoxetine, were measured at the end of the treatment period.

Five patients were dropped out of the trial; three subjects (14 percent) had intolerable side effects (nausea, insomnia, and arthralgias) and two patients did not comply with the requirements of the study. The remaining 16 patients had an average age of 38 years and premenstrual symptoms for at least three years prior to entering the study. Previous treatments included trials of diuretics, vitamins, and evening primrose oil. During the baseline observation period, all patients had premenstrual somatic complaints such as weight gain, clumsiness, and breast swelling; 15 of the 16 patients also had substantial affective disturbance, manifested mainly as irritability, depressed mood, and impairment of concentration and memory.

After three months of treatment, fluoxetine produced marked symptomatic improvement in 94 percent of the subjects studied. Statistically significant advantages over placebo were observed in the patients' daily ratings for mood swings, depression, impulsivity, abdominal bloating, breast tenderness, and abdominal pain. Fluoxetine was no better than placebo with regard to symptoms of anxiety and food cravings, but both symptoms decreased substantially during the trial. Patients reported a decrease in their family turbulence and the regressing behavior of their children. For the half of the study group who decided to continue fluoxetine treatment, the beneficial effects of fluoxetine persisted throughout the 18-month follow-up period. The plasma levels of fluoxetine and norfluoxetine showed significant variation across the group; a dose-response effect was not observed. Overall, fluoxetine was well tolerated by 88 percent of the subjects who completed the trial; however, transient side effects including nausea, insomnia, headache, tremor, urinary frequency, sour taste, dysmenorrhea, and early menstruation were reported by 63 percent of the subjects. In one case, fluoxetine therapy appeared to cause the absence of a midcycle increase in libido.

Sertraline

A naphtalenamine derivative structurally unrelated to the other currently used selective serotonin reuptake inhibitors (American Hospital Formulary Service, 1997, p. 1711), sertraline has been tested in the treatment of premenstrual syndrome in a recent multi-center trial (Yonkers et al., 1996). The research was supported by a grant from the drug's manufacturer. Patients were recruited at 12 university-affiliated centers in the United States; eligibility criteria required an age of 24 to 45, regular menstrual cycles 24 to 36 days in duration, and the absence of concurrent psychiatric, gynecologic, and general medical conditions. A laboratory panel including a urine drug screen, complete blood cell count, chemistry profile, and pregnancy test were performed for all patients prior to the start and repeated at the end of the study. The diagnosis was made if the patients had at least five symptoms of premenstrual dysphoric disorder for at least two years, and at least a 75 percent difference in the severity of symptoms recorded during the five worst luteal phase days as compared with the first five postmenstrual days. Patients meeting these criteria were given placebo in a single-blinded manner and asked to keep daily ratings of their symptoms and had their ovulation confirmed using a urinary luteinizing hormone predictor test. All subjects were reevaluated during the late luteal phase of this cycle; those who continued to meet the symptom severity criteria were randomly assigned to receive either placebo or sertraline for three consecutive menstrual cycles. The initial dose of sertraline was 50 mg every day. In contrast to the trials of fluoxetine (Stone, Pearlstein, and Brown, 1991; Steiner et al., 1995), which used fixed doses of the selective serotonin reuptake inhibitor, in this study the dose of sertraline could be increased by 50 mg/day each cycle to a maximum dose of 150 mg/day if symptoms did not improve. Outcome measures included clinical global impression and severity of depression.

Of the 162 women who participated in the study, 79 were assigned to the sertraline group and 83 to the placebo group. The groups were well matched for age (average at intake 36 years), duration of illness (10 years), number of pregnancies, history of major depression (38 percent of patients), and pretreatment functional impairment scores regarding work, housework, social and leisure activities, and relationships with partner and children. By the third and last cycle of treatment, the dose of sertraline had remained 50 mg/day for only 18 percent of patients; 48 percent were receiving 100 mg/day and 34 percent were on 150 mg/day. The attrition rates were 13 percent in the sertraline-treated group and 10 percent in the placebo group.

The efficacy of the sertraline administration was demonstrated for all of the outcomes measured. By the third treatment cycle, the clinical global impression indicated that 68 percent of the patients receiving sertraline were very much or much improved; the similar figure in the placebo group was 40 percent, a statistically significant difference. Premenstrual depressive symptoms were also significantly improved by sertraline by the first cycle of treatment and the gains maintained for the remainder of the study period. Treatment with sertraline was well tolerated; only five of the 79 patients (5 percent) withdrew from the trial because of intolerable side effects of the drug.

Recently, the authors expanded their study groups to a total of 200 patients who completed the trial; 99 were treated with sertraline and 101 received placebo (Yonkers et al., 1997). The global ratings indicated substantial improvement in 62 percent of those treated with sertraline, as compared with 34 percent of those given placebo, due to significant decrease, in the severity of the physical, depres-

sive, and anger/irritability symptom clusters. The symptoms showing the greatest favorable change in response to sertraline as
compared with placebo treatment were hopelessness, mood swings,
conflicts, feeling rejected, feeling out of control, anhedonia, and
food cravings. The improvement recorded for the symptoms of joint
and muscle pain, hypersomnia, increased appetite, breast tenderness, abdominal bloating, and breast tenderness were similar in the
placebo and sertraline-treated patients. Functional data supported
the efficacy of sertraline-for the domains of occupational productivity
(38 percent of sertraline-treated patients improved versus 13 percent of
patients in the placebo group), hobbies and social activities (38 percent
versus 17 percent), and relationships (42 percent versus 15 percent).
Adverse reactions leading to withdrawal from the study were more
prevalent in the sertraline group (8 percent as compared with 2 percent
in the placebo group); among the milder side effects nausea, diarrhea,
and decreased libido were significantly more common among the
patients given sertraline.

Recent work by members of the same group (Halbreich and
Smoller, 1997) has also addressed the important issue of treatment
duration by studying the effect of the drug given only during the
luteal (premenstrual) phase. This effort was the first well-designed
test of the efficacy of intermittent serotonin reuptake inhibition in
women with premenstrual syndrome, which had been suggested by
an investigation of fluoxetine (Steiner et al., 1997) that did not use a
placebo phase. The study of intermittent sertraline therapy was
conducted by researchers from the State University of New York at
Buffalo with support from the manufacturer of sertraline. The subjects were recruited by advertisements offering free treatment. The
60 responders invited for initial screening had to have regular
menstrual cycles 25 to 34 days in duration, fulfill standard criteria
for premenstrual dysphoric disorder (American Psychiatric Association, 1994), have no other psychiatric or physical diagnoses, and
take no medications. Prospective assessments using daily rating
forms for at least two menstrual cycles confirmed moderate or
severe late luteal phase symptoms in 32 subjects. After structured
psychiatric and psychometric evaluations, physical examination,
and extensive laboratory testing, 27 subjects were found eligible for

the study and 15 accepted entry into a single-blind treatment with 100 mg sertraline daily for one menstrual cycle.

One of these patients dropped out and three showed no improvement. The remaining 11 patients (79 percent) had a favorable response to continuous administration of sertraline and were randomized to a double-blind crossover during which placebo or sertraline (100 mg/day) were given only during the 14 days preceding menstruation for two consecutive cycles each. Two patients who started the trial with placebo dropped out before entering the sertraline phase. Of the nine remaining patients, all reported good symptom control with intermittent sertraline, but only two responded well to placebo. The statistical significance of improvement in symptom severity was demonstrated by posthoc analyses for the full-cycle sertraline treatment versus baseline and for luteal-phase sertraline treatments versus placebo. The improvement obtained by treatment with sertraline during the luteal phase was quantitatively similar to that produced by full-cycle administration of the serotonin reuptake inhibitor drug. Luteal-phase sertraline treatment was frequently associated with headache (six of nine patients), dry mouth and insomnia (five patients each), sedation, urinary frequency, and fatigue (four patients each), and nausea and flatulence (three patients each), but none of these events were considered severe.

The effectiveness of sertraline therapy administered only during the luteal phase was confirmed by researchers from Walter Reed Army Medical Center, Washington, DC, in a small but well-designed crossover trial (Young et al., 1998). Participants were recruited through advertisements placed in military media, and diagnostic screening using standard criteria (American Psychiatric Association, 1994) was conducted by telephone. The 31 eligible women were then entered into a two-month data collection period during which a structured calendar of premenstrual experiences was utilized to document the difference in overall severity of symptoms in the luteal phase as compared with the first week following the onset of menstrual bleeding. Seventeen subjects demonstrated the required 30 percent difference and were randomly assigned to start the trial with sertraline (50 mg) or placebo given from day 15 of the cycle to the first day of menses for two consecutive cycles. This phase was followed by a washout cycle, after which the patients received the alternate therapy for two additional cycles.

Three of the 17 patients dropped out for personal reasons and three women discontinued their participation due to side effects consisting of nausea (two patients treated with sertraline) and nervousness and tremulousness (one patient taking placebo). In the group of 11 patients who completed the trial, treatment with sertraline during the luteal phase was clearly superior to placebo. Severity of behavioral symptoms decreased an average of 58 percent with sertraline but only 22 percent with placebo. Similarly, a substantial reduction in physical symptoms was observed only during the sertraline phase of the trial.

The direct comparison of full- or half-cycle treatment has been performed only once at this writing (Freeman et al., 1999). Working at the University of Pennsylvania Medical Center, Philadelphia, the investigators recruited 31 women who had just completed a trial of sertraline administered daily for three months. Daily symptom reports had confirmed the presence of severe premenstrual symptomatology and had established that symptoms were significantly (50 percent or more) worse during the luteal phase of the cycle. At the onset of the current trial, 16 of the 31 patients had responded to the previous trial of sertraline, and had symptom scores significantly lower than those of the other 15 participants.

Eighteen randomly selected patients were assigned to receive the half-cycle sertraline therapy. The starting dose was one placebo capsule daily for the first 14 days of the cycle, followed by an identical-looking capsule containing 50 mg of sertraline ingested daily through the end of the cycle. Unless the condition improved or the patient complained of adverse effects, the daily dose was increased to two capsules (100 mg sertraline) on day 14 of the second cycle and to three capsules (150 mg sertraline) on day 14 of the last cycle of the trial. At end point, nine of the 18 (50 percent) patients had remained at the 50 mg/day dose, seven had increased the dose to 100 mg/day, and two were taking 150 mg/day. The full-cycle treatment group (n = 13) had dosage adjustments made in the same manner as in the half-cycle treatment group; four (31 percent) took 50 mg/day throughout the trial, six advanced to 100 mg/day, and three were receiving 150 mg/day during the last cycle of the treatment period.

Side effects were common (81 percent of patients) but led to withdrawal from the trial in only three cases (10 percent). The most common treatment-related symptoms were nausea (46 percent in the full-cycle group and 11 percent in the half-cycle group), dry mouth (15 percent versus 22 percent), headache (8 percent versus 22 percent), dizziness (15 percent versus 11 percent), fatigue (8 percent versus 17 percent), and decreased libido (8 percent versus 11 percent); all of these frequencies were statistically similar.

Half-cycle treatment with sertraline was better than the full-cycle regimen with regard to improvement in mood symptoms, and equally effective in improving the pain, appetite, and behavioral manifestations of the syndrome. The individual symptoms most favorably influenced by half-cycle treatment with sertraline were confusion, mood swings, nervous tension, and feeling out of control. The overall severity of the condition improved in 89 percent of patients given the half-cycle sertraline regimen but in only 46 percent treated full cycle, a statistically significant difference. The half-cycle treatment led to improvement in 80 percent of patients whose condition had not responded to the previous three-cycle trial of daily sertraline administration.

Paroxetine

Methodologies similar to those used to study the effect of fluoxetine and sertraline on the symptoms of premenstrual syndrome have also been employed by investigators from the University of Göteborg, Sweden, to assess the potential benefit of paroxetine, another widely available selective serotonin reuptake inhibitor (Eriksson et al., 1995). The compound is a phenylpiperidine derivative structurally different from fluoxetine and sertraline (American Hospital Formulary Service, 1997, p. 1707). For the study presented here the recruiting effort targeted women with substantial premenstrual dysphoria or irritability starting predictably during the two weeks prior to the onset of menstrual bleeding. Subjects with ongoing somatic or psychiatric disorders and those with current alcohol abuse, irregular menstruation, pregnancy or plans for pregnancy, or with a history of previous treatment with antidepressants for premenstrual symptoms were excluded.

The patients selected for the study were randomized to receive placebo or paroxetine for three consecutive menstrual cycles. Treatment was started on the first day of menstruation with a daily tablet of 10 mg paroxetine. Two weeks later, the paroxetine dose was increased to 20 mg daily, a regimen that was maintained for the rest of the trial. Starting with the fourth week of treatment, patients who perceived an unsatisfactory reduction of symptoms were allowed to increase the paroxetine or placebo dose to three tablets daily, while patients with significant side effects were instructed to decrease their dose to one daily tablet of paroxetine or placebo. Outcome assessments compared the placebo and paroxetine-treated groups with respect to global improvement and the relative symptomatic improvement, expressed as percent change of baseline score.

The trial involved 27 patients who were given paroxetine and 26 who were treated with placebo tablets. Three patients treated with paroxetine and two treated with placebo dropped out because of intolerable side effects. Two other patients in each group were excluded during the trial, one each because of pregnancy, irregular menstruation, onset of another illness, and lack of compliance. Thus, 22 patients in each group completed the trial. Two of the patients in the placebo group and one patient in the paroxetine group had been previously treated for a depressive disorder. In the paroxetine group, a majority of patients (14 of 22) received two 10 mg tablets daily; four subjects were treated with one 10 mg tablet daily and four subjects required three 10 mg tablets daily. However, serum concentrations of the active compound did not correlate with the clinical effect. Most of the placebo-treated patients chose a plateau dose of three tablets daily. The side effect profile of paroxetine was satisfactory; dry mouth, nausea, and yawning occurred more frequently than in the placebo group during the first treatment cycle and sexual dysfunction was reported by 30 percent of patients during the third treatment cycle.

As assessed by the patients, global improvement was noted by 90 percent of paroxetine-treated patients and 41 percent of the patients receiving placebo. The self-perceived magnitude of the effect was rated as "enormously improved" by 29 percent of patients in the paroxetine group, but by none of the placebo-treated patients. In contrast, 55 percent of the patients in the placebo group reported "no change," as compared with 10 percent in the paroxetine group. Individual symptom reductions were significantly larger in the paroxetine group compared with the patients taking placebo: paroxetine-associated decreases in median severity values were tenfold for depressed mood, sevenfold for irritability, fivefold for breast tenderness, and fourfold for anxiety/tension and bloating.

Citolapram

Citolapram, the newest addition to the family of selective serotonin reuptake inhibitors available in the United States, has been tried in patients with premenstrual syndrome in a carefully designed study executed by investigators from Göteborg University, Göteborg, and Molndals Wardcentral, Molndal and Lund University, Lund, Sweden (Wikander et al., 1998). Subjects were recruited from among the 123 individuals who responded to a newspaper advertisement and who indicated in subsequent interviews that they fulfilled the standard diagnostic criteria (American Psychiatric Association, 1987). The cyclic nature of the symptoms was then prospectively confirmed in 78 women over a two-month period prior to the start of the three-month drug trial. The eligible subjects were randomly assigned to one of four groups: continuous treatment with the same dose of citolapram throughout the cycle (20 mg daily); low-dose citolapram (5 mg daily) during the follicular phase and a higher dose (20 mg daily) during the luteal phase; placebo during the follicular phase and citolapram (20 mg daily) during the luteal phase; or placebo throughout the cycle. A total of 58 patients were treated with one of the three citolapram regimes, and 20 subjects received placebo. Follow-up data was obtained by recording daily the severity of premenstrual symptoms on visual analog scales; at the end of the trial, the subjects were also asked to rate the global change in their condition.

Adverse effects requiring the discontinuation of the trial developed in five patients (9 percent) treated with citolapram. Two complained of headache and three patients remonstrated because of anxiety, tension, and sedation. Three of the patients (15 percent) treated with placebo dropped out because of tension, anxiety, and increased affective lability. Among the milder side effects recorded during the trial, the most common were decreased libido, dry mouth, and diaphoresis. The frequency of decreased libido varied from a high of 41 percent in the first follicular phase in the group treated continuously with citolapram to a low of 6 percent during the third cycle of treatment in the group receiving the citolapram therapy only during the luteal phase. The frequency of decreased libido during treatment with placebo fell from 12 percent in the first cycle to none in the third cycle of the trial.

Compared with placebo, the administration of citolapram during the luteal phase of patients with premenstrual syndrome significantly improved the overall severity of illness. The two continuous modalities of treatment, i.e., a fixed dose throughout the cycle or a low dose during the follicular phase, were not better than placebo in this trial. With regard to specific symptoms citolapram was demonstrably better than placebo only for irritability.

Chapter 20

Controversial Therapies

GONADOTROPIN-RELEASING HORMONE AGONISTS

Gonadotropin-releasing hormone (GnRH) agonists are synthetic products that prevent ovulation and other ovarian hormonal functions by suppressing the release of naturally occurring gonadotropins, an action termed "medical ovariectomy" (Muse et al., 1984). The interest in using GnRH agonists in premenstrual syndrome is actually an expansion of studies performed in the 1980s reporting the effectiveness of pharmacological suppression of the normal cyclical hormonal ovarian activities with estradiol implants (Magos, Brincat, and Studd, 1986) and danazol (Sarno, Miller, and Lundblad, 1987) on the clinical manifestations of premenstrual symptoms and the success of surgical ovariectomies in Canadian patients with severe and refractory presentations of the syndrome (Casson et al., 1990; Casper and Hearn, 1990).

The first trial of a GnRH agonist was conducted at the University of California, San Diego (Muse et al., 1984). The eight patients participating in the study had been selected from among 50 women with premenstrual syndrome to form a homogenous group of employed white women with unequivocal symptoms occurring only during the last two weeks of the cycle. None of the subjects were taking medications or had detectable organic illnesses, a history of suicide attempts, a history of drug or alcohol abuse, and none had been undergoing psychotherapy during the three months preceding the study. All participants were judged to be reliable enough to comply with the requirements of a complex trial.

The study compared the effect of subcutaneous injections of the GnRH agonist D-Trp9-Pro9-NEt (50 micrograms daily) with a normal saline placebo administered for 90 consecutive days each in a crossover, random-sequence, double-blind design. The baseline and outcome variables were 15 symptoms considered by the authors to be consistent and prominent features of the premenstrual syndrome, including five physical symptoms (breast tenderness, breast fullness, abdominal distention, headache, and fatigue) and 10 behavioral symptoms (depression, fearfulness, mood swings, inability to concentrate, nervousness, irritability, tendency toward violence, increased appetite, craving for sweets, and craving for salty foods). The subjects scored the symptoms each day on a four-point scale ranging from absent to severe. The principal measurement was the mean daily symptom score calculated for the luteal and follicular phases of the second and third cycle of the placebo and GnRH agonist treatment periods.

The placebo treatment did not appreciably change the cyclic pattern of the occurring symptoms, peak scores being recorded as expected late during the luteal phase. On the other hand, the GnRH agonist abolished the cyclicity of the symptoms and significantly decreased their severity, usually at levels comparable to the follicular phase, therapeutic actions indicating the disappearance of the premenstrual syndrome. The favorable effect was similar for both physical and behavioral symptoms.

The successful use of a GnRH agonist in this study was remarkable also for the absence of significant side effects and the rapid resumption of normal ovarian function upon cessation of treatment. However, the authors questioned the long-term utility of this therapeutic modality, given the documented decrease in estradiol levels and the subsequent risk of specific complications, such as early or accelerated osteoporosis.

Buserelin

The favorable effect of GnRH agonist treatment was confirmed in a study of intranasal buserelin, a drug not approved for use in the United States, conducted at the University Hospital of Umeå, Sweden, with support from the drug's manufacturer (Hammarback and Backstrom, 1988). The 26 patients participating in the trial had requested evaluation for "premenstrual tension" and had been qualified for inclusion on the basis of daily ratings of their symptoms over two menstrual cycles, which showed cyclical mood changes and specified increases in the severity of the rated symptoms during the nine premenstrual days as compared with the nine preovulatory days. A subgroup of 12 of the 26 subjects had symptoms only during the premenstrual period and were thus considered to have the "pure" form of the syndrome; the remaining 14 patients had symptoms during the follicular phase and constituted the "premenstrual aggravation" subgroup. The study design required the administration of either 400 micrograms of buserelin or placebo intranasally for 90 days, after which the patient crossed over to the alternative treatment. Patients rated on visual analog scales the severity of their symptoms every day for the entire six-month duration of the trial. Blinding was compromised in two patients who became amenorrheic during treatment with buserelin.

Three of the 26 patients (12 percent) were withdrawn from the study because of major side effects. In two cases, the adverse reaction consisted of the appearance of severe premenstrual-type symptoms within two weeks of starting treatment with the GnRH agonist; the reaction disappeared quickly after the discontinuation of the drug, but recurred after a subsequent buserelin challenge. The third patient was withdrawn because of menopausal symptoms induced by buserelin.

The administration of placebo and GnRH agonist produced significant improvement compared with the pretreatment cycle. The GnRH agonist was superior to placebo for all the symptoms recorded. Compared with placebo, the GnRH agonist improved markedly the overall well-being of 61 percent of patients; 13 percent of patients felt significantly worse and 26 percent reported no change. Among the individual symptoms, buserelin had its most favorable effect on depression, breast tenderness, and irritability. The effect of the GnRH agonist increased over time and correlated with the presence of anovulatory cycles. Symptom cyclicity, as recorded during the pretreatment evaluation, influenced the outcome, as shown by the buserelin-induced improvement of 75 percent of the patients with "pure" premenstrual syndrome, but of only 45 percent of the "premenstrual aggravation" subgroup.

Leuprolide

The efficacy of the GnRH agonist leuprolide was tested in a well-designed study performed by a multidisciplinary group at the University of Tennessee at Memphis (Brown et al., 1994). The drug is a synthetic nonapeptide formulated to replicate the structure of the porcine and ovine GnRH but with molecular substitutions that make it at least ten times more active than the naturally occurring substance (American Hospital Formulary Service, 1997, p. 807). In the study presented here, the subjects were 36 women diagnosed with premenstrual symptoms (American Psychiatric Association, 1987) after at least two months of prospective symptom ratings. Structured psychiatric interviews were used to establish the absence of a past or current history of bipolar or psychotic disorders, major depression, panic disorder, or acute suicidal ideation in the six months preceding the study. None of the subjects had uncontrolled medical disorders or clinically significant abnormalities on routine laboratory testing, were pregnant or breast-feeding, or were taking psychotropic medications or hormones.

After the baseline evaluation, the 36 subjects were enrolled in a one-month single-blind placebo trial. Five patients who responded to placebo were excluded from the study. The remaining 31 subjects were randomized to receive depot leuprolide (3.75 mg diluted in 0.5 ml solvent) or 0.5 ml normal saline intramuscularly for three consecutive cycles and then crossed over to the alternative treatment. The only additional intervention was the administration of calcium supplementation (1 g/day) to protect against bone demineralization. Outcome measures included scales assessing the severity of premenstrual symptoms, the presence and severity of depression, and the overall change in condition after the second and third cycle of leuprolide and placebo treatments.

Of the 31 patients enrolled in the double-blind trial, two withdrew because of intolerable side effects of insomnia, headaches, and nausea and four for reasons not related to treatment. The 25 subjects who completed the study had a mean age of 37 years and had premenstrual symptoms for an average of ten years. Most patients were white, well-educated, and employed on a full-time basis. At baseline, seven patients had no significant premenstrual depressive symptomatology, 11 were moderately depressed, and seven had severe depressive symptoms.

Depot leuprolide was significantly superior to placebo on all outcome measures. The symptoms showing the most substantial improvement were irritability, fatigue, breast tenderness, and neurologic symptoms. The effectiveness of leuprolide was inversely correlated with the severity of premenstrual depression, i.e., reporting "much" or "very much" improvement were five of the seven patients without premenstrual depression, six of 11 subjects with moderate depression, and two of the seven women with severe depressive symptomatology. Side effects were more frequent during the leuprolide than during the placebo treatment (13 percent versus 3 percent) and commonly included night sweats, hot flashes, headaches, and nausea. The overall incidence of leuprolide-specific side effects was directly correlated with the severity of premenstrual depression; women without it had an overall incidence of side effects of 9 percent (not different than placebo), while the incidence of side effects among the most severely depressed was 21 percent.

Partial improvement was reported in a study that sought to evaluate prospectively the effect of the GnRH agonist leuprolide in women with premenstrual syndrome with or without ongoing dysphoric symptoms throughout the menstrual cycle (Freeman, Sondheimer, and Rickels, 1997). The study started with 40 women who had requested treatment for premenstrual syndrome at the University of Pennsylvania Medical Center in Philadelphia and whose daily symptom reports confirmed the diagnosis. They were administered a single placebo intramuscular injection and were reevaluated after one month, at which time five patients withdrew for various reason and two had a significant placebo response. After randomization to double-blind treatment, three additional subjects dropped out without providing data. The 30 patients who completed the study were found to be in good physical health. With regard to psychiatric disorders, the inclusion criteria allowed the diagnoses of major depression or dysthymia, but no other psychiatric disorder. None of the patients were considered at significant risk of suicide or had a clearly identifiable personality disorder. The subjects were not pregnant or intending pregnancy, had no history of hysterectomy, and were required to stop all psychotropic or hormonal treatments.

Fifteen of the 30 patients formed the "pure" premenstrual syndrome subgroup, i.e., had symptom criteria consistent with the standard definition of the late luteal phase dysphoric disorder (American Psychiatric Association, 1987) and no detectable dysphoric symptoms during the postmenstrual phase. The remaining 15 patients formed the "premenstrual exacerbation" subgroup, i.e., had ongoing dysphoric symptoms in the postmenstrual phase. Six patients with "premenstrual exacerbation" met criteria for current major depression and one patient was given the diagnosis of dysthymia. The mean age of the total sample (n = 30) was 37 years, and the average duration of the premenstrual syndrome was 14 years. Structured psychiatric interviews demonstrated past psychiatric disorders in 73 percent of patients. Except for past family psychiatric history, which was significantly more common among patients with "premenstrual exacerbation" compared to those with "pure" premenstrual syndrome (93 percent versus 56 percent), the two subgroups were similar with regard to all background variables.

The study design required random assignment to three monthly intramuscular injections of depot leuprolide (3.75 mg) or placebo; the procedure resulted in 21 patients receiving the GnRH agonist and nine patients receiving placebo. The outcome measures were the patient-rated daily symptom scores and the clinician-rated premenstrual depression scores.

A majority of patients reported side effects and one-third of study participants discontinued the trial. Eighteen of the 21 patients (86 percent) treated with leuprolide but only three of the nine patients (33 percent) receiving placebo experienced hot flashes, a significant difference. Three patients (14 percent) given leuprolide but none of those given placebo reported increased premenstrual symptoms. Other side effects of leuprolide reported with some frequency in the double-blind treatment included joint pains (24 percent), headache (24 percent), and vaginal dryness/irritation (19 percent). Overall, all patients treated with leuprolide but only 55 percent of placebo-treated subjects had at least one reportable adverse reaction to treatment, a significant difference. Eight patients from the "pure" premenstrual syndrome subgroup discontinued the trial; all of them were receiving leuprolide. In contrast, only three patients from the "premenstrual exacerbation" subgroup withdrew from the study; two were receiving placebo and one leuprolide.

Leuprolide treatment was superior to placebo only with regard to mood symptoms in the "pure" premenstrual syndrome subgroup. A favorable trend was noted also for physical symptoms in the same subgroup, but the difference did not reach statistical significance. By the end of the third cycle of treatment, only three of the 17 daily rated symptoms were unequivocally improved in the leuprolide-treated patients with the pure variant of the syndrome, i.e., anxiety, depression, and feeling out of control. Clinician-rated depression scores were more robustly changed, as indicated by the fact that treatment with leuprolide abolished premenstrual dysphoria in the "pure" subgroup, whereas the placebo-treated patients and those with "premenstrual exacerbation" remained at baseline dysphoric levels. Global improvement in the "pure" premenstrual syndrome, based on at least 50 percent reduction in symptoms, was reported for 67 percent of subjects treated with leuprolide and 17 percent of patients treated with placebo. Leuprolide treatment improved only 8 percent of the patients from the "premenstrual exacerbation" sub-group. These results, however, must be interpreted with caution for two important reasons. First, as mentioned, only slightly over half of the patients assigned to treatment with the GnRH agonist completed the treatment. Second, all leuprolide-treated patients were amenor-rheic by the second cycle of treatment and therefore potentially unblinded with regard to the type of treatment they had been given.

Important data regarding the efficacy of ovarian suppression were provided in a complex and only partially double-blind study of differential behavior effects of gonadal steroids in women with and without premenstrual syndrome (Schmidt et al., 1998). The 20 women enrolled in the study were referred or self-referred for evaluation and treatment of premenstrual syndrome at the National Institute of Mental Health, Bethesda, Maryland. Careful screening ensured that none of the subjects had current medical illnesses or had ever had a psychiatric disorder. All had a normal physical examination and all were confirmed to meet criteria for the diagnosis of premenstrual syndrome (American Psychiatric Association, 1994) on the basis of daily ratings of their symptoms over a period of three months.

The study design required the double-blinded random assignment to either the GnRH agonist leuprolide acetate (3.75 mg monthly by intramuscular injection) or placebo (injections of normal saline). The women who continued to have normal menstrual cycles and did not experience hot flashes were considered to be in the placebo group and the code was broken after two treatment cycles. They were then treated with leuprolide acetate in an open-label manner for an additional three months. Main measurements included daily ratings of the severity of common symptoms of premenstrual syndrome and a global assessment of well-being, and monthly standard questionnaires for assessing depression and anxiety.

Two of the 20 participants withdrew from the study. Compared with baseline symptomatology, the treatment with placebo had no significant effect. In contrast, some symptom scores improved after treatment with leuprolide by the end of the first cycle of treatment, i.e., impaired function, irritability, food cravings, sadness, and anxiety. A favorable trend was also noted for breast pain and bloating, but the differences did not reach statistical significance. With leuprolide treatment there was no difference in severity between the symptoms recorded in the second week and the fourth week of the cycle, indicating the elimination of the cyclicity characteristic of the premenstrual syndrome. However, by global impression of patients and clinicians, only six of the ten patients who had received leuprolide under double-blind conditions and only four of the eight treated under open label were considered to have responded to GnRH agonist therapy.

In contrast with studies indicating various degrees of effectiveness of GnRH agonists in the treatment of premenstrual syndrome stand negative findings published by researchers from the Division of Reproductive Endocrinology, University of South Alabama, Mobile (Helvacioglu et al., 1993). Thirty-two women were recruited through an advertisement in the local newspaper. The diagnosis of premenstrual syndrome was established in 17 of them after the completion of validated symptom questionnaires and diaries over two menstrual cycles. The women were included in the trial if their symptoms were severe and if they had no history of psychiatric illness and were otherwise in good health. None of the patients were taking hormonal or psychotropic medications. Although no patient had a history of addiction to drugs or alcohol, seven subjects (41 percent) had a family history of substance use disorder.

The design of the trial required double-blind, crossover treatment with depot leuprolide (7.5 mg) or normal saline placebo, administered by injection at 30-day intervals; two injections of each agent were given over the six-month study period. Symptom diaries were collected at biweekly intervals and a "follicular" and a "luteal" score calculated for the baseline, placebo, and leuprolide phases of the trial. The outcome was assessed by subtracting the scores computed for the cycles during which the subjects received placebo and leuprolide from the baseline scores.

Of the 17 subjects who entered the trial, five patients dropped out because they felt that the treatment was ineffective. The decision to withdraw was made after placebo-only treatment by three patients and after leuprolide-only treatment by two subjects. With the exception of amenorrhea, the reported side effects were mild. Both leuprolide and placebo treatments produced significant improvement in the luteal-phase scores as compared with the pretreatment phase of the study.

Goserelin

West and Hillier (1994) studied the effect of the GnRH agonist goserelin, a drug available in the United States, in a trial conducted at the Centre for Reproductive Biology, University of Edinburgh, with support from the product's manufacturer. The 32 participants had been referred by their primary care physician for evaluation of cyclical mood changes of at least two years' duration and had the diagnosis of premenstrual syndrome established on the basis of a two-month record of daily symptoms. Prior to inclusion in the study, all women had regular menstrual cycles. The main measurements during the trial were the presence and severity of depression, anxiety, irritability, tension, menstrual bleeding, breast discomfort, and swelling as recorded daily by the subjects and a nurse-administered monthly questionnaire for symptoms of anxiety and depression.

The 32 subjects were randomly assigned to receive three doses of 3.6 mg of goserelin (incorporated in a biodegradable rod) or placebo administered at four-week intervals via subcutaneous injection from identical-looking syringes. Four of the 16 patients treated with placebo were withdrawn from the study after the second injection because of generalized rashes (two patients), new onset of panic attacks (one patient), and newly diagnosed breast mass (one patient). Of the goserelin-treated patients, one withdrew prior to the completion of the trial after developing a severe exacerbation of preexistent urticarial dermatitis. Another patient treated with goserclin failed to provide the research data. Therefore, the analysis of the three cycles of treatment and the three-month follow-up was based on information from 14 patients treated with the GnRH agonist and 12 treated with placebo.

All 14 goserelin-treated patients stopped menstruating after the first injection and 11 of them had an episode of vaginal bleeding a median of two weeks after the onset of treatment, a side effect with potential for unblinding the study. Analysis of patients' records indicated that, compared with placebo, GnRH agonist therapy had a clear-cut favorable effect with regard to breast discomfort, swelling, and irritability. Symptoms of anxiety and depression lost their cyclicity during GnRH therapy, but the decrease in severity did not reach statistical significance.

ALPRAZOLAM

Alprazolam, a high-potency triazolobenzodiazepine, has been tried in patients with premenstrual syndrome in a number of methodologically valid studies, allowing an evidence-based assessment of the drug's efficacy. The interest in the agent is justified by the fact that it improves neurotransmissions mediated by gamma-aminobutyric acid, a substance found to be deficient in the late luteal phase of women with premenstrual dysphoric disorder (Halbreich et al., 1996).

The effectiveness of alprazolam in patients with premenstrual syndrome was first tested by researchers from the Brigham and Women's Hospital, Harvard Medical School, Boston, with partial support from the drug's manufacturer (Smith et al., 1987). The study group included 19 patients with luteal phase symptoms serious enough to disrupt work and social functioning. The patients were selected from among a thirty-member inception cohort on the basis of high scores on the Premenstrual Tension Self-Rating Scale, an instrument devised for the assessment of the severity of the syndrome (Steiner, Haskett, and Carroll, 1980). All subjects had regular menses and used only nonhormonal contraceptive methods. Screening procedures ensured that none of the subjects had significant medical or gynecologic pathology, and past or current psychiatric disorders including drug and alcohol abuse.

The study was very well designed; after one month of baseline observation and documentation of symptoms, the patients entered the four-cycle randomized, placebo-controlled, multiple crossover trial of alprazolam (0.25 mg three times daily) or identical-looking placebo tablets. Treatment was administered from cycle day 20 until the second day of menstruation, after which it was rapidly tapered and discontinued. The patients were allowed to decrease their dose from three to two tablets each day if daytime sedation occurred. Data collected during the five-month trial were extracted from diaries recording the presence and severity of 22 symptoms classified as physical (headache, weight gain, edema, abdominal distention, abdominal cramping, breast tenderness, back pain, and generalized aches), depression-related (depression, tiredness, forgetfulness, confusion, insomnia, increased appetite, and craving for sweets), and anxiety-related (anxiety, nervous tension, irritability, mood swings, dizziness, and palpitations).

The trial was completed by 14 of the 19 original participants. The withdrawals were due to anxiety disorders discovered during the baseline period (two patients), insufficient severity of luteal phase symptomatology (one patient), and personal decision to discontinue participation (two patients). The mean age of the subjects who completed the study was 33 years; nine of the 14 were married and eight had children. The symptom scores during the follicular phase were low during all of the five monthly cycles and significantly lower than the corresponding luteal scores during the baseline cycle.

Treatment with alprazolam was associated with significant symptomatic improvement. Compared with the untreated, baseline cycle as well as with the two placebo-treated cycles, a clear favorable change was noted for the symptoms of abdominal distention and cramping, headaches, craving for sweets, mood swings, crying spells, forgetfulness, fatigue, depression, anxiety, irritability, and nervous tension. The premenstrual symptoms were not influenced by placebo, although partial responses were recorded for forgetfulness and nervous tension. The treatment produced no significant adverse effects and alprazolam-induced daytime sedation was noted in only two cases and resolved after dose reduction.

Alprazolam was also found to be superior to placebo for the treatment of premenstrual symptoms in a study performed at the

New York Psychiatric Institute by faculty members from the College of Physicians and Surgeons, Columbia University, with support from the drug's manufacturer (Harrison, Endicott, and Nee, 1990). The 130 patients recruited for the trial had clear-cut symptoms of anxiety, depression, and irritability persisting for more than five days prior to menses as documented on daily rating forms for two consecutive menstrual cycles; at least moderate decrease in occupational or social functioning premenstrually; no current physical illness; and no history of suicide attempt or psychiatric hospitalization in the previous two years. The study candidates were further evaluated and 65 were considered ineligible because of concurrent medical illness (five patients), current depressive disorder (20 patients), current substance abuse (six patients), current other psychiatric disorder (nine patients), mild severity of premenstrual symptoms (six patients), current use of hormone therapy (two patients), unwillingness to take a benzodiazepine (ten patients), and inability to comply with the study's requirements (seven patients).

The 65 remaining patients entered a single-blind placebo trial for one menstrual cycle. The subjects who reported themselves to be much improved were treated for another month with placebo and those who continued to respond were removed from the study (nine patients). In addition, four patients withdrew from the trial at this stage. The 52 continuing subjects were randomly assigned to receive alprazolam (0.25 mg/tablet) or placebo tablets for three cycles and then crossed over to take the alternate therapy for three more cycles. The subjects were instructed to start taking medications at the onset of symptoms in the luteal phase, to begin treatment with three tablets daily, and to increase the dose as needed or until they developed side effects. The maximum permitted dose was 16 tablets each day (4 mg alprazolam). After the start of each menstruation, the treatment was carefully tapered off to avoid withdrawal symptoms (a reduction of 25 percent in dose each day if the daily dose was less than 12 tablets and one tablet each day for daily doses of 12 or more tablets). Of the patients in the "placebo first" phase of the study, seven dropped out because of lack of effect and two because of intolerable side effects. Six patients in the "alprazolam first" phase withdrew because of side effects. Three patients declined to complete the study and four patients failed to complete required data forms.

Thirty subjects finished at least two cycles with each treatment. Their mean age was 34 years and the average duration of their illness was eight years. The majority of patients were white, well educated, and employed outside the home. Most patients reported substantial pretreatment depression (80 percent of the group), irritability (67 percent), and anxiety (47 percent). At least one episode of major depression had been diagnosed in 22 of the 30 patients, but only four patients had a history of anxiety disorders. Family histories indicated depression in at least one parent in 12 patients and in a sibling in eight of the 30 patients. Social functioning was marred in 93 percent and vocational functioning was impaired in 59 percent of patients.

The average daily dose of alprazolam was 2.25 mg. The side effects of alprazolam were drowsiness (mild in 40 percent of patients, moderate to severe in 17 percent of patients) and headache (10 percent). Four patients (13 percent) developed mildly increased anxiety during the alprazolam taper, but none of them had any other significant withdrawal symptoms. Compared with placebo, alprazolam therapy improved the clinical global impression scored by the investigators with regard to severity of illness, side effects, and level of functional impairment. The patients' daily recordings demonstrated that alprazolam was significantly better than placebo in reducing symptoms of dysphoria and loss of pleasure, social withdrawal, fatigue, anxiety, impulsivity, and lability. The effect of treatment was not better than placebo for the physical symptoms of the syndrome and for hostility, anger, and atypical depressive features.

The confirmation of alprazolam's efficacy was attempted in a trial conducted at the Montreal General Hospital by investigators from McGill University and Concordia University, Montreal, Quebec, with support from the Canadian subsidiary of the drug's manufacturer (Berger and Presser, 1994). The 48 subjects entered in the study had regular menstrual cycles, no current psychiatric disorder, and were off all psychotropic and hormonal treatments. The patients were randomly assigned to receive placebo or alprazolam for three consecutive cycles and then were crossed over to the alternative treatment, which was given for another three cycles. Alprazolam was dispensed as 0.25 mg tablets. Patients started the treatment with one tablet twice a day and were instructed to increase the dose up to a total of 12 tablets daily until their premenstrual symptoms improved without significant side effects. Postmenstrual cessation of treatment was gradual to avoid withdrawal symptoms.

Thirty-one of the 48 original participants completed all of the study's requirements. Among those who completed the trial, the authors identified 17 patients who had been found on baseline testing to have dysphoric or anxiety symptoms only during the luteal phase. This group was similar with respect to occupational status, educational level, marital status, age, and age at onset of the premenstrual syndrome to the 14 patients who in addition to luteal symptoms also had dysphoric or anxiety symptoms during the follicular phase. Treatment with alprazolam (0.25 mg three times daily) was clearly superior to placebo and produced significant improvement in the severity of premenstrual irritability, anxiety, feelings of tension, and the feeling of being out of control in the group of 17 patients whose symptomatology was restricted to the luteal phase. Side effects were few and dose-related; sedation was reported by four patients (24 percent) during the alprazolam phase and by two patients during the placebo phase of the study. The gradual tapering at menses required an average of three days and resulted in minimal symptoms of anxiety. In contrast, among patients with symptoms of anxiety and depression throughout their menstrual cycles, higher average daily doses of alprazolam (1.25 mg) did not reduce premenstrual symptoms.

Additional data regarding the action of alprazolam on premenstrual symptoms resulted from a large-scale trial conducted by investigators from the Departments of Obstetrics and Gynecology and Psychiatry, University of Pennsylvania, Philadelphia (Freeman et al., 1995). The study included a trial of oral progesterone that will be presented separately in this monograph.

Recruitment of subjects started with a pool of 444 women who had requested treatment for premenstrual syndrome. The patients were required to maintain daily symptom reports and underwent evaluations at premenstrual and postmenstrual times. The 284 patients who fulfilled the diagnostic criteria for premenstrual syndrome (American Psychiatric Association, 1994), had experienced the syndrome for at least six months and reported moderate to severe functional impairment, and had regular menstrual cycles with no evidence of serious health problems, including current major psychiatric disorders, were entered into a single-blind placebo trial for one cycle.

During this cycle, 56 women (20 percent) experienced a response strong enough so that they no longer fulfilled the study's symptom criteria. In addition, 43 women dropped out of the study, leaving 185 participants for the double-blind therapeutic trial.

A randomization procedure assigned 56 patients to receive alprazolam and 55 patients to receive placebo premenstrually for three consecutive cycles. Treatment was administered as identical capsules containing placebo or 0.25 mg alprazolam from day 18 of the menstrual cycle to the first day of menses, followed by a two-day taper. The initial dose was one capsule four times daily, but the dosing schedule was flexible, with gradual increases allowed to a maximum of 12 capsules daily. The outcome measures were global severity ratings provided by patients and clinicians and the scores assigned to the clusters of mood symptoms (irritability, depression, mood swings, anxiety, nervous tension, crying, and feeling out of control), mental function (fatigue, poor coordination, confusion, and insomnia), pain symptoms (headache, cramps, and aches), physical symptoms (breast tenderness and swelling), and food craving on the patients' daily symptom reports.

Placebo and alprazolam-treated patients were well matched with regard to age (average 34 years), duration of premenstrual syndrome (average ten years), and baseline premenstrual symptom scores and all of the other demographic and clinical variables. Previous history of major depression was identified in 36 percent of patients assigned to receive alprazolam and 38 percent of those assigned to the placebo arm of the trial. A family history of mental illness was present in 64 percent of patients who took alprazolam and 60 percent of the placebo-treated subjects.

Alprazolam was considered superior to placebo after three months of treatment on account of the significant differences noted for the physical and pain symptoms. A moderate improvement was reported for mental function, mood symptoms, and for the patient-rated global severity scores. However, using the stringent criterion of a 50 percent change in the daily symptom ratings, improvement was confirmed in 37 percent of the alprazolam-treated patients, but also in 30 percent of the patients given placebo. Side effects were reported by 79 percent of patients receiving alprazolam and 55 percent of those receiving placebo. Seven percent of patients invoked side effects as the reason for dropping out of the study. The most common side effects were fatigue and sedation, which were experienced by 59 percent of patients receiving alprazolam and 25 percent of placebo-treated patients, a statistically significant difference; breast tenderness, swelling, and bloating (18 percent versus 15 percent); and insomnia (9 percent versus 4 percent). Thirteen percent of patients developed mild and transient symptoms of insomnia, anxiety, and depression associated with the postmenstrual alprazolam taper.

Negative results of alprazolam therapy in premenstrual syndrome have also been reported (Schmidt, Grover, and Rubinow, 1993). The setting of the study was an outpatient clinic staffed by researchers from the Biological Psychiatry Branch at the National Institute of Mental Health, Bethesda, Maryland, and the subjects 22 women (mean age 38 years) with premenstrual symptoms who met diagnostic criteria for late luteal phase dysphoric disorder (American Psychiatric Association, 1987). Clinical evaluations and structured psychiatric interviews established the absence of current mental and physical disorders. Five patients had a history of anxiety disorder, which was specified as panic disorder in one case; five patients had a history of mood disorder. All participants had negative mood symptoms (depression, anxiety, and irritability) that were at least 30 percent more severe during the week before menses than during the first postmenstrual week, and none of the women had notable mood symptoms during the follicular phase of the cycle.

The participants were randomly assigned to receive tablets containing placebo or alprazolam (0.25 mg per tablet) for four consecutive cycles. The starting dose was one tablet three times daily, administered on day 16 of the cycle and continued to the onset of menses, after which the drug was tapered off over the next three days. For the second cycle, the dose was increase to 0.5 mg alprazolam or two placebo tablets three times daily, and in the third cycle the subjects received 0.75 mg alprazolam or three placebo tablets three times daily. The last dose was continued in the fourth cycle, and the trial ended with a one-week taper of the study drug. Baseline and outcome measures included daily ratings of mood and physical symptoms and bimonthly standardized questionnaires assessing the presence and severity of depression, anxiety, and premenstrual tension.

Only 20 women completed the trial; one subject withdrew for personal reasons and one because of excessive sedation. Ten subjects could not tolerate alprazolam doses greater than 0.25 mg three times daily. Seven subjects were able to advance their regimen to the full alprazolam dose of 0.75 mg three times daily. The side effect of sedation required dosage decreases in nine women while receiving alprazolam and five women while on placebo. Postmenstrual withdrawal symptoms (headache, irritability, and restlessness) were mild and similarly frequent after alprazolam and placebo.

Compared with baseline ratings, a favorable trend was observed for the severity of premenstrual depression treated with both placebo and alprazolam, with the latter being statistically superior as measured by changes in a standardized depression inventory. For symptoms of anxiety, the improvement over baseline reached statistical significance only during treatment with placebo. The two treatments were not different with regard to impaired functional status, cravings, mood swings, irritability, and physical symptoms.

The disappointing conclusions reached in the previous study have been recently confirmed by an elegant experimental study performed at the New York State Psychiatric Institute, an affiliate of the College of Physicians and Surgeons of Columbia University, New York (Evans et al., 1998). Using double-blind conditions, the investigators tested the effect of acute administration of alprazolam during the follicular and luteal phases of 20 women with premenstrual syndrome. Care was taken to exclude subjects who had a mood, anxiety, or substance use disorder within the year prior to the study. On study days, patients completed the assessment battery before taking placebo or alprazolam at dosages that varied from 0.25 to 0.75 mg. Measurements were then repeated five times at hourly intervals. The acute administration of alprazolam did not improve the negative premenstrual mood changes or the impaired task performance. These results were explained by the increased severity of fatigue and confusion produced by this benzodiazepine.

BROMOCRIPTINE

Bromocriptine (2-bromo-α-ergocryptine), a semisynthetic ergot alkaloid, inhibits the release of prolactin from the anterior pituitary gland, most likely by stimulating the postsynaptic dopamine receptors of the hypothalamus, and is also considered able to enhance the hypothalamic production of the luteinizing hormone-releasing factor and thereby initiate menses; to act directly on the ovarian dopaminergic receptors that contribute to ovulation; and to increase renal sodium excretion (American Hospital Formulary Service, 1997, p. 2850). These properties have led to the testing of bromocriptine in patients with premenstrual syndrome by Andersen et al. (1977), but the outcome of their trial was quite disappointing, because it indicated that the agent was not better than placebo for any of the main clinical manifestations of the syndrome except breast tenderness. Yet despite this modest accomplishment, the effort to identify a therapeutic role for bromocriptine in premenstrual syndrome has continued for more than a decade (Ylostalo et al., 1981; Andersch and Hahn, 1982; Meden-Vrtovec and Vujic, 1992).

In the first of these trials, researchers from the University of Oulu, Oulu, Finland, supported by a grant from the drug's manufacturer, designed a parallel placebo-controlled clinical study of bromocriptine and norethisterone (Ylostalo et al., 1981). To retain the homogeneity of this presentation, only the bromocriptine portion of the trial, which involved 17 patients, will be reported here. To qualify for entry into the study, the subjects had to have a history of recurrent premenstrual distress due to at least two moderate or severe symptoms, the most common of which were breast engorgement, edema, irritability, and depression. The trial consisted of single-blind administration of placebo, starting on the twelfth day of the first and fourth cycles treated and continuing until the onset of menses. During the third and fourth cycles the subjects were treated with 2.5 mg of bromocriptine daily from the twelfth through the fourteenth day of the cycle and 5 mg daily from the fifteenth day until menstruation. This phase of the trial was considered double-blinded as the investigators did not know whether the subject was taking bromocriptine or norethisterone. Outcome data were collected on the first day of each menstruation on 24-item self-evaluation forms that recorded the symptoms present during the preceding cycles. A face-to-face interview with the investigators took place at the end of each cycle and aimed at ensuring accurate recording of the clinical data relevant to the premenstrual syndrome and direct evaluation of the four main symptoms of premenstrual distress, i.e., depression, irritability, breast engorgement, and edema. The list of symptoms included all of the standard manifestations of premenstrual syndrome (American Psychiatric Association, 1994) but also symptoms suggestive of adverse drug effects such as nausea, vomiting, urinary frequency, dryness of the mouth, increased salivation, tachycardia, numbness of the hands, and muscle cramps.

Six of the 17 patients (35 percent) entered into the bromocriptine trial reported at least one adverse drug reaction, and three of these subjects (18 percent) dropped out of the study. These side effects included nausea (four patients or 24 percent of the sample), vomiting (24 percent), weakness (18 percent), visual field defects (6 percent), and recurrence of paroxysmal tachycardia (6 percent). No side effects were reported during the placebo-treated cycles.

Bromocriptine was found to be more effective than placebo in alleviating premenstrual irritability and breast engorgement but not the severity of depression and edema. Data generated by patients' self-assessment were interpreted to indicate a therapeutic effect with regard to depression, sleep disturbance, and breast tenderness, but the level of statistical significance of the differences was not adjusted to reflect multiple comparisons with the response to placebo. Overall, 11 patients (65 percent) considered bromocriptine more effective than placebo. There was no correlation between the response to treatment with bromocriptine and the prolactin levels measured during the follicular and luteal phases of the cycles included in the trial.

The second of these investigations was carried out at the East Hospital, Götenborg, Sweden (Andersch and Hahn, 1982). The authors recruited 40 subjects with premenstrual syndrome, defined as a combination of "mental" symptoms and swelling that occurred cyclically in the luteal phase and were judged severe enough to require medical intervention. The subjects were otherwise healthy, had regular menstrual cycles, and were not taking any medications or hormonal contraceptive agents. After a baseline observation cycle the patients entered the four-cycle therapeutic trial, during which they received bromocriptine (2.5 mg daily) for three cycles and placebo for one cycle. The medication was started at the onset of premenstrual symptomatology and continued until the onset of menstrual bleeding. Outcome data were self-collected and included ratings of the premenstrual symptoms and of the severity of swelling in the face, breasts, abdomen, and fingers. In addition, the levels of prolactin were measured during the premenstrual phase of the five cycles studied.

Five patients (12.5 percent) developed nausea during treatment with bromocriptine and withdrew from the trial. Among the remaining 35 patients bromocriptine was no better than placebo with regard to six of the seven main features of premenstrual syndrome assessed in this study, i.e., abdominal, facial, and breast swelling; anxiety; irritability; and sadness. Treatment with placebo led to greater improvement in the premenstrual edema of upper and lower extremities as compared with therapy with bromocriptine. As expected, the administration of bromocriptine led to significant decreases in prolactin levels, but the magnitude of this effect and the baseline prolactin concentrations did not affect the therapeutic outcome of bromocriptine.

A more recent attempt to clarify the potential therapeutic role of bromocriptine in premenstrual syndrome was carried out at the University Hospital Center, Ljubljana, Slovenia, with direct involvement of the drug's manufacturer (Meden-Vrtovec and Vujic, 1992). The study cohort comprised 21 patients who had moderate or severe premenstrual symptoms; regular cycles; normal or high baseline prolactin levels; and no evidence of gynecologic or psychiatric disorders. After confirmation of eligibility the subjects were observed off medications for one cycle and then assigned to receive bromocriptine (2.5 mg) or placebo twice daily from the tenth day of the cycle until the start of menstruation. This treatment phase comprised two consecutive cycles, after which the patients crossed over to treatment with the alternate agent. Baseline and outcome data were obtained by continuous self-assessments of six symptoms (depression, irritability, anger, headache, abdominal distention, and breast tenderness). Global assessments and an evaluation of the severity of psychological (e.g., depression, apathy, pessimism, diminished libido), general (e.g., fatigue, pain, weight gain), and local (e.g., headache, diplopia, mastodynia, abdominal distention, edema) somatic symptoms were performed by the physician investigators.

One of the 21 patients (5 percent) enrolled in the study developed severe hypotension during bromocriptine therapy and was withdrawn from the trial. Five subjects dropped out due to pregnancy, poor compliance, or other causes not related to adverse effects of the treatment.

According to the assessments made by the investigators, therapy with bromocriptine was not better than placebo for any of the main psychological manifestations of premenstrual syndrome. With the exception of mild improvement of edema, the efficacy of bromocriptine was equally disappointing with regard to general or localized somatic symptoms because, with the exception of edema, none of these complaints improved significantly more than during treatment with placebo. These data were confirmed by the analysis of self-assessed severity of symptoms, which indicated no difference between the effects of bromocriptine and placebo.

DANAZOL

Danazol is a synthetic derivative of ethinyl testosterone that inhibits the production, metabolic clearance, and activity of several sex hormones by a decrease in steroidogenesis and competitive binding to progesterone and androgen receptors; it has no specific antigonadotropic effect in normal women (Barbieri and Ryan, 1981). The agent's variable effect on premenstrual symptoms is attributed to the elimination of hormonal cyclicity and is considered dependent on achieving anovulatory cycles (Halbreich, Rojansky, and Palter, 1991).

The first controlled trial of danazol for premenstrual syndrome was designed and conducted by researchers from the Fitzsimmons Army Medical Center, Denver, Colorado (Sarno, Miller, and Lundblad, 1987). Candidates (n = 30) for participation in the study were referred to one of the investigators by professionals delivering care in the outpatient gynecology unit of this military facility. Eligibility for the trial required symptoms consistent with premenstrual syndrome, authenticated by prospective diaries kept for at least one full cycle. A severity gradient between the follicular and luteal phases of the cycle was specified and measured for all of the 19 symptoms graded, a procedure that excluded patients with moderate or severe symptoms during the follicular phase. None of the participants had a currently active psychiatric disorder or history of suicide attempts or illicit drug use; chronic physical disorders; and history of gynecological disorders or surgery of the reproductive tract. Only women who were not pregnant and were not using hormonal contraception were included in the final study group. A total of 17 patients fulfilled these requirements and were assigned to receive danazol (200 mg) or placebo (mixture of cornstarch, lactose, talc, and magnesium stearate) once daily for two consecutive cycles, after which they crossed over to the alternate treatment. Symptom diaries were kept throughout the study and the variable duration of the symptomatic phase standardized according to an acceptable mathematical maneuver relying on the scores recorded for the last three days of the cycle.

Three of the 17 patients dropped out of the trial for personal reasons. No side effects were reported and cycle length, menstrual flow, and serum levels of estradiol and gonadotropins were not affected by either danazol or placebo therapy. Danazol was no better than placebo for any of the 19 individual symptoms measured during the trial. However, global severity scores were lower after treatment with danazol as compared to the placebo phase of the crossover trial in 11 of the 14 subjects (79 percent).

The danazol therapy was next studied at the Birmingham and Midland Hospital for Women, Birmingham, United Kingdom, by a team of investigators who had received financial support from the drug's manufacturer (Watts, Butt, and Edwards, 1987). A total of 40 women were recruited for the trial; the diagnosis of premenstrual syndrome was established by examining the presence and severity of 13 symptoms (breast pain, abdominal distention, swollen fingers, headache, increased appetite, increased thirst, clumsiness, tearfulness, aggression, irritability, lethargy, depression, and anxiety) recorded daily during two successive cycles. The trial was not open to subjects who were pregnant nor to those with any chronic physical disorders or history of alcohol or drug abuse. The study design required random assignment for treatment with one of three dosages of danazol (100 mg, 200 mg, or 400 mg) or placebo daily for three months. The double-blind was ensured by having all patients take two identical-looking capsules twice each day (e.g., the patient assigned to treatment with danazol 100 mg took one danazol capsule and three placebo capsules). The four treatment groups were well matched with regard to age and duration of menstrual cycle. Outcome assessments relied on the comparison between the baseline severity of premenstrual symptoms and that recorded for each of the three months of the trial; symptoms were considered "improved" if the treatment had been associated with a greater than 50 percent decrease in severity.

Eight of the 30 patients (27 percent) assigned to receive danazol withdrew from the trial because of adverse effects, which consisted of nausea (three patients), rash (two patients), drowsiness (two patients), and musculoskeletal pain (one patient). Four additional patients taking danazol dropped out because of lack of improvement. Of interest is the fact that patients who discontinued danazol therapy on account of adverse effects or for want of a positive effect had significantly more severe baseline symptoms than those who completed the trial. One patient treated with placebo dropped out due to lack of improvement.

Treatment with danazol was better than placebo only for four of the 13 symptoms whose severity was scored during the trial, i.e., breast pain, irritability, anxiety, and lethargy. An analysis of the median scores recorded in the premenstrual week of the third month of treatment indicated improvement only for breast pain and irritability. The effect did not seem dose-related, as the end-of-trial severity of anxiety and lethargy improved only among the patients treated with the lowest dose of danazol. Breast pain improved significantly with all three dosages of danazol.

The small-scale investigations continued four years later with a trial conducted by gynecologists working at Stobhill General Hospital, Glasgow, United Kingdom (Deeny, Hawthorn, and Hart, 1991). Participants were recruited from among women receiving care through the hospital's premenstrual syndrome clinic. The diagnosis was confirmed prospectively over a two-month baseline period during which patients kept diaries recording the characteristics of 11 symptoms commonly described for this syndrome. Eligibility for the trial required premenstrual symptomatic worsening leading to impairment in social functioning and significant improvement soon after the onset of menses; weight between 45 and 80 kg;

absence of significant medical pathology; and no hormonal or anti-coagulant treatment of any kind within three months of the trial. The 37 patients selected for the study were assigned to receive danazol (100 mg) or placebo twice daily for three cycles and then were crossed over to the alternate treatment. The order of the treatment sequence was established in a random manner; the danazol-first and placebo-first groups were well matched with respect to age and age at menarche, length of menstrual cycle and bleeding, and number of pregnancies. Symptom diaries were kept all through the trial, and an assessment of the overall condition was made after each treatment.

Four of the 37 patients withdrew without explanation. Therapy with danazol was associated with 29 reported side effects in 21 of the 33 patients (64 percent) treated and led to the discontinuation of the drug in four patients (12 percent), who developed weight gain (two subjects), irregular bleeding (one patient), and psychosexual problems (one patient). Overall, change in menstrual pattern (28 percent), nausea (18 percent), and acne (15 percent) were the adverse effects reported by more than two subjects each; other drug-related events included headache, abdominal distention, exacerbation of duodenal ulcer, flushing, and edema. Because of danazol-related withdrawals, only 31 patients received the course of treatment with placebo; 11 patients (33 percent) reported side effects that included altered menses (10 percent) and nausea (6 percent).

Treatment was followed by symptomatic improvement in 89 percent of patients who completed three months of danazol therapy. In contrast, treatment with placebo led to improvement in only 22 percent of the patients, a statistically significant difference. These overall assessments are supported by the severity scores given each of the 11 symptoms during the last cycle of treatment, which indicated a superior effect of danazol for breast discomfort, abdominal distention, irritability, anxiety, depression, mood swings, and depressed libido. For the symptoms of premenstrual headaches, fluid retention, increased appetite, and crying spells the effect of danazol and placebo were statistically identical.

The investigative effort continued with a study conducted at Queen's University, Kingston, Ontario (Hahn, Van Vugt, and Reid, 1995). Supported by the drug's manufacturer, researchers attempted to test the effectiveness of a relatively high dose of danazol (400 mg daily) and to determine whether the intervention would be accompanied by a high dropout rate due to iatrogenic symptoms or amenorrhea. The subjects were recruited from among referrals to a reproductive endocrinology unit. The diagnosis was prospectively confirmed by data collected over two cycles and by clinical evaluation seeking to confirm that the potential participants were otherwise free of another physical or psychiatric disorder. Of the 53 subjects screened, 31 met inclusion criteria and were randomly assigned to receive danazol (200 mg) or placebo twice daily for three cycles. This phase was followed by three cycles of treatment with the alternate therapy. Data were collected by patients every third day throughout the trial with instruments assessing the core symptoms of premenstrual syndrome, the clinical manifestations of depression, and the impact of the illness on interpersonal relationships and work performance.

Only 11 of the 16 patients assigned to start the trial with danazol completed this phase of the trial. Although adverse effects were not presented in detail, danazol appears to have produced gastric irritation and hot flashes that led to withdrawal from the study in one patient each. Amenorrhea occurred in six patients and a significant change in menstrual pattern was indicated by three other patients. In contrast, none of the patients treated with placebo developed any important change in menstrual flow and cycle. These data suggest that most of the subjects (nine of 11, or 82 percent) treated first with danazol may have been able to identify the treatment sequence of the trial.

Danazol and placebo therapy produced significant improvement in the overall symptom scores as compared with the baseline period. The effect of danazol was better than that of placebo only for comparisons taking into account the symptoms recorded in the third cycle of treatment. Seven patients became asymptomatic after danazol therapy, as opposed to only one patient treated with placebo. Again, the "unblinding" potential of the danazol-induced menstrual abnormalities must be considered in interpreting this finding. The treatments were similar in their effect on the symptoms of depression, and data were not presented to judge the effect of danazol on social and occupational functioning.

The latest attempt to document a therapeutic role for danazol in premenstrual syndrome was made by investigators from North Staffordshire Hospital, Keele University in Stoke on Trent, United Kingdom, with the help of a research fellowship from the drug's manufacturer (O'Brien and Abukhalil, 1999). Based on earlier work reviewed in this chapter (Sarno, Miller, and Lundblad, 1987), this trial sought to test the effect of danazol administered only during the luteal phase of 100 women recruited from among the patients followed in a clinic specializing in premenstrual syndrome. The diagnosis required the presence of somatic, psychological, or behavioral symptoms during at least four of the previous six menstrual cycles. All subjects were described as mentally and physically fit, were not pregnant or intending to become pregnant, were not considered near menopause, and were not taking cortico-steroids, oral contraceptives, or anticoagulants. After carrying out a prospective self-evaluation of their symptoms, the participants were assigned to receive danazol (200 mg) or placebo once daily during days 14 through 28 of three consecutive cycles. Diaries were used to record on visual analog scales the severity of the six most promi-nent symptoms during the baseline cycle, the three treatment cycles, and the two posttreatment cycles.

Ten of the 100 participants withdrew from the study; eight had been assigned to take placebo. One patient from each treatment group invoked abdominal distention as the reason for discontinuing the study medication. Luteal phase treatment with danazol was no better than placebo with regard to the main symptoms of irritability, depression, anxiety, and abdominal distention and did not prove superior with regard to the overall discomfort created by the pre-menstrual syndrome.

Chapter 21

Ineffective Therapies

PROGESTERONE AND PROGESTOGENS

Progesterone

The therapeutic effectiveness of progesterone suppositories was well tested in a large trial conducted by an experienced group of investigators from the University of Pennsylvania's School of Medicine, Philadelphia (Freeman et al., 1990). The initial population sample consisted of 630 women who passed a screening telephone interview and kept a one-month diary of their symptoms. Of these, 320 women were confirmed to have premenstrual syndrome; were not pregnant, lactating, or desiring pregnancy; had regular menstrual cycles; had no serious medical illnesses; and were not taking psychotropic or hormonal treatments. Although the precise way in which the diagnosis of premenstrual syndrome was made is not indicated or referenced, the authors based it on the evaluation of severity ratings of 17 symptoms and required also that the illness be present for at least six months and be the cause of significant impairment in major occupational and social activities. "Most" patients were subsequently found to fulfill criteria for late luteal phase dysphoric disorder (American Psychiatric Association, 1987). A four-month washout period that included two single-blind placebo-treated cycles confirmed the eligibility of 168 subjects. The double-blind treatment consisted of vaginal suppositories containing progesterone or placebo administered from the sixteenth through the twenty-eighth day of two cycles each. The dosage employed was one suppository each day in the first cycle and one suppository twice daily in the second cycle of each treatment phase. Suppositories contained placebo or 400 mg of progesterone.

Thirty of the 168 patients (18 percent) discontinued their participation in the trial. Side effects were reported by eighty-five of the patients (51 percent) and led to withdrawal of five subjects (3 percent), but no clinical details were provided with regard to these five cases. The most common side effects were menstrual timing changes (noted in 15 percent of patients after treatment with progesterone and 20 percent after placebo therapy), flow changes (12 percent versus 16 percent), abdominal distention/weight gain (8 percent versus 5 percent), and breast tenderness (6 percent versus 7 percent).

Therapy with progesterone was no better than placebo for the alleviation of the 17 symptoms of premenstrual syndrome recorded throughout the study period. Clustering these symptoms into an emotional symptom factor (which included nervous tension, irritability, mood swings, and depression), a cognitive-physical symptom factor (consisting of poor coordination, confusion, aches, and fatigue), and a physical symptom factor (computed from the ratings given for swelling and breast tenderness) indicated the same lack of difference between the placebo and progesterone therapy. A significant worsening was noted in the symptom severity of patients treated with progesterone after receiving placebo therapy. The observation did not represent a "time effect," as no such worsening was noted among patients treated with placebo after the progesterone phase of the trial. Symptoms improved with doubling of the dose in equal measure during treatment with placebo and progesterone. The study did not identify any pretreatment variables that correlated with the effectiveness of the treatment with progesterone.

Vaginal suppositories containing progesterone were also tested for efficacy in alleviating the "nervous" symptoms of patients with premenstrual syndrome in a study performed by investigators from the University of South Carolina School of Medicine, Columbia, South Carolina, and the Milton S. Hershey Medical Center, Pennsylvania State University, Hershey, Pennsylvania (Baker et al., 1995). The authors recruited 47 women registered for care with the premenstrual clinic of the University of South Carolina and determined that 25 of them met the study's requirements. Two-month diaries of symptoms and basal temperature recordings were used to establish cycle length and to approximate the time of ovulation. A comprehensive evaluation established the absence of chronic illnesses and psychiatric disorders. The participants had not been treated with a hormonal preparation within three months of the trial, were not dependent on alcohol or drugs, and were not pregnant or anovulatory. Psychometric data were collected by a psychiatrist at baseline and during the luteal phase of each cycle treated and included structured and validated inventories of depression, anxiety, mood states, and personality.

The study started with placebo therapy for one cycle, after which the patients were randomly assigned to treatment with progesterone (200 mg) or placebo suppositories for the following two cycles. At this point, all the patients were again treated with placebo for one cycle, then crossed over to the alternate therapy for two additional cycles. The suppositories were inserted vaginally once daily beginning 12 days prior to the next anticipated menstruation during the first cycle and twice daily during the second cycle treated with the same agent. The protocol was completed by 17 of the 25 eligible subjects; the reasons for the withdrawal of 32 percent of the sample, as well as the type and severity of any adverse reactions, were not reported.

Progesterone was no better than placebo for any of the measures used to determine the severity of depression, anxiety, and anger. Similarly, no differences were observed between the two treatments with regard to interpersonal sensitivity, hostility, fatigue/inertia, somatization, and confusion/bewilderment. Progesterone therapy was associated with improvement of a subcategory of symptoms related to guilt and self-image.

Finally, the efficacy of vaginal or rectal administration of progesterone was evaluated by the Progesterone Study Group in a trial organized and funded by the drug's manufacturer, which involved the participation of 45 general practitioners from throughout the United Kingdom (Magill, 1995). The participating physicians recruited patients with complaints suggestive of premenstrual syndrome during the previous three months who did not have evidence of psychosis, suicidal tendency, drug or alcohol abuse and who had not been treated with antidepressants, benzodiazepines, or medication modifying the function of the ovaries. From a diagnostic standpoint, the authors decided that eligibility for the trial required at least one symptom consistently present during the luteal phase but not the follicular phase of the two cycles preceding the trial. Of the 281 subjects recruited for the screening phase of the study, 141 were found eligible for the trial and were randomly assigned to treatment with a suppository containing 400 mg of progesterone (n = 80) or placebo (n = 61), administered vaginally or rectally twice daily starting 14 days before the predicted date of the onset of menses for four consecutive cycles. Outcome measurements consisted of ratings given the symptoms recorded during the seven days prior to menses and first three days of menstrual bleeding.

Adverse effects were reported by 41 of the patients (51 percent) treated with progesterone and 26 (43 percent) of those assigned to the placebo group. Menstrual abnormalities, primarily changes in the duration of the cycle, were noted by 11 patients (17 percent) in the progesterone group but only 2 patients (3 percent) receiving placebo, a statistically significant difference. The frequency of the other side effects was statistically similar in the two groups: vaginal itching (10 percent in the progesterone group versus 4 percent in the placebo group), headache (10 percent versus 3 percent), nausea (7 percent versus 6 percent), abdominal pain (5 percent versus 2 percent), flu-like symptoms (4 percent versus 1 percent), dysmenorrhea (4 percent versus 1 percent), and breast pain (4 percent versus none). No patients appear to have been withdrawn because of side effects.

The study protocol was completed by 93 of the 141 patients; the other 48 patients did not comply with data collection or had luteal symptoms of insufficient severity. Analysis by intention to treat of the entire sample indicated that progesterone was no better than placebo with regard to the reduction of luteal symptom scores after the second, third, and fourth cycle treated. When the analysis was repeated only for those who completed the study, progesterone treatment was superior to placebo during the first three of the four cycles treated. However, a statistical correction for multiple comparisons is not indicated in the report, raising doubts with regard to the significance of the difference. The adjustment of data, using as covariates the most common premenstrual symptoms (abdominal distention, depression, tension, and irritability), produced only a marginal change in the assessment of overall treatment effect.

The most recent attempt to validate a therapeutic role for progesterone in premenstrual syndrome was made by a group of Australian investigators from the Key Centre for Women's Health, University of Melbourne, Carlton, Victoria, with technical and financial support from the drug's manufacturer and in collaboration with researchers based at La Trobe University, Melbourne, and Hôpital Necker, Paris (Vanselow et al., 1996). The study was the first trial to compare the effect of progesterone administered orally and vaginally and to assess the correlation between therapeutic response and serum concentrations of 5α- and 5β-pregnanolone, active metabolites of progesterone considered to have sedative-hypnotic properties.

The study cohort was recruited from among 200 women who called the research unit after the trial was described in lay and medical media. Pretreatment assessments carried out over two consecutive cycles identified 39 subjects eligible for the trial, i.e., women who had the required symptoms during the luteal phase for at least six months; impairment in occupational activities and interpersonal relationships; and no evidence of psychiatric, medical, or gynecological disorder, menstrual migraine, or current therapy with psychotropic drugs or hormonal preparations. The study cohort was treated for ten days premenstrually during six consecutive cycles with oral capsules and vaginal suppositories. Treatment was started on the third day after the ovulation, as anticipated by cycle length and basal temperature charts. Capsules and suppositories contained 100 mg of progesterone or placebo, which were administered in the following combinations: oral and vaginal placebo; oral progesterone (daily total 300 mg) and vaginal placebo; and oral placebo and vaginal progesterone (daily total 200 mg). Therapeutic outcome was measured on the twenty-sixth day of each treated cycle.

Only 22 of the 39 subjects (56 percent) provided complete data sets. Side effects led three patients (8 percent) to withdraw from the trial. Two of these were treated with vaginal progesterone at the time of developing depression and amenorrhea, respectively. One patient developed severe nausea during treatment with placebo. Other side effects included relapse of thyrotoxicosis in a patient with history of same who had been euthyroid at the onset of the trial, and frequent but not significant complaints of fatigue, drowsiness, and dizziness. Eleven patients dropped out for other reasons.

Three patients were noncompliant with the outcome assessments. The 22 patients who completed the study had a mean age of 36 years and an average duration of illness of eight years. Their most common symptoms were irritability (59 percent), depression (56 percent), breast tenderness and swelling (26 percent), and tiredness (26 percent). Half of the sample gave a history of psychiatric or psychological treatment, and 45 percent of patients had a family history of psychiatric illness, primarily mood disorder.

Although statistically significant improvement was noted for most of the symptoms assessed (i.e., depression and negative affect, anger, anxiety, ability to concentrate, pain, and water retention), the treatment with vaginal or oral progesterone was no better than placebo for any of these clinical variables. Treatment with vaginal suppositories produced a substantial increase in the serum levels of progesterone but only minimal change in the titers of 5α- and 5β-pregnanolone, while the opposite was observed following the administration of oral progesterone. Statistically significant correlations between these active metabolites and the outcome variables after oral treatment with progesterone were observed only between 5α-pregnanolone and anxiety and 5β-pregnanolone and lack of control.

Medroxyprogesterone

Medroxyprogesterone (acetoxymethylprogesterone), a widely preprescribed synthetic derivative of 17 α-hydroxyprogesterone with slight androgenic and anabolic activity but devoid of any detectable estrogenic activity (American Hospital Formulary Service, 1997, pp. 2468-2469), has been tested for efficacy in a group of patients with premenstrual syndrome treated at Falu Hospital, Falun, Sweden (Hellberg, Claesson, and Nilsson, 1991). The 43 subjects enrolled first in an observation period during which they recorded the presence and severity of ten symptoms (i.e., depression, tension, sadness, loss of libido, lethargy, anxiety, aggression, abdominal distention, headache, and breast tenderness) every day and were then treated according to a crossover design with medroxyprogesterone (5 mg) or placebo, taken twice daily from the nineteenth through the twenty-sixth day of the cycle.

The trial was not associated with significant adverse effects of the two treatments and was completed by 38 of the 43 original participants. Medroxyprogesterone was better than placebo only with regard to improvement in the severity of premenstrual depression; for the other nine symptoms rated the treatment effect was similar to that of placebo. In line with these observations is also the fact that medroxyprogesterone was identified as the best treatment by 12 women (36 percent), while placebo was considered to have the best effect by 11 subjects (29 percent).

Dydrogesterone

Dydrogesterone is a synthetic progestogen (6-dehydro-retroprogesterone) which has been tested in patients with premenstrual syndrome in several well-designed and executed trials with identical dosages performed in Australia, England, and Denmark (Dennerstein et al., 1986; Sampson et al., 1988; Hoffman et al., 1988). The drug is not available for clinical use in the United States.

In the first of these efforts, researchers from the University of Melbourne, Parkville, Victoria, Australia, recruited 32 women who were receiving care through the premenstrual tension clinic of a teaching hospital (Dennerstein et al., 1986). Eligibility for the trial required an unspecified number of mood and physical symptoms during the luteal phase of the cycle and improvement within three days of the onset of menses, followed by at least one week free of symptoms; impairment of occupational and social functioning while symptomatic; and no current psychiatric disorder or psychotropic or hormonal therapy. After a baseline observation cycle during which the symptoms and their severity were recorded every day, the patients entered the double-blind trial of dydrogesterone (10 mg) or placebo, administered from the twelfth through the twenty-sixth day of two consecutive cycles each. Daily ratings were continued throughout the trial and in-person follow-up interviews performed during the luteal phase of each treatment cycle.

Six of the 30 patients (20 percent) with prospectively confirmed premenstrual syndrome entered in the study failed to complete the trial. One patient developed abdominal pain and menorrhagia during treatment with placebo; two patients dropped out during the dydrogesterone phase of the trial because their symptoms were unchanged or worse; and three patients dropped out for reasons not related to the effect of treatment.

Dydrogesterone was no better than placebo for any of the ten main symptoms rated during the trial. A treatment effect was observed after the first two cycles on therapy (placebo or dydrogesterone), with a marked fall in the severity of symptoms compared with the pretreatment period.

The second trial of dydrogesterone was conducted by investigators from the Whitely Wood Clinic and the Family Planning Association, Sheffield, United Kingdom, with research funding from the drug's manufacturer (Sampson et al., 1988). The authors recruited 110 subjects who had been referred to a hospital-based clinic for specialized treatment by their general practitioners and 105 women who sought care from a self-referral clinic. Eligibility for the trial required the absence of current gynecological or psychiatric disorder. The treatment consisted of dydrogesterone (10 mg) or placebo, administered twice daily from the twelfth through the twenty-sixth day of the cycle. During the four consecutive cycles treated, the subjects crossed over to the alternate agent after each cycle of treatment. Outcome data were the daily symptom ratings made throughout the trial and the monthly assessment of the most bothersome symptoms and global rating of response to therapy.

Of the 108 patients found eligible for the trial, 39 (36 percent) failed to complete the study but only five patients (4.6 percent) were withdrawn because of side effects. The specific adverse effects leading to withdrawal were not indicated. Overall, side effects were reported by 73 (68 percent) of the 108 patients who started the trial, the most common being breast tenderness, which occurred in 20 patients (18 percent) who developed the adverse effect during progesterone therapy and eight patients (7 percent) while taking placebo. Other frequent side effects were nausea, change in menstrual bleeding pattern, urinary frequency, and headache.

Global rating of illness severity indicated improvement during at least one of the four treated cycles by 65 patients (94 percent) who completed the trial. The effect of placebo was similar to that of dydrogesterone in bettering the duration and severity of all premenstrual symptoms rated by the participating patients. Placebo therapy appeared more effective in reducing the duration but not severity of breast tenderness. The impact of illness on work, home, and social activities was similarly affected by placebo and dydrogesterone, with a trend toward improvement observed as the trial progressed, most notably among self-referred patients.

Finally, dydrogesterone was also tested in a trial organized by the Central Research Unit of General Practice and Rigshospitalet, Copenhagen, Denmark (Hoffman et al., 1988). The investigators obtained the participation of 59 Danish general practitioners, who enrolled 199 women with premenstrual complaints. A total of 161 patients fulfilled the authors' definition of premenstrual syndrome (i.e., had at least one postovulatory symptom, which improved substantially with the onset of menses); had no drug therapy for a psychiatric disorder within two years of the trial; and had no significant gynecologic pathology, systemic disorder, or regular use of prescribed medications. After one month of observation, the subjects were randomly assigned to treatment with 10 mg of dydrogesterone (n = 89) or placebo (n = 72) twice daily from the twelfth day of the cycle until the first day of menstrual bleeding. The treatment was administered for three consecutive cycles during which the subjects kept comprehensive symptom diaries. The global effect of treatment and the potential side effects were assessed at monthly intervals during scheduled visits with the general practitioner.

Three of the 89 patients (3.4 percent) treated with placebo developed side effects (abdominal pain, disturbed sleep, headache) considered serious enough to require the discontinuation of the trial. Overall, 15 patients (17 percent) assigned to treatment with dydrogesterone and 23 patients (32 percent) treated with placebo failed to complete the trial, but the group-specific reasons for withdrawal were not made available. The dropouts had baseline demographic and clinical characteristics similar to those of subjects who finished the three months of treatment and complied with all of the study's requirements. Side effects were reported by 25 patients (31 percent) from the dydrogesterone group and 19 (26 percent) of those treated with placebo.

Global improvement was reported by 49 percent of patients treated with dydrogesterone and 47 percent of those who received placebo. With regard to the 18 individual symptoms rated throughout the trial, dydrogesterone was more effective than placebo only for decreased libido. The authors note that dydrogesterone's effect on the symptoms of irritability and headache was just short of statistical significance; however, the judgment on the value of these observations must be negative in view of the absent statistical correction for multiple comparisons.

ESTROGENS

Conjugated Estrogens

The effect of estrogen therapy was tested in a trial organized by investigators from Montreal General Hospital and McGill University, Montreal, Quebec, Canada (Dhar and Murphy, 1990). A total of 11 patients were entered in the study; none of the subjects had evidence of pregnancy, hepatic dysfunction, arterial hypertension, breast cancer, endometrial cancer or hyperplasia, or history of cerebrovascular accidents, myocardial infarction, thrombophlebitis, or migraine headache. The sample was treated according to a crossover design with conjugated estrogens (0.625 mg) or placebo administered as identical-looking tablets once daily for the last 14 days of the menstrual cycle. All patients took estrogens or placebo for at least two cycles each and used no other medications throughout the study period. Outcome data were collected by patients daily during the treatment period of each cycle using a rating scale addressing mental and physical symptoms characteristic of premenstrual syndrome.

Therapy with conjugated estrogens was well tolerated by this group of patients and no significant adverse reactions were noted from a clinical or laboratory standpoint. Compared with placebo, estrogen therapy produced a statistically significant worsening of both mental and physical manifestations of the premenstrual syndrome.

Estradiol

Estradiol treatment of premenstrual syndrome has been proposed and tested by a group of British investigators affiliated with Kings

College, London (Magos, Brincat, and Studd, 1986; Watson et al., 1989). The first trial studied the efficacy of suppressing ovulation with subcutaneous estradiol implants combined with cyclical oral administration of norethisterone, a progestogen agent, to produce withdrawal bleeding (Magos, Brincat, and Studd, 1986). Although premenstrual symptoms were successfully treated, long-term adverse effects led to severely symptomatic myometrial hypertrophy requiring hysterectomy in 16 percent of the subjects included in the study (Watson et al., 1990). This unacceptable rate of complications of estradiol implants and cyclical oral progestogen therapy was similar to that observed in postmenopausal patients treated for symptoms of estrogen deficiency (Gangar et al., 1990) and is probably the explanation for the cessation of efforts with regard to the testing of this therapeutic modality in patients with premenstrual syndrome.

To prevent the adverse effects produced by subcutaneous implants, Watson et al. (1989) have used transdermal administration of estradiol to suppress ovulation in a well-designed trial for which they recruited 45 patients receiving care through a specialized outpatient unit at Dulwich Hospital, London. All patients had distressing premenstrual symptoms, regular cycle length, and normal pelvic examinations and were not currently taking any other medications or hormonal contraceptive agents. After confirmation of eligibility, 40 patients agreed to participate in the six-month trial and were assigned to treatment with estradiol (200 μg) or placebo patches (renewed at three-day intervals) for three consecutive cycles, after which patients crossed over to the alternate treatment. Norethisterone (5 mg daily) was administered orally from the nineteenth through the twenty-sixth day of the six cycles treated with transdermal estradiol or placebo. Outcome data was self-collected daily by using standardized premenstrual distress questionnaires.

Five patients (12 percent) failed to complete the trial; four of these patients dropped out after developing skin reaction to the medicated (two patients) or placebo (two patients) patches. The other dropout was noncompliant with the study protocol. No other significant adverse effects were reported, but 12 patients (30 percent) were noted to have transient rashes.

Treatment with transdermal estradiol was better than placebo with regard to six of the ten premenstrual distress symptoms recorded, i.e., improvement of abdominal distention, weight gain, irritability, mood swings, tension, and loss of efficiency. Estradiol and placebo had similar effects on the symptoms of depression, restlessness, tiredness, and difficulty concentrating.

NONSTEROIDAL ANTI-INFLAMMATORY DRUGS

Mefenamic Acid

Mefenamic acid, an anthranilic acid derivative with analgesic, anti-inflammatory, and antipyretic effects thought to be mediated by an inhibitory effect on prostaglandin synthesis and release (American Hospital Formulary Service, 1997, p. 1532), was first tried in patients with premenstrual syndrome by investigators from Monash University, Queen Victoria Medical Centre, Melbourne, Australia, with technical and conceptual support from the drug's manufacturer (Wood and Jakubowicz, 1980). The trial was advertised in a commercial radio broadcast, and about 100 women called the research unit. Fifty-nine callers reported for an initial meeting with the investigators, and 39 agreed to participate in the placebo-controlled trial. Although the diagnostic criteria were not described, the authors did indicate that all of the participants had confirmed the presence of premenstrual symptoms, the most common of which were tension (41 percent), irritability (33 percent), depression (31 percent), headache or other pain (23 percent), and breast tenderness (20 percent). After a drug-free control cycle the subjects were assigned to take mefenamic acid (500 mg) or placebo three times daily after meals for one cycle and then crossed over to the alternate therapy for another cycle. Outcome data were self-collected daily on a checklist of 18 symptoms.

Adverse reactions to mefenamic acid were recorded in four of the 39 participants (10 percent) and consisted of worsened premenstrual symptoms reported by two patients and rash and delayed menstruation in one patient each.

A statistical comparison of the individual symptoms' response to mefenamic acid and placebo was either not performed or not disclosed in this report, except to indicate that breast symptoms and fluid retention were never helped by mefenamic acid. The authors chose to emphasize only the fact that of the 37 participants who provided analyzable data 23 (62 percent) preferred mefenamic acid, as compared with six (16 percent) who favored placebo and 20 percent without a drug predilection. From this standpoint, the difference between mefenamic acid and placebo did reach statistical significance.

Australian researchers have also conducted the second trial of mefenamic acid in premenstrual syndrome, in a carefully designed investigation carried out as a collaborative effort between the University of Sydney and Macquarie University, Sydney (Mira et al., 1986). The subjects recruited for the study had all been referred by their gynecologist or primary care provider and had suffered severe premenstrual distress for at least two years. After excluding the women with significant physical disorders or past psychiatric history, the authors enrolled the remaining subjects in a baseline observation period lasting three cycles, during which the participants kept diaries recording the presence and severity of 22 psychological and 41 physical symptoms. The subjects were then randomly assigned to start treatment with capsules of mefenamic acid (250 mg) or placebo (lactose). The patients were instructed to take one capsule every eight hours for the sixteenth through the nineteenth day of the cycle and double the dose for the remaining days until the onset of menstrual bleeding. The initial treatment was given for two cycles, after which the subjects crossed over to the alternate treatment for two cycles and then back to the first treatment for two additional cycles. Differences in cycle length were appropriately standardized by planned collapsing of the data.

Of the 54 subjects who entered the preliminary phase of the trial, 17 chose not to participate in the placebo-controlled experiment and 18 decided to join another study. Two of the 19 women (11 percent) treated with mefenamic acid developed adverse reactions, i.e., nausea and giant urticaria that led to withdrawal from the trial. One patient complained of nausea and dropped out during treatment with placebo and another relocated, so that the group completing the trial consisted of 15 individuals. The frequency of the mild side effects of diarrhea, rashes, chest pain, and abdominal pain was similar during the placebo and mefenamic acid treatment periods.

Mefenamic acid was clearly better than placebo with regard to premenstrual fatigue, generalized aches and pains, headache, and mood swings. On the other hand, the effect of mefenamic acid was statistically similar to that of placebo for symptoms of breast pain, tenderness, or swelling; abdominal distention, discomfort, or pain; changes in appetite; craving for specific foods; back pain; inability to concentrate; indecisiveness and confusion; difficulty in sleeping; and feeling tense, inefficient, and disappointed in self.

Finally, the third placebo-controlled trial to study this issue found no evidence that the administration of mefenamic acid improves any of the symptoms associated with premenstrual syndrome (Gunston, 1986). This investigation was conducted at Groote Schuur and Somerset Hospitals, teaching units of the University of Cape Town, Cape Town, South Africa, and involved 42 patients receiving care through the premenstrual syndrome clinics of these institutions. After a month-long observation period, the participants were assigned to treatment with mefenamic acid (250 mg) or placebo administered three times daily at mealtimes from the eleventh through the twenty-sixth day of the cycle. After two cycles, patients crossed over to treatment with the other agent for two additional cycles. Data collection relied on symptom diaries kept by the patients for the entire duration of the study.

There were no significant adverse effects and 30 of the 42 participants completed all the data-gathering requirements of the study. Mefenamic acid was no better than placebo with regard to depression, irritability, bloating, breast tenderness, headache, lack of concentration, tension, and insomnia. Nonetheless, 16 patients (53 percent) reported global improvement after mefenamic acid therapy, as compared with 3 (10 percent) who felt better only during therapy with placebo.

Naproxen

The efficacy of the nonsteroidal anti-inflammatory agent naproxen in the treatment of premenstrual syndrome was studied in a placebo-controlled trial by investigators from the University of Modena and University of Pavia, Italy (Facchinetti et al., 1989). The 34 women recruited into the study had been suffering from premenstrual syndrome for at least two years and had significant impairment in their occupational and social function as a consequence of this disorder. Mood swings, difficulty with concentration, breast discomfort, migraine headache, and edema were noted as the most common symptoms, but the criteria used to diagnose premenstrual syndrome were not described or referenced. The subjects had no concurrent medical disorders and were not taking any medications or using hormonal contraceptive methods. After a two-month observation period during which the patients collected daily data on a structured self-administered questionnaire, they were randomly assigned to treatment with naproxen (550 mg) or placebo, to be taken twice daily starting one week prior to the expected onset of menses and continuing until the fourth day of menstruation for three consecutive cycles. After completing this phase of the trial, the patients crossed over to the alternate medication, which was administered for three more cycles. Outcome measurements relied upon questionnaire data collected at least ten times during each cycle treated.

Two of the 34 patients (6 percent) stopped their participation after developing epigastric pain and nausea, respectively; the report does not indicate whether these complaints occurred during treatment with naproxen. Four other subjects withdrew voluntarily for reasons not related to adverse drug effects.

Only pain symptoms improved with naproxen, and the magnitude of the response was commensurate with the decrease in the severity of premenstrual and perimenstrual headache. A trend toward improvement in premenstrual "behavioral changes" was observed only toward the end of the trial and was appropriately considered a consequence of the pain-relieving effect.

BETA-ADRENERGIC BLOCKING AGENTS

Atenolol

Atenolol, a widely used beta-adrenergic blocking agent, has been the object of study in two controlled therapeutic trials (Rausch et al., 1988; Parry, Rosenthal, et al., 1991). The first group of authors hypothesized that a beneficial effect can be expected given atenolol's potential to inhibit excessive mineralocorticoid activity, which was considered by them to explain some of the physiologic and behavioral manifestations of the syndrome. The second research team used the experience of a single case of seasonal premenstrual syndrome (Parry et al., 1987) to postulate that atenolol inhibits melatonin synthesis and thus leads to changes of the sleep/wake cycle, resulting in the improvement of the premenstrual dysphoric manifestations.

The first trial was conducted by investigators from the School of Medicine, University of California at San Diego, La Jolla, California, and the University of North Carolina, Chapel Hill, North Carolina, (Rausch et al., 1988). The 16 subjects were recruited through advertisements from among the students and employees of the California site and the diagnosis was made in accordance with standard criteria (American Psychiatric Association, 1987). Treatment consisted of atenolol (50 mg) or placebo taken once daily for the ten days prior to menses and continuing until the fourth day after the onset of menses. After one cycle of treatment the subjects crossed over to the alternate therapy, which was administered for an identical duration. Outcome measures relied on data generated by well-validated instruments assessing menstrual distress, depression, and anxiety.

Side effects were reported by nine patients (56 percent) during treatment with atenolol and five (31 percent) during the placebo phase of the trial. Atenolol therapy was associated with headache in three patients (19 percent), insomnia in two patients (12 percent), and depression, dizziness or lightheadedness, and frequency of urination in one patient (6 percent) each. The frequency and severity of adverse drug reactions were not different between atenolol and placebo and none of these complications required the discontinuation of the study medication.

The measures of anxiety and depression showed no significant therapeutic effect of atenolol. A favorable result was noted only with regard to premenstrual irritability. In addition, atenolol was better than placebo in preventing premenstrual reductions in friendliness, elation, and vigor. A separate analysis that evaluated only the data generated by the subjects who had premenstrual symptoms for more than five years suggested a differential improvement for this group. Atenolol therapy did not influence the expected luteal phase increase in the plasma renin and aldosterone activity.

The second trial was the result of a collaboration between researchers from the University of California at San Diego, La Jolla, California; Yorba Hills Hospital, Yorba Hills, California; and the Clinical Psychobiology Branch, National Institute of Mental Health, Bethesda, Maryland (Parry, Rosenthal, et al., 1991). Recruitment relied on advertisements in local newspapers and on referrals from practicing gynecologists and psychiatrists. The diagnosis of premenstrual syndrome was made on the basis of data collected during a two-month prospective observation period as required by the accepted definition of the syndrome (American Psychiatric Association, 1987), and appropriate investigations ruled out significant medical, gynecologic, or psychiatric morbidity. Of the 60 subjects evaluated, 13 agreed to participate and were randomly assigned to treatment with atenolol (100 mg daily) or placebo for the seven days preceding their menses. The alternate treatment was administered in a similar fashion during the following cycle. The outcome of therapy was based on data produced by double-blind assessments made daily by patients and weekly by clinicians.

No side effects were reported and all 13 subjects completed the trial. Atenolol was not better than placebo with regard to depression scores given by clinicians. The daily mood and sleep ratings made by patients also failed to indicate a therapeutic benefit of atenolol. The melatonin level did decrease during treatment with atenolol, but the number of patients tested (five of 13) was insufficient to reach a statistically meaningful conclusion.

Propranolol

The effect of propranolol on the clinical manifestations of patients with severe premenstrual symptoms was studied in a complex trial executed by investigators from the University of São Paolo, São Paolo, Brazil (Diegoli et al., 1998). In addition to propranolol, this double-blind, placebo-controlled study evaluated the therapeutic efficacy of alprazolam, fluoxetine, and pyridoxine. The diagnosis was based on data collected with structured questionnaires, and specific thresholds were used to select patients with the most severe form of illness. Patients with severe headache were assigned to receive propranolol (20 mg daily between menses and 40 mg daily during menses) or placebo for three months and then crossed over to the alternate therapy for an additional three months. Outcome data were collected at the end of each treatment cycle.

No adverse drug reactions were reported. A clinically meaningful change, i.e., more than 50 percent improvement, was recorded for 73 percent of patients after treatment with atenolol and 40 percent of patients at the end of the placebo phase of the trial, a statistically significant difference. However, with the exception of headache and backache, the improvement observed for the important premenstrual symptoms (e.g., nervous tension, mood swings, irritability, anxiety, breast tenderness, abdominal distention, and fatigue) were statistically similar after treatment with propranolol and placebo.

SPIRONOLACTONE

Spironolactone, a synthetic steroid that inhibits the physiologic effect of aldosterone on the distal renal tubules and has an antiandrogenic action by decreasing testosterone concentration and increasing estradiol levels (American Hospital Formulary Service, 1997, p. 2055) was first tested in patients with premenstrual syndrome more than 20 years ago and was reportedly followed by improvement in the psychological symptoms of more than 80 percent of the sample (O'Brien et al., 1979). The mechanism for the drug's intervention has not been defined, and later research has identified normal levels of aldosterone and increased levels of estradiol in subjects with premenstrual syndrome (Munday, Brush, and Taylor, 1981), in patients whose premenstrual syndrome was associated with demonstrable fluid retention (Davidson, Rea, and Valenzuela, 1988), and in cases in which the renal handling of water and electrolytes was abnormal during the luteal phase of the menstrual cycle (Piccoli et al., 1993). A well-controlled investigation has even demonstrated decreased aldosterone plasma levels throughout the cycle in women with premenstrual syndrome (Cerin et al., 1993).

The first large trial of spironolactone was organized at St. Thomas' Hospital, London, with the collaboration of researchers employed by the drug's manufacturer (Vellacott et al., 1987). Premenstrual syndrome was diagnosed on the basis of cyclical recurrence of at least two of the following six symptoms: depression, anxiety, irritability, abdominal distention, edema, and breast tenderness. The illness had to have a duration of at least six months and symptoms had to be relieved within two days after the onset of menses. Subjects with endogenous depression, a history of psychiatric illness, or evidence of renal, hepatic, or hematologic pathology were not included in the study cohort. Using a double-blind parallel design, the 63 eligible patients were assigned to receive spironolactone (100 mg) or placebo once daily from the twelfth day of the cycle through the first day of the next menstrual bleeding for two consecutive cycles.

The groups treated with spironolactone (n = 31) and placebo (n = 32) were well matched with respect to all important demographic and clinical characteristics. No intergroup differences were noted with regard to arterial blood pressure or weight variations. The frequency and type of adverse treatment effects were not reported. Four patients from the spironolactone group and five patients assigned to treatment with placebo dropped out for personal reasons or were withdrawn due to lack of compliance with research protocol. Two patients treated with placebo discontinued the trial because of lack of improvement.

Spironolactone was no better than placebo in producing improvement in any of the 12 symptoms surveyed after the first treatment cycle. This observation was confirmed after the second treatment cycle, when placebo therapy was just as effective as spironolactone for all symptoms except abdominal distention. At the end of the trial, 56 percent of patients treated with spironolactone and 30 percent of patients from the placebo group felt that the treatment had improved their overall condition for at least one of the two cycles treated; the difference did not reach statistical significance.

The lack of efficacy of spironolactone demonstrated by the preceding study was confirmed by investigators from the Royal Adelaide Hospital, Adelaide, Australia (Burnet et al., 1991). The subjects were selected from among women who contacted the research center in response to a newspaper article, but the report does not indicate the criteria used to diagnose premenstrual syndrome. The data collected included daily recordings of symptoms and their severity. Blood pressure, weight, and bust size measurements, an inventory of depressive symptomatology, and comprehensive bio-chemical and hormonal testing were performed at baseline and at six-week intervals for the duration of the trial. After a drug-free baseline observation cycle, the 61 subjects entered in the study were randomly assigned to start the trial with spironolactone (100 mg) or placebo each morning after breakfast from the fifth through the twenty-fith day of the menstrual cycle for three consecutive cycles, after which the subjects crossed over to the alternate therapy. The placebo and spironolactone tablets were identical in appearance, smell, and taste.

Three patients (5 percent) withdrew from the trial because of adverse effects of spironolactone consisting of nausea and irregular menses. Nausea led to the discontinuation of the trial by two patients during treatment with placebo. The treatment was stopped in one case after a renal colic. Twenty-two other patients dropped out for a variety of reasons including lack of compliance (14 patients), dislike of the trial (seven), and social reasons (one patient).

Among the 41 women with premenstrual syndrome who completed the trial, treatment with spironolactone was no better than placebo with regard to the self-reported severity of depression, irritability, headache, breast swelling, abdominal distention, and swelling of the hands or feet. Structured assessments of depressive symptomatology also failed to indicate a positive therapeutic effect of spironolactone. Objective measurements of weight and chest circumference demonstrated no significant changes between the two therapeutic modalities. A comparison of the 17 patients (41 percent) who improved after treatment with spironolactone with the 24 subjects whose condition did not change suggested that response to spironolactone was predicted by a rise in androgen levels from the follicular to the luteal phase of the baseline (untreated) cycle.

A similar daily dose of spironolactone (100 mg) was tried in a group of patients enrolled in a controlled crossover trial by investigators from Sweden (Hellberg, Claesson, and Nilsson, 1991). The trial compared the effect of spironolactone with that of medroxyprogesterone and placebo on seven psychologic symptoms (depression, tension, sadness, loss of libido, lethargy, anxiety, and aggression) and three somatic symptoms (abdominal distention, headache, and breast tenderness). The 43 subjects were required to have at least four of the ten symptoms listed above during the luteal phase of the cycle with swift regression at the start of menses. After a baseline observation cycle the subjects were assigned to treatment with spironolactone (50 mg) or placebo, administered as nonidentical tablets twice daily from the nineteenth through the twenty-sixth day of the cycle. This was followed by a 20-day drug-free period, after which the patients were treated with the alternate agent. Outcome data consisted of self-assessed severity of each of the ten symptoms on visual analog scales performed daily from the nineteenth through the twenty-sixth day.

One patient (2 percent) withdrew because of dizziness that developed during treatment with spironolactone, one stopped the trial after becoming pregnant, and three subjects failed to submit the outcome data. The 38 subjects who completed the trial had a mean age of 36 years and had been experiencing the symptoms of premenstrual syndrome for an average of seven years.

The effect of spironolactone and placebo was similar with respect to nine of the ten symptoms evaluated during this investigation. Abdominal distention was the only manifestation of premenstrual syndrome that appeared to respond to spironolactone therapy. Cluster analyses of the psychological and somatic symptoms failed to reveal a difference between placebo and spironolactone. A "mood index" obtained by summing up the visual analog scores of the symptoms (not including the scores given to the severity of headache and breast tenderness) was statistically lower after spironolactone therapy, a difference used by the authors to claim therapeutic efficacy for this drug. However, including abdominal distention in this composite score of mood changes is rather odd and raises the question of a post-hoc stratagem.

The effect of spironolactone was also studied in a crossover trial conducted by investigators from Umeå University Hospital, Umeå, and Uppsala Academy Hospital, Uppsala, Sweden, with grant support from the drug's manufacturer (Wang et al., 1995). The trial included 35 women with cyclic mood changes who fulfilled standard diagnostic criteria (American Psychiatric Association, 1987). After a baseline observation period lasting two months, during which the presence and severity of 12 symptoms was recorded using structured diaries, the participants were assigned to daily treatment with spironolactone (100 mg) or a matching placebo tablet during the last two weeks of each of the following three cycles and then crossed over to the alternate treatment.

Thirty-three of the 35 subjects completed the trial; two women dropped out because of the long duration of the trial. Spironolactone was better than placebo with respect to the improvement noted in social interactions and in the severity of five of the 12 symptoms surveyed, i.e., irritability, depression, breast tenderness, feeling of swelling, and craving for carbohydrates, but not for headache, anxiety and tension, fatigue, feeling of well-being, and work performance.

PYRIDOXINE

The use of pyridoxine (vitamin B6) in the treatment of premenstrual syndrome was justified by researchers employed by one of this vitamin's manufacturers on the basis of its participation in the production of serotonin (Williams, Harris, and Dean, 1985), a position supported by experimental data that has indicated a regulatory role of pyridoxine on the tryptophan decarboxylation step, which in turn controls the synthesis rate of serotonin in the rat (Dakshinamurti, Sharma, and Bonke, 1990) and monkey brain (Hartvig et al., 1995). However, premenstrual syndrome is not a pyridoxine-deficient state, as no evidence of impaired activities of the red cell enzymes which are known to depend on pyridoxine was found in women with this condition (Mira, Stewart, and Abraham, 1988). To prove the clinical utility of pyridoxine, Williams, Harris, and Dean (1985) assembled 724 subjects referred by 93 British general practitioners. Of these subjects, 617 were considered to have premenstrual syndrome, defined by the authors as the presence during the menstrual cycle of at least one of the following 11 symptoms: breast tenderness, edema, bloating, acne, lack of coordination, headache, depression, lethargy, tension, irritability, and violent feelings. This definition is overinclusive and constitutes a serious methodological flaw of this work. No additional physical or psychiatric evaluations were performed and no changes were made in the patients' current drug regimen. The subjects were enrolled in the study at presentation to their physicians, and the treatment was continued for three full cycles after their next menstruation. The trial required random assignment to therapy with pyridoxine (50 mg twice daily) or placebo. Adjustments in dosage were allowed in the event of side effects or lack of effect. Symptom ratings were performed daily by patients and monthly by their physicians. A global assessment was made at the end of the trial.

Of the 313 patients assigned to treatment with pyridoxine, 109 (35 percent) failed to complete the trial. The dropouts included 76 subjects (24 percent) who violated the research protocol, 22 (7 percent) who withdrew because they felt that their symptoms were not helped, and 11 (4 percent) who developed intolerable side effects. In the placebo group (n = 304), the total number of dropouts was 74 (24 percent), with 53 subjects (17 percent) being withdrawn for noncompliance, 13 women (4 percent) because of insufficient effect, and eight (3 percent) due to severe side effects. Details were not offered for any of the cases in which pyridoxine or placebo produced serious adverse reactions. The dosage of medication was increased by 29 percent of patients from the pyridoxine group and 35 percent of placebo group; the dosage was decreased by 3 percent of patients in each group.

Placebo therapy was just as effective as pyridoxine therapy for all of the symptoms recorded. The global assessment of the condition at the end of the trial indicated improvement for 82 percent of the patients treated with pyridoxine and of 70 percent of the placebo group. Predictors of treatment failure were the presence of severe breast tenderness at baseline and the use of analgesics during the trial. The authors conclude that "there is indeed significant benefit to be gained from pyridoxine treatment" (Williams, Harris, and Dean, 1985, p. 178). To this writer, such an assertion lacks clinical merit given the fact that a very substantial majority of patients improved after treatment with placebo; the 12 percent net improvement rate obtained by pyridoxine over placebo is statistically significant only because of the large sample size.

A contemporary effort to determine the therapeutic properties of pyridoxine in premenstrual syndrome was made by investigators from the Central Institute for Industrial Research, Akershus Central Hospital, and University of Oslo, Oslo, Norway (Hagen, Nesheim, and Tuntland, 1985). Employees of four companies known to have a large female workforce were invited to volunteer for a trial concerning premenstrual tension. Eligibility criteria required the presence of regularly occurring symptoms of premenstrual syndrome, absence of predominantly menstrual complaints, and regular periods. Subjects taking other drugs and those previously treated with pyridoxine for premenstrual syndrome were excluded. The patients were not informed what type of treatment was studied nor that the study had a crossover design during which they would be taking placebo. The 42 participants received pyridoxine (50 mg) or placebo twice daily for two cycles, and then crossed over to the alternate treatment for a similar interval. Visual analog scales were used to obtain patients' assessments of the overall status of their condition and ratings of the severity of six symptoms (breast tenderness, fatigue, headache, bloating/weight gain, depression, and irritability) at the end of each treatment period.

Eight of the 42 patients did not complete the trial, four because they proved unable to comply with the study's requirements and the remaining four (10 percent) on account of adverse reactions. One of these four patients developed fatigue while being treated with pyridoxine; three patients stopped their participation during the placebo phase of the trial because of irregular menstrual bleeding, nervousness, and fatigue. Within the group completing the trial (n = 34), five patients (15 percent) complained of mild nausea during treatment with pyridoxine, a side effect noted in the placebo phase by only one patient.

The baseline symptomatology of the 34 subjects who completed the trial was dominated by irritability (62 percent of women), depression (38 percent), breast tenderness (26 percent), bloating (21 percent), headache (18 percent), and fatigue (15 percent). On the 0-10 scale used to measure the aggregate severity of these symptoms, the median score was 6.6 at baseline, 5.8 after treatment with pyridoxine, and 4.9 after placebo. Pyridoxine was no better than placebo in any of the patients studied. A period effect was consistently noted, as the subjects indicated preference for the treatment used in the second half of the trial; the finding provides further support for the conclusion that pyridoxine did not have a distinctive therapeutic effect for premenstrual symptoms in this population.

The third study that attempted to elucidate a possible contribution of pyridoxine to the alleviation of premenstrual syndrome was conducted by investigators from the University of Massachusetts, Amherst, Massachusetts, and Dartmouth Medical School, Hanover, New Hampshire (Kendall and Schnurr, 1987). The starting point for this research effort was the authors' anecdotal experience indicating that 40 percent of women attending a local premenstrual syndrome clinic had tried pyridoxine for their symptoms. For their controlled study, the authors evaluated 110 women who responded to advertisements placed in local media. Seventy-four subjects with premenstrual symptoms noticeable to friends and relatives met the study's diagnostic criteria, which included the confirmation of their premenstrual symptomatology and postmenstrual improvement with structured instruments assessing the previous three menstrual cycles. The participants were also required to have regular menstrual cycles, to have no intention of becoming pregnant during the trial period, and to avoid all other medications. Eligible women were then entered in a baseline observation cycle during which a standardized questionnaire was used daily for data collection. After this cycle, the participants were paired according to severity of physical and dysphoric manifestations of premenstrual syndrome and members of each pair randomly assigned to receive pyridoxine (50 mg) or placebo three times daily for two consecutive cycles. Outcome was assessed by data collected daily by the participants and monthly by research assistants.

Fifty-five women completed the study; data regarding the reasons for withdrawal of one-quarter of the initial participants were not provided. Similarly, the report does not contain information about the adverse effects of therapy. The demographic characteristics of the dropouts were similar to those of patients who finished the trial. Therapy with pyridoxine was not better than placebo for the following six of eight clusters of symptoms evaluated: impaired concentration (forgetfulness, distractibility, confusion); negative affect (irritability, anxiety, mood swings, sadness); control (feelings of suffocation, palpitations, chest pain, numbness); arousal (feelings of well-being, orderliness, affection); pain (headache, cramps, fatigue); and water retention (breast tenderness, edema). A favorable trend attributed to treatment with pyridoxine was noted with respect to premenstrual autonomic reaction (dizziness, vomiting) and behavior change (staying in bed, decreased social interactions, poor performance). Nonetheless, improvement in these latter dimensions of the illness was considered insufficient to justify a therapeutic role of pyridoxine in premenstrual syndrome.

Finally, the latest effort to demonstrate that pyridoxine has therapeutic benefit in women with premenstrual syndrome was made by faculty from the Department of Community Medicine and General Practice, Oxford University, Oxford, United Kingdom (Doll et al., 1989). The vitamin trial was originally designed as part of a community-based survey of menstrual patterns of women (n = 2,000) registered for care with two general practices; 220 subjects were considered eligible for starting treatment with a daily dose of 200 mg of pyridoxine. However, physicians from one of these practices expressed concerns with regard to the potential for a neuropathic side effect of high-dose pyridoxine therapy and declined participation; therefore, only 70 women were entered in the study. The diagnosis of premenstrual syndrome was based on a review of illness experience at intake. The study started with an observation period lasting one cycle, during which the subjects kept a structured diary grading the severity of nine symptoms that are common among patients with premenstrual syndrome. Treatments with placebo or pyridoxine (50 mg daily) were then administered for three consecutive cycles after which the participants crossed over to therapy with the alternate agent. Outcome data consisted of the self-scored severity of the nine symptoms during the week prior to menses in each of the treatment cycles.

Only 32 of the 70 participants (46 percent) completed the trial. Efforts to determine the reasons for the withdrawal of the majority of participants were unrewarding. Pyridoxine was no better than placebo for any of the nine symptoms commonly described by patients with premenstrual syndrome, but a favorable statistical trend was noted for the group of symptoms comprising depression, irritability, and tiredness. Of note is the fact that treatment with placebo first led to a 57 percent decrease in the overall severity of the syndrome, a statistically significant effect.

EVENING PRIMROSE OIL

The justification for the therapeutic use of essential free fatty acids in premenstrual syndrome is based on a single, uncontrolled study of the plasma levels of linoleic acid and its metabolites in a group of 42 women with this disorder (Brush et al., 1984). Measured during the follicular and luteal phases, the titers of linoleic acid were found to be above normal limits, while the concentration of its metabolites was subnormal. The findings suggested normal dietary intake and absorption, coupled with incomplete transformation of the linoleic acid to gamma-linoleic acid. The metabolite's deficiency was considered a contributory factor to an abnormal response to the hormonal changes that characterize the luteal phase of the menstrual cycle.

This assumption appeared to receive confirmation in a clinical trial of a compound containing linoleic and gamma-linoleic acids on the premenstrual symptoms of 30 women performed at the University of Oulu, Oulu, and University of Helsinki, Helsinki, Finland (Puolakka et al., 1985). The subjects had a mean age of 38 years and had been suffering premenstrual symptoms for an average of nine years. Although the diagnostic criteria were not described, data provided indicate that a majority of the subjects had experienced moderate or severe premenstrual breast tenderness and engorgement, abdominal distention, generalized edema, weight gain, depression, and irritability. Treatment consisted of placebo or oil extracted from the seeds of a unique variety of evening primrose (*Oenothera biennis*) administered as three capsules twice daily starting on the fifteenth day of the cycle and continuing until the onset of menses. The evening primrose oil contained 2.16 g of cis-linoleic acid and 0.27 g of gamma-linoleic acid. After two cycles patients crossed over to the alternate therapy. Outcome measurements relied on self-scored severity of symptoms and global change in condition on the last day of each of the four cycles treated. All subjects completed the trial, apparently without any significant adverse effects.

Treatment with the evening primrose oil extract containing linoleic and gamma-linoleic acids was no better than placebo with regard to eight of the nine most common premenstrual symptoms experienced by these patients, dysphoria being the only symptom for which the plant extract seemed to be beneficial. A secondary analysis that trebled the weight of the three most bothersome symptoms indicated marginal superiority of the extract over placebo, but statistical significance as calculated by the authors is very much in doubt, given the lack of correction for multiple comparisons. Marked improvement was reported for 28 percent of the cycles treated with the plant extract and for 14 percent of the cycles treated with placebo, and slight improvement for 34 percent and 26 percent of cycles, respectively; neither difference was statically significant.

The same preparation of evening primrose oil was studied in a trial conducted by investigators from the Royal Brisbane Hospital and the Royal Women's Hospital, Herston, Queensland, Australia (Khoo, Munro, and Battistutta, 1990). Enrollment was open to patients and female hospital staff who had premenstrual syndrome characterized by at least one symptom of fluid retention and one of breast discomfort and two symptoms indicating mood changes. The trial design required assignment to placebo (liquid paraffin) or evening primrose oil for three cycles and crossover to the alternate treatment after a three-week washout period. The daily dose of the plant extract contained 2.88 g of linoleic acid and 0.36 g of gamma-linoleic acid, administered as four capsules twice daily.

All 38 participants completed all the requirements of the trial, and no adverse reactions were mentioned in the published report. Treatment with evening primrose oil was no better than placebo for any of the clinical manifestations of premenstrual syndrome. A "carryover" effect of the evening primrose oil into the placebo phase of the trial was not observed. A significant placebo response was inferred from the fact that subjects' symptoms improved rapidly after the start of the trial and worsened slightly by the third cycle following the crossover, regardless of the sequence in which the plant extract or placebo had been administered.

The third trial designed to test the effectiveness of the same evening primrose seed extract was carried out by investigators from the Karolinska Institute, Stockholm, Sweden, with financial and technical support from the drug's manufacturer (Collins et al., 1993). Eight thousand women living in two districts of Stockholm County were invited to participate in this controlled investigation;

340 individuals responded indicating interest in treatment for premenstrual syndrome and 30 women volunteered for the symptom-free control group. The diagnosis was established in accordance with the criteria proposed by the American Psychiatric Association (1987). A total of 68 subjects with premenstrual syndrome entered the ten-cycle trial. After one cycle of baseline assessments, the subjects were treated with placebo in a single-blinded manner, then randomly assigned to receive placebo (liquid paraffin) or the evening primrose oil preparation at a dose of four capsules three times daily. The daily dose of the plant extract contained 4.32 g of linoleic acid and 0.54 g of gamma-linoleic acid. Each treatment was administered for four cycles, after which the subjects crossed over to the other treatment. The healthy control subjects were enrolled in the baseline assessment cycle only. Outcome data were collected daily by all subjects by rating on visual analog scales the severity of four physical and 12 psychological symptoms.

Analyzable data were available from 27 subjects with premenstrual syndrome and 22 healthy women. Of the 68 women with premenstrual syndrome entered in the trial, nine dropped out during the baseline evaluation, 21 withdrew during the double-blind treatment phase, seven were excluded because of lack of symptom cyclicity, and four because of anovulatory cycles. Women with premenstrual syndrome were similar to healthy control subjects with regard to marital, educational and occupational status, age at menarche, and cycle length. Significant differences between groups were noted only for a much lower frequency of dysmenorrhea and a family history of premenstrual symptoms in the control group.

No adverse effects of treatment with evening primrose oil were noted, but an unspecified number of women reported weight gain. Evening primrose oil was no better than placebo for any of the 16 premenstrual symptoms surveyed in this trial. However, for 13 out of the 16 symptoms a significant time effect was noted; regardless of whether they were taking placebo or the plant extract, the subjects felt better the longer they continued the treatment. Symptoms not improved by time in trial were breast tenderness, level of energy, and headache.

MAGNESIUM

A clinical use for magnesium supplementation in patients with pre-menstrual syndrome is justified by a small and relatively homogenous body of work demonstrating a magnesium deficiency in this condition. The first controlled study showed that although serum levels were within normal limits, the red cell magnesium concentration was signif-icantly lower (Abraham and Lubran, 1981). This report was followed by the publication of findings of lower plasma levels of magnesium during the luteal phase compared with the follicular phase in patients with premenstrual "tension" syndrome (Posaci et al., 1994). The lower concentration of magnesium in the red blood cell was confirmed in a study that demonstrated that a deficiency of similar magnitude can be identified in the mononuclear blood cell; however, neither of these abnormalities was limited to the luteal phase (Rosenstein et al., 1994). Finally, a cyclical variation in the ionized magnesium levels was pres-ent in sera collected from women with premenstrual syndrome, with high titers identified in the early follicular phase, and a significant decrease in the luteal phase, which coincided with the peak of the progesterone concentration (Muneyvirci-Delale et al., 1998). Nonethe-less, an explanatory model for these findings and the specific contribu-tion of a magnesium-deficient state to the production of premenstrual symptoms has not been elucidated.

The earliest clinical trial of magnesium supplementation in pre-menstrual syndrome was conducted by investigators from academic centers in Modena and Pavia, Italy (Facchinetti et al., 1991). The 32 otherwise healthy subjects had premenstrual symptoms that were se-vere enough to interfere with social and occupational activities and had the formal diagnosis confirmed by data collected prospectively over two consecutive cycles with a standardized structured questionnaire. Psychiatric evaluations established the absence of mood or anxiety disorders. Treatment consisted of magnesium tablets (administered as a pyrrolidone carboxylic acid salt containing 120 mg of elemental mag-nesium) or placebo three times daily for two complete cycles. Magne-sium and sex hormone levels were measured in the luteal phase of the second treatment cycle.

Two patients dropped out because of side effects; one of them had been assigned to receive magnesium and developed diarrhea. Two other subjects could not comply with the requirements of the trial. The remaining 28 patients were equally distributed into well-matched magnesium and placebo groups. At the end of the double-blind trial, neither magnesium nor placebo therapy had a detectable effect on the severity on symptoms of cognitive dysfunction, behavioral changes, autonomic reaction, and water retention. Both placebo and magnesium improved the pain symptoms of the premenstrual syndrome. Changes in symptom scores did not correlate with magnesium or sex hormone levels.

Explicitly inspired by the research effort of the Italian team (Facchinetti et al., 1991), investigators from Royal Berkshire Hospital and University of Reading, Reading, United Kingdom, have carried out a double-blind trial of magnesium that involved the administration of the mineral throughout the menstrual cycle, rather than just during the premenstrual half of it (Walker et al., 1998). The 54 subjects were students and employees who responded to poster advertisements and were shown on a symptom analysis of their last menstrual cycle to have significant discomfort during the luteal phase, with marked reduction (more than 30 percent) after the onset of menses. Therapy was initiated on the first day of menstrual bleeding with magnesium oxide (200 mg) or placebo (microcrystalline cellulose) once daily for two complete cycles, followed by treatment with the alternate agent for a similar period of time. Outcome data were collected daily throughout the study by using a well-validated 22-symptom questionnaire.

Only 24 of the 54 subjects completed the trial and the reasons for withdrawal were not followed up for fear of breaking promised confidentiality. Data analysis included symptom scores provided by the 38 subjects who complied with the research protocol for at least the first phase (two cycles) of the trial. The oral preparation of magnesium was well absorbed, as evidenced by a daily urinary output of 101 mg of magnesium during the supplementation, as compared with a baseline output of 72 mg/day and an output of 74 mg/day during therapy with placebo. Outcome analyses indicated that the administration of magnesium was no better than placebo for 20 of the 22 premenstrual symptoms scored by the subjects; the only improvement was recorded for breast tenderness and abdominal distention during the second month of magnesium supplementation.

Chapter 22

Unreplicated Trials

CALCIUM CARBONATE

The effect of calcium supplementation has been the object of two clinical trials conducted by Thys-Jacobs and her collaborators (1989, 1998), which have not been independently replicated. The mechanism of action of calcium in premenstrual syndrome has not been defined, and the scant literature exploring the relationship offers somewhat inconsistent findings. On one hand, total and ionized calcium levels were found to decline significantly at midcycle in women with and without evidence of premenstrual syndrome (Thys-Jacobs and Alvir, 1995). On the other hand, a cyclic alteration of the ionized calcium level was not found in another group of healthy female volunteers (Muneyvirci-Delale et al., 1998). Calcium levels may influence serotonergic neurotransmission, but the available literature does not support such a mechanism, first because the intracellular calcium levels of patients with subsyndromal affective disorder were shown to be similar to those of healthy control subjects both at baseline and after stimulation with serotonin (Berk, Mitchell, and Plein, 1998), and second because serotonin reuptake inhibition leads to a decrease in intracellular calcium (Jagadeesh and Subhash, 1998).

The first trial was carried out at Metropolitan Hospital, a teaching affiliate of the New York Medical College in New York City with limited material support from the manufacturer of a popular brand of calcium carbonate tablets (Thys-Jacobs et al., 1989). The project was brought to the attention of patients, physicians, and hospital staff, and 78 women volunteered for the study. Sixty subjects were found eligible for the trial because they had moderate or severe symptoms in the second half of the menstrual cycle that were at least 50 percent more severe than in the days immediately following their menstruation. None of them were pregnant or had active major depression or a history of psychosis, renal insufficiency, nephroli-thiasis or renal colic, active peptic ulcer disease or inflammatory bowel disease, evidence of malabsorption or history of endometrio-sis, and all had normal levels of calcium in the blood. The subjects were not being treated with thiazide diuretic, digitalis preparations, or calcium channel blocking agents at the time of the study and agreed to refrain from using nonsteroidal anti-inflammatory agents and to avoid changing their diet during the trial. After one cycle of baseline measurements the subjects were randomly assigned to treat-ment with calcium carbonate (500 mg of elemental calcium) or pla-cebo twice daily for three menstrual cycles, then crossed over to the alternate treatment for an equal duration. Outcome data were col-lected during the first cycle following the end of the trial.

Twenty-seven (45 percent) of the 60 participants dropped out of the study before the crossover; 19 of these 27 patients did not comply with the research protocol, three withdrew because of lack of improvement, and one each was dropped out because of preg-nancy and alcoholism, respectively. Two patients treated with calcium carbonate dropped out because of adverse effects (peptic ulcer symp-toms in one case and rash in another), while one patient treated with placebo discontinued participation after developing renal stones.

Treatment with calcium carbonate was associated with side effects in 11 of the 33 patients (33 percent) who completed the trial. The side effects were constipation (four patients), nausea (three patients), other gastrointestinal discomfort (three patients), and flatulence (one patient). In contrast, treatment with placebo was associated with only two (6 percent) complaints of nausea. Calcium carbonate was better than placebo as measured by degree of improvement in the overall severity of the luteal phase symptoms with the exception of in-creased appetite and craving for carbohydrates.

A larger trial of the effect of calcium carbonate on premenstrual symptoms was coordinated by the same author at St. Luke's-Roosevelt Hospital Center and Columbia University, New York (Thys-Jacobs et al., 1998). The study was supported by a grant from the consumer health care division of a large pharmaceutical company and employees of the medical and regulatory division of this company were among the authors of the publication reporting the findings. Subjects were recruited through a variety of means (e.g., advertisements, physicians referrals, and word of mouth) at six "northern" clinical sites located in the states of New York, Connecticut, Ohio, and Utah and six "southern" locations in South Carolina, Florida, Alabama, Louisiana, and Texas. Altogether, 720 subjects with premenstrual complaints were given a screening evaluation aimed to confirm the diagnosis of premenstrual syndrome and the absence of organic disorder. The clinical manifestations of premenstrual syndrome were documented by structured diaries recording 17 symptoms for two consecutive menstrual cycles, while the absence of organic disorder was confirmed by comprehensive physical and laboratory evaluations. Exclusion criteria were similar to those applied in the authors' previous work (Thys-Jacobs et al., 1989).

Of the 720 women recruited, 497 were eligible for the trial and were randomly assigned to treatment with calcium carbonate (600 mg elemental calcium) or placebo twice daily for three consecutive cycles. Outcome data were collected with a structured diary and compliance with the study's requirements ascertained by telephone contact and monthly follow-up visits. Ibuprofen was the only rescue drug permitted during the trial.

Analyzable data were provided by 466 subjects. Adverse effects were reported by 422 (91 percent) of the participants; their frequency was similar in the two treatment groups. Eleven of the 231 patients (5 percent) treated with calcium supplements discontinued the trial due to adverse side effects. The complete list of these adverse reactions is not presented in the published report, which indicated only that five patients stopped their participation because of nausea and that one patient developed symptomatic nephrolithiasis. Side effects led to the withdrawal of five (2 percent) of patients treated with placebo.

The majority of patients included in the trial showed substantial (more than 50 percent change) improvement in the global severity of their premenstrual syndrome. The rate of improvement was 84 percent in the calcium group and 52 percent in the placebo-treated group. The proportion of patients reporting superior (more than 74 percent improvement) results was 29 percent in the calcium-treated group and 16 percent among the patients who had completed treatment with placebo. With regard to individual symptoms, calcium carbonate was better than placebo for tension/irritability, anxiety/nervousness, anger/short temper, breast tenderness/fullness, abdominal distention, abdominal cramping, diffuse pain, and low back pain.

ALPHA-TOCOPHEROL

A controlled trial of alpha-tocopherol (vitamin E) was conducted by investigators associated with North Charles Hospital, a Johns Hopkins Health Systems Institution, Baltimore, Maryland (London et al., 1987). The authors had previously noted a favorable effect of vitamin E on the premenstrual symptoms of a group of women with benign breast disease (London et al., 1983) and aimed at replicating those findings in a large population of self-referred women seeking treatment for premenstrual syndrome. The authors postulated that the mechanism of action of vitamin E was either regulation of "aberrant" prostaglandin synthesis or its effect on abnormalities in central nervous system neurotransmission. However, it is important to point out that controlled research studies performed at the University of Sydney, Sydney, Australia (Mira, Stewart, andAbraham, 1988) and University of Texas Medical Branch, Galveston, Texas (Chuong, Dawson, and Smith, 1990) have convincingly shown that vitamin E levels in women with premenstrual syndrome were normal during the luteal and follicular phases of the menstrual cycle.

The trial was brought to the attention of the general population in Baltimore, Maryland, through print and television announcements and informal means (i.e., word of mouth). Eligibility criteria included the presence of premenstrual syndrome; no history of psychiatric disorder or current major physical disorder; normal scores on a standard personality inventory administered during the follicular phase of the menstrual cycle; and willingness to avoid all other prescribed and over-the-counter drugs and vitamins for the duration of the trial. The diagnostic criteria for premenstrual syndrome were not specified. A total of 46 women were found eligible for the trial and were randomly assigned to receive vitamin E (400 IU) or an identical placebo capsule once a day for three consecutive menstrual cycles. Data were collected at baseline and during the follicular and luteal phases throughout the study and consisted of a structured questionnaire used by patients to score the severity of the symptoms known to be part of the premenstrual syndrome.

Five of the 46 participants were unwilling to complete the trial because of lack of efficacy of the study medication. Four of these patients had been treated with placebo; one of them also developed headache, chest pain, and paranoid ideation. The placebo group (n = 19) and the vitamin E group (n = 22) of subjects were well matched with regard to the baseline severity of the symptoms experienced during the luteal and follicular phases of the menstrual cycle.

The effect of treatment was first determined by the intragroup (baseline versus posttreatment) and intergroup (vitamin E versus placebo) differences for the cumulative scores calculated for the following four symptom clusters: nervous tension, mood swings, irritability, and anxiety; weight gain, breast tenderness, edema, and abdominal distention; headaches, fatigue, palpitations, increased appetite, and carbohydrate craving; and depression, crying, confusion, forgetfulness, and insomnia. In intragroup comparisons, neither vitamin E nor placebo therapy produced a statistically significant decrease in the severity scores of premenstrual symptoms. A second analysis evaluated the same symptoms grouped this time in 11 categories, and found that vitamin E was not better than placebo for irritability, tension, efficiency, dysphoria, cognitive ability, eating habits, sexual drive, and the common somatic manifestations of the syndrome.

L-TRYPTOPHAN

The amino acid L-tryptophan was recently tried in a group of patients with premenstrual syndrome by investigators from St. Mary's Hospital and McGill University, Montreal, Quebec, Canada (Steinberg et al., 1999). The premise of this attempt was the established relationship between L-tryptophan depletion and the severity of premenstrual symptoms (Menkes, Coates, and Fawcett, 1994) and the implied effect of L-tryptophan on serotonergic neurotransmission (Bancroft et al., 1991). However, it is important to point out that the available L-tryptophan was similar in the plasma of women with and without premenstrual syndrome (Rapkin et al., 1991) and that the concentration of L-tryptophan in the cerebrospinal fluid does not differ between the follicular and luteal phases of the cycle in this condition (Parry, Gerner, et al., 1991). For their study, the Canadian investigators had access to a pool of 240 women who were either referred by a gynecological care provider or who responded to a newspaper announcement describing the trial. Prospective assessments were carried out to establish the diagnosis of premenstrual syndrome according to the standard definition (American Psychiatric Association, 1987). Subjects who had a current psychiatric disorder or had been treated for such a disorder in the previous two years were excluded, as were the women with cyclical disorders such as dysmenorrhea, migraine, and endometriosis, and those who needed concomitant medications, were lactating, or planned to become pregnant.

A total of 80 women who were eligible for the three-month trial were randomly assigned to treatment with L-tryptophan (6 g daily in divided doses) or placebo for 17 days starting on the day of ovulation through the third day after the onset of menses. The primary outcome instruments were visual analog scales measuring the global severity of the condition and the symptoms of irritability, dysphoria, tension, mood swings, headache, bloating/edema, and breast tenderness. Other data were obtained by using psychometric scales and structured psychiatric interviews. All follow-up data were collected during visits scheduled to coincide with the follicular and luteal phase of each cycle treated.

Sixty-three of the 80 participants completed the trial. The majority of dropouts (14 of 17 cases) failed to comply with the research protocol. Two patients withdrew after developing intercurrent illnesses. One patient discontinued her participation after an adverse drug reaction, but clinical details were not disclosed in the report. Common (i.e., encountered in more than 20 percent of patients) side effects included dizziness (37 percent in the tryptophan group versus 14 percent in the placebo group, a statistically significant difference), nausea or vomiting (26 percent versus 14 percent), skin conditions (26 percent versus 11 percent), hypotension (21 percent versus 5 percent), and dry mouth (21 percent versus 16 percent).

Overall, 68 percent of patients treated with tryptophan and 62 percent of the placebo-treated group had at least one adverse drug reaction, which were described as transient and of mild or moderate severity. None of the patients showed evidence of the eosinophilia-myalgia syndrome that has been reported to follow the oral administration of certain commercial preparations of L-tryptophan (Horwitz and Daniels, 1996).

Treatment with L-tryptophan produced a 35 percent decrease in the self-assessed severity score of an index comprising dysphoria, mood swings, tension, and irritability, while therapy with placebo was associated with a 10 percent reduction, a statistically significant difference. The therapeutic effect was evident by the end of the first cycle treated and did not change thereafter. Psychometric measures of depression, anxiety, and hostility did not produce significant differences between L-tryptophan and placebo. Treatment with L-tryptophan was no better than placebo with regard to changes in the physical symptoms of headache, breast tenderness, and bloating/edema.

Chapter 23

Evidence-Based Therapy
of Premenstrual Syndrome

The analysis of the evidence regarding the effect of pharmacological interventions in premenstrual syndrome indicates decisively that selective serotonin reuptake inhibitors are safe, well tolerated, and clearly better than placebo in all of the trials to date. We are in complete agreement with the consensus expressed by Pearlstein (1998, p. 87) when she wrote that "most clinicians now consider serotonergic antidepressants the first line treatment for this condition." As indicated in our presentation, it is reasonable to initiate the treatment with a modest dose administered only during the luteal phase of the menstrual cycle and to titrate carefully dosage and duration of treatment according to response and reported side effects over the next two to three months. General experience with this class of drugs indicates that adverse effects will require treatment discontinuation in as many as 15 percent of patients because of iatrogenic symptoms, the most common being nervousness, anxiety, insomnia, headache, dizziness, nausea, and skin reactions (American Hospital Formulary Service, 1997, p. 1699). These drugs should not be prescribed to women who are or who plan to get pregnant, and to those who are nursing or plan to breast-feed. The presence of systemic disorder (e.g., hepatic or renal dysfunction), hemodynamic impairment, or history of seizures must also be considered contraindications for this use of serotonin reuptake enhibitors. The prescribing physican and dispensing pharmacist must ensure that the potential for drug-drug interactions has been carefully addressed before the initiation of therapy.

When serotonin reuptake inhibitors are contraindicated or have failed, the symptoms of premenstrual syndrome may be treated with one of the agents described as controversial in our review (i.e., agonists of gonadotropin-releasing hormone, alprazolam, bromocriptine, or danazol). However, the potential for substantial side effects, such as premature menopause or physiologic benzodiazepine dependence, suggests that extreme caution must be exercised in choosing to proceed with one of these agents.

Referral for cognitive-behavioral therapy should be considered for all patients whose premenstrual syndrome leads to impairment in family life and social or occupational functioning. The effectiveness of intervention is supported by a small but congruent body of work. Controlled trials of this therapeutic method in Australia have shown significant positive effects after one month of treatment (Morse et al., 1991); reduction in premenstrual symptomatology and irrational thinking persisting nine months after treatment (Kirkby, 1994); and amelioration of anxiety, depression, negative thoughts, and physical symptoms by interventions aimed at cognitive restructuring and assertion training (Christensen and Oei, 1995). These findings were supported by data obtained in an investigation conducted at John Radcliffe Hospital, Headington, Oxford, United Kingdom (Blake et al., 1998) which compared the effect of 12 weekly sessions of cognitive-behavioral therapy with the outcome of an untreated sample. With the caveat prompted by the absence of a placebo intervention, this study confirmed the fact that cognitive-behavioral therapy leads to a substantial improvement of the clinical manifestations of the syndrome and a significant increase in functional ability.

Conclusions

And if you find her poor, Ithaka won't have fooled you
Wise as you will have become, so full of experience
you will have understood by then what these Ithakas mean

C. P. Cavafy, *Ithaka*

The research efforts described in detail in the preceding sections have produced evidence indicating that effective drug therapy is available for fibromyalgia, irritable bowel syndrome, and premenstrual syndrome but not for chronic fatigue syndrome, (see Table 1). The drugs that worked were the tricyclic antidepressants amitriptyline and dothiepin in fibromyalgia; the tricyclic antidepressants amitriptyline, trimipramine, and desipramine in irritable bowel syndrome; and the selective serotonin reuptake inhibitor antidepressants fluoxetine, sertraline, paroxetine, and citolapram for patients with premenstrual syndrome.

TABLE 1. Effective Therapies for Common Functional Syndromes

	CFS	FM	IBS	PMS
Serotonergic antidepressants	−/−	+/−		+/+
Tricyclic antidepressants		+/+	+/+	
Cognitive-behavioral psychotherapy	+/+	−/−	−/−	+/+
Graded aerobic exercise	+/+	+/−		

+/+   effective therapy
+/−   controversial therapy
−/−   ineffective therapy

271

The effectiveness and specificity of these pharmacological interventions reflect the application of two scientific paradigms. The first consists of pursuing an etiologic hypothesis to the limit permitted by the most modern investigative tools followed by aggressive therapy targeted at the functional abnormalities identified in the process. This paradigm explains the success story of premenstrual syndrome, which has been carefully defined as a serotonergic-deficient state (Ashby et al., 1988; Bancroft et al., 1991; Menkes, Coates, and Fawcett, 1994; FitzGerald et al., 1997) and then treated with a class of drugs able to correct the neurotransmitter aberrance of the central nervous system. The logic of the investigative progress is remarkably easy to follow, as the approach has been refined from using fixed, low doses of the long-acting drug fluoxetine (Stone, Pearlstein, and Brown, 1991) to luteal-phase therapy with individualized dosages of the short-acting drugs sertraline (Halbreich and Smoller, 1997; Young et al., 1998) or citolapram (Wikander et al., 1998).

The contrasting paradigm is that employed in trials of tricyclic antidepressants for patients with fibromyalgia and irritable bowel syndrome. Although the definition of these syndromes describes the major role of chronic pain in their clinical presentation, researchers have not explicitly employed the chronic pain model in the design of clinical trials. Without exception, the trials have used very small doses of these drugs, e.g., 10 to 50 mg/day of amitriptyline in fibromyalgia (Carette et al., 1986; Goldenberg, Felson, and Dinerman, 1986; Carette et al., 1994; Goldenberg et al., 1996; Hannonen et al., 1998) and 50 mg/day of amitriptyline (Steinhart, Wong, and Zarr, 1981), trimipramine (Myren et al., 1982; Myren et al., 1984), or desipramine (Greenbaum et al., 1987) in irritable bowel syndrome. The reason for this timid approach is not entirely clear, but appears to have been based on the belief that low-dose tricyclic therapy is effective when the target of pharmacologic intervention is not a mood disorder. At least with regard to alleviation of pain, support for this view has been provided in only one controlled study, in which amitriptyline (25 mg/day) was found to be superior to placebo for chronic nonmalignant pain (McQuay, Carroll, and Glynn, 1992). All other placebo-controlled trials have allowed the individualization of therapy so that patients used 75 mg/day of amitriptyline for painful diabetic and nondiabetic polyneuropathy (Vrethem et al., 1997), 100 mg/day of amitriptyline to treat neuropathic pain following therapy for breast cancer (Eija, Tiina, and Pertti, 1996), 150 mg/day of amitriptyline for the management of acute low back pain (Stein et al., 1996), and an average of 167 mg/day of desipramine for relief of postherpetic neuralgia (Kishore-Kumar et al., 1990). Therefore, the research community may need to explore the effect of full doses of tricyclic agents in these syndromes and to compare them with other agents useful in the treatment of chronic pain, such as gabapentin (Hunter et al., 1997) and carbamazepine (Kudoh, Ishihara, and Matsuki, 1998).

Compared with the other three common functional illnesses, chronic fatigue syndrome has not been shown to respond favorably to drug therapy, but patients with this frustrating condition are clearly helped by graded aerobic exercise (Fulcher and White, 1997; Wearden et al., 1998) and by some programs of cognitive-behavioral therapy (Sharpe et al., 1996; Deale et al., 1997). It is quite likely that chronic fatigue syndrome will remain a drug-resistant illness and that greater efforts must be made to understand its psychosocial rather than biological characteristics.

The examination of controversial (see Table 2) and ineffective (see Table 3) therapies reveals two common denominators. First is that of the etiology-driven trial, evident in work postulating chronic fatigue syndrome as an immunologic dysfunction responsive to intravenous immunoglobulin; fibromyalgia as a condition of abnormal sleep amenable to the effect of a variety of hypnotic agents; irritable bowel as a disorder of intestinal motility that should be influenced by smooth muscle relaxants, calcium channel blockers, ondansetron, and cisapride; and premenstrual syndrome as an endocrinologic problem correctable with estrogen, progesterone, GnRH agonists, bromocriptine, spironolactone, and danazol. The discouraging results of these trials was not unexpected, given the shaky theoretical framework and the paucity of experimental support of the etiological models mentioned. The conceptual error contained in these studies is correctable, but the approach will require the scientific realism, commitment, and courage to "unpack" the assumption of categorical structure of disorder (Sonuga-Barke, 1998) into hypotheses that will be then put to empirical test before pro-

TABLE 2. Controversial Therapies for Common Functional Syndromes

	CFS	FM	IBS	PMS
Benzodiazepines		$-/-$		$+/-$
Free fatty acids	$+/-$			$-/-$
Immunoglobulin	$+/-$			
Cyclobenzaprine		$+/-$		
S-adenosylmethionine		$+/-$		
Smooth muscle relaxants			$+/-$	
Bulking agents			$+/-$	
Calcium channel blockers			$+/-$	
Cisapride			$+/-$	
GnRH agonists				$+/-$
Bromocriptine				$+/-$
Danazol				$+/-$

$+/-$ controversial therapy
$-/-$ ineffective therapy

ceeding to a treatment study. We may also have to overcome scientific rituals and repeated behaviors in which researchers, clinicians, and patients alike engage so often to promote the feeling of self-efficacy (Franzblau, 1997).

The second of the common denominators of ineffective or controversial drug therapies is the focus on remedies that can be bought over the counter, such as dietary fiber supplements, bulking agents, and lactase for irritable bowel syndrome; nonsteroidal analgesics for fibromyalgia and premenstrual syndrome; plant and fish oils for chronic fatigue syndrome and premenstrual syndrome; and vitamins and minerals for premenstrual syndrome. This may reflect a situation in which clinical reality influences scientific design, as over-the-counter drug prescribing by physicians is substantial (Pradel et al., 1999) and consists most often of nonsteroidal analgesics, vitamins and minerals, and laxatives (Stoehr et al., 1997). Research has also identified the fact that over-the-counter medication use is

TABLE 3. Ineffective Therapies for Common Functional Syndromes

	CFS	FM	IBS	PMS
Nonsteroidal anti-inflammatory		$-/-$		$-/-$
Hypnotic drugs		$-/-$		
Dietary fiber			$-/-$	
Lactase			$-/-$	
Ondansetron			$-/-$	
Progesterone				$-/-$
Estrogen				$-/-$
Beta-blockers				$-/-$
Spironolactone				$-/-$
Pyridoxine				$-/-$
Magnesium				$-/-$

$-/-$ ineffective therapy

directly correlated with female gender, higher education, and the presence of bodily pain (Johnson and Ried, 1996; Stoehr et al., 1997), all too common features of patients with chronic fatigue syndrome (Gunn, Connell, and Randall, 1993), fibromyalgia (Wolfe et al., 1995), irritable bowel syndrome (Talley, Zinmeister, and Melton, 1995), and premenstrual syndrome (Halbreich and Smoller, 1997). Here again we witness the interdependence between biological concepts of disease and social conceptions of health (Fulford, 1993), a relationship bridged by the illness experience of patients with common functional somatic syndromes and most deserving of our wisdom, discernment, and compassion.

References

Introduction

Abeles, M. (1998). "Fibromyalgia syndrome," in Manu, P. (Editor) *Functional Somatic Syndromes.* New York: Cambridge University Press, 32-57.

Barsky, A. J. and Borus, J. F. (1999). "Functional somatic syndromes," *Annals of Internal Medicine,* 130(11):910-921.

Demitrack, M. A. (1998). "Chronic fatigue syndrome and fibromyalgia. Dilemmas in diagnosis and clinical management," *Psychiatric Clinics of North America,* 21(3):671-692.

Drossman, D. A., Whitehead, W. E., and Camilleri, M. (1997). "Irritable bowel syndrome: A technical review for practice guideline development," *Gastroenterology,* 112(6):2120-2137.

Freeman, E. W. and Halbreich, U. (1998). "Premenstrual syndromes," *Psychopharmacology Bulletin,* 34(3):291-295.

Glasziou, P., Guyatt, G. H., Dans, A. L., Dans, L. F., Straus, S., and Sackett, D. L. (1998). "Applying the results of trials and systematic reviews to individual patients," *American College of Physicians Journal Club,* 129(3):A15-A16.

Goldenberg, D. L. (1999). "Fibromyalgia syndrome a decade later: What have we learned?" *Archives of Internal Medicine,* 159(8):777-785.

Komaroff, A. L. and Buchwald, D. S. (1998). "Chronic fatigue syndrome: An update," *Annual Review of Medicine,* 49:1-13.

Longstreth, G. F. (1998). "Irritable bowel syndrome," in Manu, P. (Editor) *Functional Somatic Syndromes.* New York: Cambridge University Press, 58-79.

Manu, P. (1998). "Definition and etiological theories," in Manu, P. (Editor) *Functional Somatic Syndromes.* New York: Cambridge University Press, 1-7.

Manu, P. and Matthews, D. A. (1998). "Chronic fatigue syndrome," in Manu, P. (Editor) *Functional Somatic Syndromes.* New York: Cambridge University Press, 8-31.

Maxwell, P. R., Mendall, M. A., and Kumar, D. (1997). "Irritable bowel syndrome," *Lancet,* 350(9902):1691-1695.

Meade, M. O. and Richardson, W. S. (1997). "Selecting and appraising studies for a systematic review," *Annals of Internal Medicine,* 127(7):531-537.

Oxman, A. D., Sackett, D. L., and Guyatt, G. H. (1993). "Users' guides to the medical literature. I. How to get started. The Evidence-Based Medicine Working Group," *Journal of the American Medical Association,* 270(17):2093-2095.

Pearlstein, T. (1998). "Premenstrual syndrome," in Manu, P. (Editor) *Functional Somatic Syndromes.* New York: Cambridge University Press, 80-97.

Pearlstein, T. and Stone, A. B. (1998). "Premenstrual syndrome," *Psychiatric Clinics of North America*, 21(3):577-590.

Sharpe, M., Bass, C., and Mayou, R. (1995). "An overview of the treatment of functional somatic symptoms," in Mayou, R., Bass, C., and Sharpe, M. (Editors) *Treatment of Functional Somatic Symptoms.* New York: Oxford University Press, 66-86.

Sharpe, M., Gill, D., Strain, J., and Mayou, R. (1996). "Psychosomatic medicine and evidence-based treatment," *Journal of Psychosomatic Research*, 41(2):101-107.

Simms, R.W. (1998). "Fibromyalgia is not a muscle disorder," *American Journal of Medical Sciences*, 315(6):346-350.

Section I

Abbott Laboratories. (1997). *Sterile Water for Injection USP.* Product Insert 06-9494-R6. North Chicago, Illinois: Abbott Laboratories.

American Hospital Formulary Service. (1997). *AHFS 97 Drug Information.* Bethesda, Maryland: American Society of Health-System Pharmacists.

Andersson, J., Britton, S., Ernberg, I., Andersson, U., Henle, W., Skoldenberg, B., and Tisell, A. (1986). "Effect of acyclovir on infectious mononucleosis: A double blind, placebo-controlled study," *Journal of Infectious Diseases*, 153(2):283-290.

Bates, D. W., Buchwald, D., Lee, J., Kith, P., Doolittle, T. H., Umali, P., and Komaroff, A. L. (1994). "A comparison of case definitions of chronic fatigue syndrome," *Clinical Infectious Diseases*, 18(Suppl 1):S11-S15.

Beck, A. T., Ward, C. H., Mendelson, M., Mock, J. E., and Rebaugh, J. K. (1961). "An inventory for measuring depression," *Archives of General Psychiatry*, 4(6):561-571.

Behan, P. O., Behan, W. M. H., and Horrobin, D. (1990). "Effect of high doses of essential fatty acids on the postviral fatigue syndrome," *Acta Neurologica Scandinavica*, 82(3):209-216.

Bennett, A. L., Fagioli, L. R., Schur, P. H., Schacterle, R. S., and Komaroff, A. L. (1996). "Immunoglobulin subclass levels in chronic fatigue syndrome," *Journal of Clinical Immunology*, 16(6):215-320.

Birkmayer, J. G. (1996). "Coenzyme nicotinamide adenine dinucleotide: New therapeutic approach for improving dementia of the Alzheimer type," *Annals of Clinical and Laboratory Science*, 26(1):1-9.

Birkmayer, W., Birkmayer, G. J., Vrecko, K., Mlekusch, W., Paletta, B., and Ott, E. (1989). "The coenzyme nicotinamide adenine dinucleotide (NADH) improves the disability of parkinsonian patients," *Journal of Neural Transmission. Parkinson Disease and Dementia Section*, 1(4):297-302.

Bou-Holaigh, I., Rowe, P. C., Kan, J., and Calkins, H. (1995). "The relationship between neurally mediated hypotension and the chronic fatigue syndrome," *Journal of the American Medical Association*, 274(12):961-967.

Clague, J. E., Edwards, R. H. T., and Jackson M. J. (1992). "Intravenous magnesium loading in chronic fatigue syndrome," *Lancet*, 340(8811):124-125.

Cleare, A. J., Bearn, J., Allain, T., McGregor, A., Wessely, S., Murray, R. M., and O'Keane, V. (1995). "Contrasting neuroendocrine responses in depression and chronic fatigue syndrome," *Journal of Affective Disorders*, 35(4):283-289.

Cleare, A. J., Heap, E., Malhi, G. S., Wessely, S., O'Keane, V., and Miell, J. (1999). "Low-dose hydrocortisone in chronic fatigue syndrome: A randomised crossover trial," *Lancet*, 353(9151):455-458.

Cleare, A. J., Murray, R. M., and O'Keane, V. (1996). "Reduced prolactin and cortisol responses to d-fenfluramine in depressed compared to healthy matched control subjects," *Neuropsychopharmacology*, 14(5):349-354.

Collins, A., Cerin, A., Coleman, G., and Landgren, B. M. (1993). "Essential fatty acids in the treatment of premenstrual syndrome," *Obstetrics and Gynecology*, 81(1):93-98.

Cox, I. M., Campbell, M. J., and Dowson, D. (1991). "Red blood cell magnesium and chronic fatigue syndrome," *Lancet*, 337(8744):757-760.

Deale, A., Chalder, T., Marks, I., and Wessely, S. (1997). "Cognitive behavior therapy for chronic fatigue syndrome: A randomized controlled trial," *American Journal of Psychiatry*, 154(3):408-414.

Deale, A., Chalder, T., and Wessely, S. (1998). "Illness beliefs and treatment outcome in chronic fatigue syndrome," *Journal of Psychosomatic Research*, 45 (1 Spec No):77-83.

Demitrack, M. A., Dale, J. K., Straus, S. E., Laue, L., Listwak, S. J., and Kruesi. M. J. P. (1991). "Evidence for impaired activation of the hypothalamic-pituitary-adrenal axis in patients with chronic fatigue syndrome," *Journal of Clinical Endocrinology and Metabolism*, 73(6):1224-1234.

Deulofeu, R., Gascon, J., Gimenez, N., and Corachan, M. (1991). "Magnesium and chronic fatigue syndrome," *Lancet*, 338(8767):641.

Dizdar, N., Kagedal, B., and Lindvall, B. (1994). "Treatment of Parkinson's disease with NADH," *Acta Neurologica Scandinavica*, 90(5):345-347.

Faber, W. R., Leiker, D. L., Nengerman, I. M., and Schellekens, P. T. (1979). "A placebo controlled clinical trial of transfer factor in lepromatous leprosy," *Clinical and Experimental Immunology*, 35(1):45-52.

Fischler, B., Dendale, P., Michiels, V., Cluydts, R., Kaufman, L., and De Meirleir, K. (1997). "Physical fatigability and exercise capacity in chronic fatigue syndrome: Association with disability, somatization and psychopathology," *Journal of Psychosomatic Research*, 42(4):369-378.

Forsyth, L. M., Preuss, H. G., MacDowell, A. L., Chiazze Jr., L., Birkmayer, G. D., and Bellanti, J. A. (1999). "Therapeutic effects of oral NADH on the symptoms of patients with chronic fatigue syndrome," *Annals of Allergy Asthma and Immunology*, 82(2):185-191.

Freeman, R. and Komaroff, A. L. (1997). "Does the chronic fatigue syndrome involve the autonomic nervous system," *American Journal of Medicine*, 102(4): 357-364.

Friedberg, F. and Krupp, L. B. (1994). "A comparison of cognitive behavioral treatment for chronic fatigue syndrome and primary depression," *Clinical Infectious Diseases*, 18(Suppl 1):S105-S110.

Fukuda, K., Straus, S. E., Hickie, I., Sharpe, M. C., Dobbins, J. C., Komaroff, A., and the International Chronic Fatigue Syndrome Study Group. (1994). "The chronic fatigue syndrome: A comprehensive approach to its definition and study," *Annals of Internal Medicine,* 121(12):953-959.

Fulcher, K. Y. and White, P. D. (1997). "Randomised controlled trial of graded exercise in patients with the chronic fatigue syndrome," *British Medical Journal,* 314(7095):1647-1652.

Gantz, N. M. (1991). "Magnesium and chronic fatigue," *Lancet,* 338(8758):66.

Graven-Nielsen, T., McArdle, A., Phoenix, J., Arendt-Nielsen, L., Jensen, T. S., Jackson, M. J., and Edwards, R. H. (1997). "In vivo model of muscle pain: Quantification of intramuscular chemical, electrical, and pressure changes associated with saline-induced muscle pain in humans," *Pain,* 69(1-2):137-143.

Harel, Z., Biro, F. M., Kottenhahn, R. K., and Rosenthal, S. L. (1996). "Supplementation with omega-3 polyunsaturated fatty acids in the management of dysmenorrhea in adolescents," *American Journal of Obstetrics and Gynecology,* 174(4):1335-1338.

Hinds, G., Bell, N. P., McMaster, D., and McCluskey, D. R. (1994). "Normal red cell magnesium concentration and magnesium loading tests in patients with chronic fatigue syndrome," *Annals of Clinical Biochemistry,* 31(Pt. 5):459-461.

Holmes, G. P., Kaplan, J. E., Gantz, N. M., Komaroff, A. L., Schonberger, L. B., Straus, S. E., Jones, J. F., Dubois, R. E., Cunningham-Rundles, C., Pahwa, S., Tosato, G., Zegans, L. S., Purtillo, D. T., Brown, N., Schooley, R. T., and Brus, I. (1988). "Chronic fatigue syndrome: A working case definition," *Annals of Internal Medicine,* 108(3):387-389.

Hovmark, A. and Ekre, H. P. (1978). "Failure of transfer factor therapy in atopic dermatitis," *Acta Dermatologica Venereologica,* 58(6):497-500.

Karnofsky, D., Abelmann, W., Craver, L., and Burchenal, J. (1948). "The use of nitrogen mustards in the palliative treatment of carcinoma," *Cancer,* 1(6):634-656.

Kaslow, J. E., Rucker, L., and Onishi, R. (1989). "Liver extract-folic acid-cyancobalamin versus placebo for chronic fatigue syndrome," *Archives of Internal Medicine,* 149(11):2501-2503.

Komaroff, A. L., Geiger, A. M., and Wormsely, S. (1988). "IgG subclass deficiencies in chronic fatigue syndrome," *Lancet,* 1(8597):1288-1289.

LaManca, J. J., Sisto, S. A., Zhou, X., Ottenweller, J. E., Cook, S., Peckerman, A., Zhang, Q., Denny, T. N., Gause, W. C., and Natelson, B. H. (1999). "Immunological response in chronic fatigue syndrome following a graded exercise test to exhaustion," *Journal of Clinical Immunology,* 19(2):135-142.

Lau, C. S., Morley, K. D., and Belch, J. J. (1993). "Effects of fish oil supplementation on nonsteroidal anti-inflammatory drug requirements in patients with mild rheumatoid arthritis. A double-blind placebo controlled study," *British Journal of Rheumatology,* 32(11):982-989.

Linde, A., Andersson, B., Svenson, S. B., Ahrne, H., Carlsson, M., Forsberg, P., Hugo, H., Karstorp, A., Lenkei, R., and Lindwall, A. (1992). "Serum levels of lymphokines and soluble cellular receptors in primary Epstein-Barr virus infection and in patients with chronic fatigue syndrome," *Journal of Infectious Diseases,* 165(6):994-1000.

Linde, A., Hammarstrom, L., and Smith, C. I. (1988). "IgG subclass deficiency and chronic fatigue syndrome," *Lancet,* 1(8590):885-886.

Lloyd, A., Gandevia, S., Brockman, A., Hales, J., and Wakefield, D. (1994). "Cytokine production and fatigue in patients with chronic fatigue syndrome and healthy control subjects in response to exercise," *Clinical Infectious Diseases,* 18(Suppl 1):S142-146.

Lloyd, A. R., Hickie, I., Boughton, C. R., Spencer, O., and Wakefield, D. (1990). "Prevalence of chronic fatigue syndrome in an Australian population," *Medical Journal of Australia,* 153(9):522-528.

Lloyd, A. R., Hickie, I., Brockman, A., Hickie, C., Wilson, A., Dwyer, J., and Wakefield, D. (1993). "Immunologic and psychologic therapy for patients with chronic fatigue syndrome: A double-blind, placebo-controlled trial," *American Journal of Medicine,* 94(2):197-202.

Lloyd, A., Hickie, I., Wakefield, D., Boughton, C., and Dwyer, J. (1990). "A double-blind, placebo-controlled trial of intravenous immunoglobulin therapy in patients with chronic fatigue syndrome," *American Journal of Medicine,* 89(5):561-568.

Lloyd, A. R., Wakefield, D., Boughton, C.R., and Dwyer, J. M. (1989). "Immunological abnormalities in the chronic fatigue syndrome," *Medical Journal of Australia,* 151(3):122-124.

Mann, J. J., Aarons, S. F., Wilner, P. J., Keilp, J. G., Sweeney, J. A., Pearlstein, T., Frances, A. J., Kocsis, J. H., and Brown, R. P. (1989). "A controlled study of the antidepressant efficacy and side effects of (-)-deprenyl, a selective monoamine oxidase inhibitor," *Archives of General Psychiatry,* 46(1):45-50.

McKenzie, R., O'Fallon, A., Dale, J., Demitrack, M., Sharma, G., Deloria, M., Garcia-Borreguero, D., Blackwelder, W., and Straus, S. (1998). "Low-dose hydrocortisone for treatment of chronic fatigue syndrome: A randomized controlled trial," *Journal of the American Medical Association,* 280(12):1061-1066.

Miller, L. L., Spitler, L. E., Allen, R. E., and Minor, D. R. (1988). "A randomized, double-blind, placebo-controlled trial of transfer factor as adjuvant therapy for malignant melanoma," *Cancer,* 61(8):1543-1549.

Mobacken, H., Hanson, L. A., Lindholm, L., and Ljunggren, C. (1980). "Transfer factor in the treatment of chronic mucocutaneous candidiasis: A controlled study," *Acta Dermatologica Venereologica,* 60(1):51-55.

Natelson, B. H., Cheu, J., Hill, N., Bergen, M., Korn, L., Denny, T., and Dahl, K. (1998). "Single-blind, placebo phase-in-trial of two escalating doses of selegiline in the chronic fatigue syndrome," *Neuropsychobiology,* 37(3):150-154.

Natelson, B. H., Cheu, J., Pareja, J., Ellis, S. P., Policastro, T., and Findley, T. W. (1996). "Randomized, double blind, controlled placebo-phase in trial of low dose phenelzine in the chronic fatigue syndrome," *Psychopharmacology,* 124(3):226-230.

National Institute of Allergy and Infectious Diseases. (1996). *Chronic Fatigue Syndrome: Information for Physicians.* Bethesda, Maryland: National Institute of Health, Public Health Service, U.S. Department of Health and Human Services.

O'Keane, V. and Dinan, T. G. (1991). "Prolactin and cortisol responses to d-fenfluramine in major depression: Evidence for diminished responsivity of central serotonergic function," *American Journal of Psychiatry,* 148(8):1009-1015.

Olarte, M. R., Gersten, J. C., Zabriskie, J., and Rowland, L. P. (1979). "Transfer factor is ineffective in amyotrophic lateral sclerosis," *Annals of Neurology,* 5(4):385-388.

Pagano, J. S., Sixbey, J. W., and Lin, J. C. (1983). "Acyclovir and Epstein-Barr virus infection," *Journal of Antimicrobial Chemotherapy,* 12(Suppl B):113-121.

Peterson, P. K., Pheley, A., Schroeppel, J., Schenck, C., Marshall, P., Kind, A., Haugland, J. M., Lambrecht, L. J., Swan, S., and Goldsmith, S. (1998). "A preliminary placebo-controlled crossover trial of fludrocortisone for chronic fatigue syndrome," *Archives of Internal Medicine,* 158(8):908-914.

Peterson, P. K., Shepard, J., Macres, M., Schenck, C., Crosson, J., Rechtman, D., and Lurie, N. (1990). "A controlled trial of immunoglobulin G in chronic fatigue syndrome," *American Journal of Medicine,* 89(5):554-560.

Read, R., Spickett, G., Harvey, J., Edwards, A. J., and Larson, H. E. (1988). "IgG1 subclass deficiency in patients with chronic fatigue syndrome," *Lancet,* 1(8579): 241-242.

Rowe, K. S. (1997). "Double-blind randomized controlled trial to assess the efficacy of intravenous gammaglobulin for the management of chronic fatigue syndrome," *Journal of Psychiatric Research,* 31(1):133-147.

Sawyer, M. H., Webb, D. E., Balow, J. E., and Straus, S. E. (1988). "Acyclovir-induced renal failure. Clinical course and histology," *American Journal of Medicine,* 84(6):1067-1071.

See, D. M. and Tilles, J. G. (1996). "Alpha interferon treatment of patients with chronic fatigue syndrome," *Immunological Investigations,* 25(1-2):153-164.

Sharpe, M. C., Archard, L. C., Banatvala, J. E., Borysiewicz, L. K., Clare, A. W., David, A., Edwards, R. H., Hawton, K. E., Lambert, H. P., and Lane, R. J. (1991). "Chronic fatigue syndrome: Guidelines for research," *Journal of the Royal Society of Medicine,* 84(2):118-121.

Sharpe, M., Hawton, K., Clements, A., and Cowen, P. J. (1997). "Increased brain serotonin function in men with chronic fatigue syndrome," *British Medical Journal,* 315(7101):164-165.

Sharpe, M., Hawton, K., Simkin, S., Surawy, C., Hackmann, A., Klimes, I., Peto, T., Warrell, D., and Seagroatt, V. (1996). "Cognitive behaviour therapy for the chronic fatigue syndrome: A randomised controlled trial," *British Medical Journal,* 312(7022):22-26.

Siever, L. J., Murphy, D. L., Slater, S., De La Vega, E., and Lipper, S. (1984). "Plasma prolactin changes following fenfluramine in depressed patients compared to controls: An evaluation of central serotonergic responsivity in depression," *Life Sciences,* 34(11):1029-1039.

Stainforth, J. M., Layton, A. M., and Goodfield, M. J. (1996). "Clinical aspects of the use of gamma linolenic acid in systemic sclerosis," *Acta Dermatologica Venereologica,* 76(2):144-146.

Steinberg, P., McNutt, B. E., Marshall, P., Schenck, C., Lurie, N., Pheley, A., and Peterson, P. K. (1996). "Double-blind placebo-controlled study of the efficacy of oral terfenadine in the treatment of chronic fatigue syndrome," *Journal of Allergy and Clinical Immunology,* 97(1, Pt. 1):119-126.

Straus, S. E. (1990). "Intravenous immunoglobulin treatment for the chronic fatigue syndrome," *American Journal of Medicine,* 89(5):551-553.

Straus, S. E., Dale, J. K., Tobi, M., Lawley, T., Preble, O., Blaese, M., Hallahan, C., and Henle, W. (1988). "Acyclovir treatment of the chronic fatigue syndrome: Lack of efficacy in a placebo-controlled trial," *New England Journal of Medicine,* 310(26):1692-1698.

Straus, S. E., Dale, J. K., Wright, R., and Metcalfe, D. D. (1988). "Allergy and the chronic fatigue syndrome," *Journal of Allergy and Clinical Immunology,* 81(5, Pt. 1):791-795.

Strayer, D. R., Carter, W. A., Brodsky, I., Cheney, P., Peterson, D., Salvato, P., Thompson, C., Loveless, M., Shapiro, D. E., Elsasser, W., and Gillespie, D. H. (1994). "A controlled clinical trial with a specifically configured RNA drug, Poly(I)-Poly (C12U), in chronic fatigue syndrome," *Clinical Infectious Diseases,* 18(Suppl 1):S88-S95.

Suhadolnik, R. J., Reichenbach, N. L., Hitzges, P., Adelson, M. E., Peterson, D. L., Cheney, P., Salvato, P., Thompson, C., Loveless, M., Muller, W. E. G., Schroder, H. C., Strayer, D., and Carter, W. A. (1994). "Changes in the 2-5A synthetase/Rnase L antiviral pathway in a controlled clinical trial with Poly(I)-Poly(C12U) in chronic fatigue syndrome," *In Vivo,* 8(4):599-604.

Sunderland, T., Cohen, R. M., Molchan, S., Lawlor, B. A., Mellow, A. M., Newhouse, P. A., Tariot, P. N., Mueller, E. A., and Murphy, D. I. (1994). "High-dose selegiline in treatment-resistant older depressive patients," *Archives of General Psychiatry,* 51(8):607-615.

Thase, M. E., Frank, E., Mallinger, A. G., Hamer, T., and Kupfer, D. J. (1992). "Treatment of imipramine-resistant recurrent depression, III: Efficacy of monoamine oxidase inhibitors," *Journal of Clinical Psychiatry,* 53(1):5-11.

Trissel, L. A. (1990). "Magnesium sulfate," in Trissel, L. A. (Editor), *Handbook on Injectable Drugs.* Bethesda, Maryland: American Society of Hospital Pharmacists, p. 457.

Tynell, E., Aurelius, E., Brandell, A., Julander, I., Wood, M., Yao, Q. Y., Rickinson, A., Akerlund, B., and Andersson, J. (1996). "Acyclovir and prednisolone treatment of acute infectious mononucleosis: A multicenter, double-blind, placebo-controlled study," *Journal of Infectious Diseases,* 174(2):324-331.

Tyrer, P., Gardner, M., Lambourn, J., and Whitford, M. (1980). "Clinical and pharmacologic factors affecting response to phenelzine," *British Journal of Psychiatry,* 136(April):359-365.

van der Horst, C., Joncas, J., Ahronheim, G., Gustafson, N., Stein, G., Gurwith, M., Fleisher, G., Sullivan, J., Sixbey, J., and Roland, S. (1991). "Lack of effect of peroral acyclovir for the treatment of acute infectious mononucleosis," *Journal of Infectious Diseases*, 164(4):788-792.

Vercoulen, J. H. M. M., Swanink, C. M. A., Zitman, F. G., Vreden, S. G. S., Hoofs, M. P. E., Fennis, J. F. M., Galama, J. M. D., van der Meer, J. W. M., and Bleijenberg, G. (1996). "Randomized, double-blind, placebo-controlled study of fluoxetine in chronic fatigue syndrome," *Lancet*, 347(9005):858-861.

Vicary, F. R., Chambers, J. D., and Dhillon, P. (1979). "Double-blind trial of the use of transfer factor in the treatment of Crohn's disease," *Gut*, (5):408-413.

Vollmer-Conna, U., Hickie, I., Hadzi-Pavlovic, D., Tymms, K., Wakefield, D., Dwyer, L., and Lloyd, A. (1997). "Intravenous immunoglobulin is ineffective in the treatment of patients with chronic fatigue syndrome," *American Journal of Medicine*, 103(1):38-43.

Warren, G., McKendrick, M., and Peet, M. (1999). "The role of essential fatty acids in chronic fatigue syndrome. A case-controlled study of red-cell membrane essential fatty acids (EFA) and a placebo-controlled treatment study with high dose of EFA," *Acta Neurologica Scandinavica*, 99(2):112-116.

Wearden, A. J., Morriss, R. K., Mullis, R., Strickland, P. L., Pearson, D. J., Appleby, L., Campbell, I. T., and Morris, J. A. (1998). "Randomised, double-blind, placebo-controlled treatment trial of fluoxetine and graded exercise for chronic fatigue syndrome," *British Journal of Psychiatry*, 172(June):485-490.

Wilson, A., Hickie, I., Lloyd, A., and Wakefield, D. (1994). "The treatment of chronic fatigue syndrome: Science and speculation," *American Journal of Medicine*, 96(6):544-550.

Yataco, A., Talo, H., Rowe, P., Kass, D. A., Berger, R. D., and Calkins, H. (1997). "A comparison of heart rate variability in patients with chronic fatigue syndrome and controls," *Clinical Autonomic Research*, 7(6):293-297.

Yatham, L. N., Morehouse, R. L., Chisholm, T., Haase, D. A., MacDonald, D. D., and Marrie, T. J. (1995). "Neuroendocrine assessment of serotonin (5-HT) function in chronic fatigue syndrome," *Canadian Journal of Psychiatry*, 40(2):93-96.

Zurier, R. B., Rossetti, R. G., Jacobson E. W., DeMarco, D. M., Liu, N. Y., Temming, J. E., White, B. M., and Laposata, M. (1996). "gamma-Linolenic acid treatment of rheumatoid arthritis. A randomized, placebo-controlled trial," *Arthritis and Rheumatism*, 39(11):1808-1817.

Section II

Abeles, M. (1998). "Fibromyalgia syndrome," in Manu, P. (Editor) *Functional Somatic Syndromes*. New York: Cambridge University Press, 32-57.

Ahles, T. A., Khan, S. A., Yunus, M. B., Spiegel, D. A., and Masi, A. T. (1991). "Psychiatric status of patients with primary fibromyalgia, patients with rheumatoid arthritis, and subjects without pain; a blind comparison of DSM-III diagnoses," *American Journal of Psychiatry*, 148(12):1721-1726.

Alfici, S., Sigal, M., and Landau, M. (1989). "Primary fibromyalgia syndrome—a variant of depressive disorder?" *Psychotherapy and Psychosomatics*, 51(3): 156-161.

American Hospital Formulary Service (1997). *AHFS 97 Drug Information*. Bethesda, MD: American Society of Health-System Pharmacists.

Basmajian, J. V. (1989). "Acute back pain and spasm. A controlled multicenter trial of combined analgesic and antispasm agents," *Spine*, 14(4):438-439.

Bengtsson A., Henriksson, K. G., and Larsson, J. (1986). "Reduced high energy phosphate levels in the painful muscles of patients with primary fibromyalgia," *Arthritis and Rheumatism*, 29(7):817-821.

Bennett, R. M., Clark, S. R., Campbell, S. M., and Burckhardt, C. S. (1992). "Low levels of somatomedin C in patients with the fibromyalgia syndrome. A possible link between sleep and muscle pain," *Arthritis and Rheumatism*, 35(10):1113-1115.

Bennett, R. M., Clark, S. C., and Walczyk, J. (1998). "A randomized, double-blind, placebo-controlled study of growth hormone in the treatment of fibromyalgia," *American Journal of Medicine*, 104(3):227-231.

Bennett, R. M., Gatter, R. A., Campbell, S. M., Andrews, R. P., Clark, S. R., and Sarola, J. A. (1988). "A comparison of cyclobenzaprine and placebo in the management of fibrositis," *Arthritis and Rheumatism*, 31(12):1535-1542.

Bessette, L., Carette, S., Fossel, A. H., and Lew, R. A. (1998). "A placebo controlled crossover trial of subcutaneous salmon calcitonin in the treatment of patients with fibromyalgia," *Scandinavian Journal of Rheumatology*, 27(2):112-116.

Borenstein, D. G., Lacks, S., and Wiesel, S. W. (1990). "Cyclobenzaprine and naproxen versus naproxen alone in the treatment of acute low back pain and muscle spasm," *Clinical Therapeutics*, 12(2):125-131.

Buckelew, S. P., Conway, R., Parker, J., Deuser, W. E., Read, J., Witty, T. E., Hewett, J. E., Minor, M., Johnson J. C., Van Male, L., McIntosh, M. J., Nigh, M., and Kay, D. R. (1998). "Biofeedback/relaxation training and exercise interventions in fibromyalgia: A prospective trial," *Arthritis Care and Research*, 11(3):196-209.

Burckhardt, C. S., Clark, S. R., and Bennett, R. M. (1991). "The fibromyalgia impact questionnaire: Development and validation," *Journal of Rheumatology*, 18(5): 728-733.

Burckhardt, C. S., Mannerkorpi, K., Hedenberg, L., and Bjelle, A. (1994). "A randomized, controlled clinical trial of education and physical training for women with fibromyalgia," *Journal of Rheumatology*, 21(4):714-720.

Carette, S., Bell, M. J., Reynolds, W. J., Haraoui, B., McCain, G. A., Bykerk, V. P., Edworthy, S. M., Baron, M., Koehler, B. E., Fam, A. G., Bellamy, N., and Guimont, C. (1994). "Comparison of amitriptyline, cyclobenzaprine, and placebo in the treatment of fibromyalgia. A randomized, double-blind clinical trial," *Arthritis and Rheumatism*, 37(1):32-40.

Carette, S., McCain, G. A., Bell, D. A., and Fam, A. G. (1986). "Evaluation of amitriptyline in primary fibrositis. A double-blind, placebo-controlled study," *Arthritis and Rheumatism*, 29(5):655-659.

Caruso, I. and Pietrogrande, V. (1987). "Italian double-blind multicenter study comparing S-adenosylmethionine, naproxen, and placebo in the treatment of degenerative joint disease," *American Journal of Medicine*, 83(Suppl 5A):66-71.

Caruso, I., Sarzi Puttini, P. C., Boccassini, L., Santandrea, S., Locati, M., Volpato, R., Montrone, F., Benvenuti, C., and Beretta, A. (1987). "Double-blind study of dothiepin versus placebo in the treatment of primary fibromyalgia syndrome," Journal of International Medical Research, 15(3):154-159.

Cathey, M. A., Wolfe, F., and Kleinheksel, S. M. (1986). "Socioeconomic impact of fibrositis: A study of 81 patients with primary fibrositis," American Journal of Medicine, 81(Suppl 3A):78-84.

Clark, S., Tindall, E., and Bennett, R. M. (1985). "A double blind crossover trial of prednisone versus placebo in the treatment of fibrositis," Journal of Rheumatology, 12(5):980-983.

Cohn, L., Feller, A. G., Draper, M. W., Rudman, I. W., and Rudman, D. (1993). "Carpal tunnel syndrome and gynecomastia during growth hormone treatment of elderly men with low circulating IGF-1 concentrations," Clinical Endocrinology (Oxford), 39(7):417-425.

Commissiong, J. W., Karoum, F., Reiffenstein, R. J., and Neff, N. H. (1981). "Cyclobenzaprine: A possible mechanism of action for its muscle relaxant effect," Canadian Journal of Physiology and Pharmacology, 59(1):37-44.

Drewes, A. M., Andreasen, A., Jennum, P., and Nielsen, K. D. (1991). "Zopiclone in the treatment of sleep abnormalities in fibromyalgia," Scandinavian Journal of Rheumatology, 20(4):288-293.

Goldenberg, D. L., Felson, D. T., and Dinerman, H. (1986). "A randomized, controlled trial of amitriptyline and naproxen in the treatment of patients with fibromyalgia," Arthritis and Rheumatism, 29(11):1371-1377.

Goldenberg, D., Mayskiy, M., Mossey, C., Ruthazer, R., and Schmid, C. (1996). "A randomized, double-blind crossover trial of fluoxetine and amitriptyline in the treatment of fibromyalgia," Arthritis and Rheumatism, 39(11):1852-1859.

Gronblad, M., Nykanen, J., Konttinen, Y., Jarvinen, E., and Helve, T. (1993). "Effect of zopiclone on sleep quality, morning stiffness, widespread tenderness and pain and general discomfort in primary fibromyalgia patients: A double-blind randomized trial," Clinical Rheumatology, 12(2):186-191.

Hannonen, P., Malminiemi, K., Yli-Kerttula, U., Isomeri, R., and Roponen, P. (1998). "A randomized, double-blind, placebo-controlled study of moclobemide and amitryptiline in the treatment of fibromyalgia in females without psychiatric disorder," British Journal of Rheumatology, 37:1279-1286.

Houvenagel, E., Forzy, G., Leloire, O., Gallois, P., Hary, S., Hautecoeur, P., Convain, L., Henniaux, M., Vincent, G., and Dhondt, J. L. (1990). "Cerebrospinal fluid monoamines in primary fibromyalgia" (in French), Revue du Rhumatisme et de Maladies Osteo-Articulaires, 57(1):21-23.

Hrycaj, P., Stratz, T., Mennet, T. P., and Muller, W. (1996). "Pathogenetic aspects of responsiveness to ondansetron (5-hydroxytryptamine type 3 receptor antagonist) in patients with primary fibromyalgia syndrome. A preliminary study," Journal of Rheumatology, 23(8):1418-1423.

Hudson J. I., Hudson, M. S., Pliner, L. F., Goldenberg, D. L., and Pope, H. G. Jr. (1985). "Fibromyalgia and major affective disorder: A controlled phenomenology and family history study," American Journal of Psychiatry, 142(4):441-446.

Jacobsen, S., Danneskiold-Samsoe, B., and Bach Andersen, R. (1991). "Oral S-adenosylmethionine in primary fibromyalgia. Double-blind clinical evaluation," *Scandinavian Journal of Rheumatology,* 20(4):294-392.

Kagan, B. L., Sultzer, D. L., Rosenlicht, N., and Gerner, R. H. (1990). "Oral S-adenosylmethionine in depression: A randomized, double-blind, placebo-controlled trial," *American Journal of Psychiatry,* 147(5):591-595.

Kameyama, S., Tanaka, R., Hasegawa, A., Tamura, T., and Kuroki, M. (1993). "Subclinical carpal tunnel syndrome in acromegaly," *Neurologia Medico-Chirurgica (Tokyo),* 33(8):547-551.

Katz, R. S. and Kravitz, H. M. (1996). "Fibromyalgia, depression and alcoholism: A family history study," *Journal of Rheumatology,* 23(1):149-154.

Keel, P. J., Bodoky, C., Gerhard, U., and Muller, W. (1998). "Comparison of integrated group therapy and group relaxation training for fibromyalgia," *Clinical Journal of Pain,* 14(3):232-238.

Kirmayer, L. J., Robbins, J. M., and Kapusta, M. A. (1988). "Somatization and depression in fibromyalgia syndrome," *American Journal of Psychiatry,* 145(8): 950-954.

Klein, R., Bansch, M., and Berg, P. A. (1992). "Clinical relevance of antibodies against serotonin and gangliosides in patients with primary fibromyalgia syndrome," *Psychoneuroendocrinology,* 17(6):593-598.

Kobayashi, H., Hasegawa, Y., and Ono, H. (1996). "Cyclobenzaprine, a centrally acting muscle relaxant, acts on descending serotonergic systems," *European Journal of Pharmacology,* 311(1):29-35.

Krag, N. J., Norregaard, J., Larsen, J. K., and Danneskiold-Samsoe, B. (1994). "A blinded, controlled evaluation of anxiety and depressive symptoms in patients with fibromyalgia as measured by standardized psychometric scales," *Acta Psychiatrica Scandinavica,* 89(6):370-379.

Kravitz, H. M., Katz, R., Kot, E., Helmke, N., and Fawcett, J. (1992). "Biochemical clues to a fibromyalgia-depression link: Imipramine binding in patients with fibromyalgia or depression and in healthy controls," *Journal of Rheumatology,* 19(9):1428-1432.

Martin, L., Nutting, A., MacIntosh, B. R., Edworthy, S. M., Butterwick, D., and Cook, J. (1996). "An exercise program in the treatment of fibromyalgia," *Journal of Rheumatology,* 23(6):1050-1053.

McCain, G. A., Bell, D. A., Mai, F. M., and Halliday, P. D. (1988). "A controlled study of the effects of a supervised cardiovascular fitness training program on the manifestations of primary fibromyalgia," *Arthritis and Rheumatism,* 31(9):1135 1141.

Mengshoel, A. M., Komnaes, H. B., and Forre, O. (1992). "The effect of 20 weeks of physical fitness training in female patients with fibromyalgia," *Clinical and Experimental Rheumatology,* 10(4):345-349.

Mengshoel, A. M., Vollestad, N. K., and Forre, O. (1995). "Pain and fatigue induced by exercise in fibromyalgia patients and sedentary subjects," *Clinical and Experimental Rheumatology,* 13(4):477-482.

Moldotsky, H., Lue, F. A., Mously, C., Roth-Schechter, B., and Reynolds, W. J. (1996). "The effect of zolpidem in patients with fibromyalgia: A dose ranging double blind, placebo controlled, modified crossover study," *Journal of Rheumatology,* 23(3):529-533.

Moldofsky, H., Scarisbrick, P., England, R., and Smythe, H. (1975). "Musculo-skeletal symptoms and non-REM sleep disturbance in patients with fibrositis syndrome, and healthy subjects," *Psychosomatic Medicine,* 37(4):341-351.

Mouret, J., Ruel, D., Maillard, F., and Bianchi, M. (1990). "Zopiclone versus triazolam in insomniac geriatric patients: A specific increase in delta sleep with zopiclone," *International Clinical Psychopharmacology,* 5(Suppl 2):47-55.

Nicassio, P. M., Radojevic, V., Weisman, M. H., Schuman, C., Kim, J., Schoenfeld-Smith, K., and Krall, T. (1997). "A comparison of behavioral and educational interventions for fibromyalgia," *Journal of Rheumatology,* 24(10):2000-2007.

Nichols, D. S. and Glenn, T. M. (1994). "Effects of aerobic exercise on pain perception, affect, and level of disability in individuals with fibromyalgia," *Physical Therapy,* 74(4):327-332.

Norregaard, J., Wolkmann, H., and Danneskiold-Samsoe, B. (1995). "A randomized controlled trial of citalopram in the treatment of fibromyalgia," *Pain,* 61(3):445-449.

Olin, R., Klein, R., and Berg, P. A. (1998). "A randomised double-blind 16-week study of ritanserin in fibromyalgia syndrome: Clinical outcome and analysis of autoantibodies to serotonin, gangliosides and phospholipids," *Clinical Rheumatology,* 17(2):89-94.

Patat, A., Trocherie, S., Thebault, J. J., Rosenzweig, P., Dubruc, C., Bianchetti, G., Court, L. A., and Morselli, P. L. (1994). "EEG profile of intravenous zolpidem in healthy volunteers," *Psychopharmacology,* 114(1):138-146.

Pattrick, M., Swanell, A., and Doherty, M. (1993). "Chlormezanone in primary fibromyalgia syndrome: A double blind placebo controlled syndrome," *British Journal of Rheumatology,* 32(1):55-58.

Quijada-Carrera, J., Valenzuela-Castano, A., Povedano-Gomez, J., Fernadez-Rodriguez, A., Hernanz-Mediano, W., Gutierrez-Rubio, A., De la Iglesia-Salgado, J. L., and Garcia-Lopez, A. (1996). "Comparison of tenoxicam and bromazepan in the treatment of fibromyalgia: A randomized, double-blind, placebo-controlled trial," *Pain,* 65(2-3):221-225.

Quimby, L. G., Gratwick, G. M., Whitney, C. D., and Block, S. R. (1989). "A randomized trial of cyclobenzaprine for the treatment of fibromyalgia," *Journal of Rheumatology,* 16(Suppl 19): 140-143.

Reynolds, W. J., Moldofsky, H., Saskin, P., and Lue, F. A. (1991). "The effects of cyclobenzaprine on sleep physiology and symptoms in patients with fibromyalgia," *Journal of Rheumatology,* 18(3):452-454.

Russell, I. J., Fletcher, E. M., Michalek, J. E., McBroom, P. C., and Hester, G. G. (1991). "Treatment of primary fibrositis/fibromyalgia syndrome with ibuprofen and alprazolam. A double-blind, placebo-controlled study," *Arthritis and Rheumatism,* 34(5):552-560.

Russell, I. J., Michalek, J. E., Flechas, J. D., and Abraham, G. E. (1995). "Treatment of fibromyalgia syndrome with Super Malic: A randomized, double blind, placebo controlled, crossover pilot study," *Journal of Rheumatology,* 22(5):953-958.

Russell, I. J., Michalek, J. E., Vipraio, G. A., Fletcher, E. M., Javors, M. A., and Bowden, C. A. (1992). "Platelet 3H-imipramine uptake receptor density and serum serotonin levels in patients with fibromyalgia/fibrositis syndrome," *Journal of Rheumatology,* 19(1):104-109.

Russell, I. J., Vaeroy, H., Javors, M., and Nyberg, F. (1992). "Cerebrospinal biogenic amine metabolites in fibromyalgia/fibrositis syndrome and rheumatoid arthritis," *Arthritis and Rheumatism,* 35(5):550-556.

Salmaggi, P., Bressa, G. M., Nicchia, G., Coniglio, M., La Greca, P., Le Grazie, C. (1993). "Double-blind, placebo-controlled study of S-Adenosyl-L-Methionine in depressed postmenopausal women," *Psychotherapy and Psychosomatics,* 59(1): 34-40.

Scudds, R. A., McCain, G. A., Rollman, G. B., and Harth, M. (1989). "Improvements in pain responsiveness in patients with fibrositis after successful treatment with amitriptyline," *Journal of Rheumatology,* 16 (Suppl 19):98-103.

Simms, R. W. (1994). "Controlled trials of therapy in fibromyalgia syndrome," *Bailliere's Clinical Rheumatology,* 8(4):917-934.

Simms, R. W., Felson, D. T., and Goldenberg, D. L. (1991). "Development of preliminary criteria for response to treatment in fibromyalgia syndrome," *Journal of Rheumatology,* 18(10):1558-1663.

Stratz, T., Samborski, W., Hrycaj, P., Pap, T., Mackiewicz, S., Mennet, P., and Muller, W. (1993). "Serotonin concentration in serum of patients with generalized tendomyopathy (fibromyalgia) and chronic polyarthritis," (in German) *Medizinische Klinik,* 88(8):458-462.

Tavoni, A., Vitali, C., Bombardieri, S., and Pasero, G. (1987). Evaluation of S-adenosylmethionine in primary fibromyalgia. A double-blind crossover trial," *American Journal of Medicine,* 83(Suppl 5A):107-110.

Vlaeyen, J. W., Teeken-Gruben, N. J., Goossens, M. E., Rutten-van Molken, M. P., van Eek, H., and Heuts, P. H. (1996). "Cognitive-educational treatment of fibromyalgia: A randomized clinical trial. I. Clinical effects," *Journal of Rheumatology,* 23(7):1237-1245.

Volkman, H., Norregard, J., Jacobsen, S., Danneskiold-Samsoe, B., Knoke, G., and Nehrdich, D. (1997). "Double-blind placebo-controlled cross-over study of intravenous S-Adenosyl-L-Methionine in patients with fibromyalgia," *Scandinavian Journal of Rheumatology,* 26(3):206-211.

White, K. P. and Harth, M. (1996). "An analytical review of 24 controlled clinical trials for fibromyalgia syndrome (FMS)," *Pain,* 64(2):211-219.

Wolfe, F., Cathey, M. A., and Hawley, D. J. (1994). "A double-blind placebo controlled trial of fluoxetine in fibromyalgia," *Scandinavian Journal of Rheumatology,* 23(5):255-259.

Wolfe, F., Russell, I. J., Vipraio, G., Ross, K., and Anderson, J. (1997). "Serotonin levels, pain threshold, and fibromyalgia symptoms in the general population," *Journal of Rheumatology,* 24(3):555-559.

Wolfe, F., Smythe, H. A., Yunus, M. B., Bennett, R. M., Bombardier, C., Goldenberg, D. L., Tugwell, P., Campbell, S. M., Abeles, M., Clark, P., Fam, A. G., Farber, S. J., Fiechtner, J. J., Franklin, C. M., Gatter, R. A., Hamaty, D., Lessard, J., Lichtbroun, A. S., Masi, A. T., McCain, G. A., Reynolds, W. J., Romano, T. J., Russell I. J., and Sheon, R. P. (1990). "The American College of Rheumatology 1990 criteria for the classification of fibromyalgia: Report of the multicenter criteria committee," *Arthritis and Rheumatism,* 33(2):160-177.

Yamadera, H., Kato, M., Tsukahara, Y., Kajimura, N., and Okuma, T. (1997). "Relationship between the effects of a hypnotic drug, zopiclone, on polysomnography and on daytime EEGs," *Neuropsychobiology,* 35(3):152-153.

Yunus, M. B., Masi, A. T., and Aldag, J. C. (1989). "Short term effects of ibuprofen in primary fibromyalgia syndrome: A double blind, placebo controlled trial," *Journal of Rheumatology,* 16(4):527-532.

Yunus, M., Masi, A. T., Calabro, J. J., Miller, K. A., and Feigenbaum, S. L. (1981). "Primary fibromyalgia (fibrositis): Clinical study of 50 patients with matched normal controls," *Seminars in Arthritis and Rheumatism,* 11(1):151-171.

Section III

American Hospital Formulary Service. (1997). *AHFS 97 Drug Information.* Bethesda, Maryland: American Society of Health-System Pharmacists.

Arffmann, S., Andersen, J. R., Hegnhoj, J., Schaffalitzky, O. B., Muckadell, D. E., Mogensen, N. B., and Krag, E. (1985). "The effect of coarse wheat bran in the irritable bowel syndrome. A double-blind cross-over study," *Scandinavian Journal of Gastroenterology,* 20(3):295-298.

Arseculeratne, S. N., Gunatilaka, A. A., and Panabokke, R. G. (1985). "Studies of medicinal plants of Sri Lanka. Part 14: Toxicity of some traditional medicinal herbs," *Journal of Ethnopharmacology,* 13(3):323-335.

Awad, R. A., Cordova, V. H., Dibildox, M., Santiago, R., and Camacho, S. (1997). "Reduction of post-prandial motility by pinaverium bromide, a calcium channel blocker acting selectively on the gastrointestinal tract in patients with irritable bowel syndrome," *Acta Gastroenterologica Latinoamericana,* 27(4):247-51.

Awad, R., Dibildox, M., and Ortiz, F. (1995). "Irritable bowel syndrome treatment using pinaverium bromide as a calcium channel blocker. A randomized double blind placebo-controlled trial," *Acta Gastroenterologica Latinoamericana,* 25(3): 137-144.

Baldi, F., Longanesi, A., Blasi, A., Monello, S., Cestari, R., Missale, G., Corazziari, E., Badiali, G., Marzio, L., Di Felice, F., Pescatori, M., Anastasio, G., Surrenti, C., Salvadori, G., Tittobello, A., Passaretti, S., Colonna, C. V., and Formica, N. (1992). "Octylonium bromide in the treatment of the irritable bowel syndrome: A clinical-functional study," *Hepato-Gastroenterology,* 39(5):392-395.

Battaglia, G., Morselli-Labate, A. M., Camarri, E., Francavilla, A., DeMarco, F., Mastropaolo, G., and Naccarato, R. (1998). "Otilonium bromide in irritable bowel syndrome: A double-blind, placebo-controlled, 15-week study," *Alimentary Pharmacology and Therapeutics,* 12(10):1003-1010.

Bensoussan, A., Talley, N. J., Hing, M., Menzies, R., Guo, A., and Ngu, M. (1998). "Treatment of irritable bowel syndrome with Chinese herbal medicine. A randomized controlled trial," *Journal of the American Medical Association,* 280(18):1585-1589.

Blanchard, E. B., Schwarz, S. P., Suls, J. M., Gerardi, M. A., Green, B., Taylor, A. E., Berreman, C., and Malamood, H. S. (1992). "Two controlled evaluations of multicomponent psychological treatment of irritable bowel syndrome," *Behaviour Research and Therapy,* 30(2):175-189.

Chan, H., Billmeier, G. J. Jr., Evans, W. E., and Chan, H. (1977). "Lead poisoning from ingestion of Chinese herbal medicine," *Clinical Toxicology,* 10(3):273-281.

Cook, I. J., Irvine, E. J., Campbell, D., Shannon, S., Reddy, S. N., and Collins, S. M. (1990). "Effect of dietary fiber on symptoms and rectosigmoid motility in patients with irritable bowel syndrome," *Gastroenterology,* 98(1):66-72.

Corney, R. H., Stanton, R., Newell, R., Clare, A., and Fairclough, P. (1991). "Behavioural psychotherapy in the treatment of irritable bowel syndrome," *Journal of Psychosomatic Research,* 35(4-5):461-469.

Dapoigny, M., Abitbol, J. L., and Fraitag, B. (1995). "Efficacy of peripheral agonist fedotozine versus placebo in treatment of irritable bowel syndrome. A multicenter dose-response study," *Digestive Diseases and Science,* 40(10):2244-2249.

Delvaux, M., Louvel, D., Lagier, E., Scherrer, B., Abitbol, J. L., and Frexinos, J. (1999). "The kappa agonist fedotozine relieves hypersensitivity to colonic distention in patients with irritable bowel syndrome," *Gastroenterology,* 116(1):38-45.

DiPaola, R. S., Zhang, H., Lambert, G. H., Meeker, R., Licitra, E., Rafi, M. M., Zhu, B. T., Spaulding, H., Goodin, S., Toledano, M. B., Hait, W. N., and Gallo, M. A. (1998). "Clinical and biologic activity of an estrogenic herbal combination (PC-SPES) in prostate cancer," *New England Journal of Medicine,* 339(12):785-791.

Drossman, D. A. (1995). "Diagnosing and treating patients with refractory functional gastrointestinal disorders," *Annals of Internal Medicine,* 123(9):688-697.

Evangelista, S., Giachetti, A., Chapelain, B., Neliat, G., and Maggi, C. A. (1998). "Receptor binding profile of otilonium bromide," *Pharmacological Research,* 38(2):111-117.

Evans, P. R., Bak, Y. T., and Kellow, J. E. (1996). "Mebeverine alters small bowel motility in irritable bowel syndrome," *Alimentary Pharmacology and Therapeutics,* 10(5):787-793.

Evans, P. R., Bak, Y. T., and Kellow, J. E. (1997). "Effects of oral cisapride on small bowel motility in irritable bowel syndrome," *Alimentary Pharmacology and Therapeutics,* 11(5):837-844.

Farup, P. G., Hovdenak, N., Wetterhus, S., Lange, O. J., Hovde, O., and Trondstad, R. (1998). "The symptomatic effect of cisapride in patients with irritable bowel syndrome and constipation," *Scandinavian Journal of Gastroenterology,* 33(2):128-131.

Fioramonti, J., Frexinos, J., Staumont, G., and Bueno, L. (1988). "Inhibition of the colonic motor response to eating by pinaverium bromide in irritable bowel syndrome patients," *Fundamental and Clinical Pharmacology,* 2(1):19-27.

Fowlie, S., Eastwood, M. A., and Prescott, R. (1992). "Irritable bowel syndrome: Assessment of psychological disturbance and its influence on the response to fibre supplementation," *Journal of Psychosomatic Research,* 36(2):175-180.

Frexinos, J., Fioramonti, J., and Bueno, L. (1985). "Effect of trimebutine on colonic myoelectrical activity in IBS patients," *European Journal of Clinical Pharmacology,* 28(2):181-185.

Gade, J. and Thorn, P. (1989). "Paraghurt for patients with irritable bowel syndrome. A controlled clinical investigation from general practice," *Scandinavian Journal of Primary Health Care,* 7(1):23-26.

Giachetti, A., Giraldo, E., Ladinsky, H., and Montagna, E. (1986). "Binding and functional profiles of the selective M1 muscarinic receptor antagonist trihexyphenidyl and dicyclomine," *British Journal of Pharmacology,* 89(1):83-90.

Goldberg, P. A., Kamm, M. A., Setti-Carraro, P., van der Sijp, J. R. M., and Roth, C. (1996). "Modification of visceral sensitivity and pain in irritable bowel syndrome by 5-HT3 antagonism (ondansetron)," *Digestion,* 57(6):478-483.

Greenbaum, D. S., Mayle, J. E., Vanegeren, L. E., Jerome, J. A., Mayor, J. W., Greenbaum, R. B., Matson, R. W., Stein, G. E., Dean, H. A., Halvorsen, N. A., and Rosen, L. W. (1987). "Effects of desipramine on irritable bowel syndrome compared with atropine and placebo," *Digestive Diseases and Science,* 32(3):257-266.

Greene, B. and Blanchard, E. B. (1994). "Cognitive therapy for irritable bowel syndrome," *Journal of Consulting and Clinical Psychology,* 62(3):576-582.

Guerot, C., Khemache, A., Sebbah, J., and Noel, B. (1988). "Electrophysiological study of intravenous pinaverium bromide in cardiology," *Current Medical Research and Opinion,* 11(2):73-79.

Halpern, G. M., Prindiville, T., Blankenburg, M., Hsia, T., and Gershwin, M. E. (1996). "Treatment of irritable bowel syndrome with Lacteol Fort; a randomized, double-blind, cross-over trial," *American Journal of Gastroenterology,* 91(8):1579-1585.

Jalihal, A. and Kurian, G. (1990). "Ispaghula therapy in irritable bowel syndrome: Improvement in overall well-being is related to reduction in bowel dissatisfaction," *Journal of Gastroenterology and Hepatology,* 5(5):507-513.

Kane, J. A., Kane, S. P., and Jain, S. (1995). "Hepatitis induced by traditional Chinese herbs; possible toxic components," *Gut,* 36(1):146-147.

Kilbinger, H. and Stein, A. (1988). "Dicyclomine discriminates between M1- and M2-muscarinic receptors in the guinea-pig ileum," *British Journal of Pharmacology,* 94(4):1270-1274.

Kjaerulff, E. and Tojner, H. (1977). "Treatment of irritable colon in general practice. A controlled study of metoclopramide" *Ugeskrift For Lager,* (in Danish), 139 (39):2322-2325.

Klein, K. B. (1988). "Controlled treatment trials in the irritable bowel syndrome: A critique," *Gastroenterology,* 95(1):232-241.

Kruis, W., Weinzierl, M., Schussler, P., and Holl, J. (1986). "Comparison of the therapeutic effect of wheat bran, mebeverine and placebo in patients with the irritable bowel syndrome," *Digestion,* 34(3):196-201.

Lacheze, C., Coelho, A. M., Fioramonti, J., and Bueno, L. (1998). "Influence of trimebutine on inflammation- and stress-induced hyperalgesia to rectal distention in rats," *Journal of Pharmacy and Pharmacology,* 50(8):921-928.

Langlois, A., Diop, L., Friese, N., Pascaud, X., Junien, J. L., Dahl, S. G., and Riviere, P. J. (1997). "Fedotozine blocks hypersensitive visceral pain in conscious rats: Action at peripheral kappa-opioid receptors," *European Journal of Pharmacology,* 324(2-3):211-217.

Langlois, A., Pascaud, X., Junien, J. L., Dahl, S. G., and Riviere, P. J. (1996). "Response heterogeneity of 5-HT3 receptor antagonists in a rat visceral hypersensitivity model," *European Journal of Pharmacology,* 318(1):141-144.

Lisker, R., Solomons, N. W., Briceno, R. P., and Mata, M. R. (1989). "Lactase and placebo in the management of the irritable bowel syndrome: A double-blind, cross-over study," *American Journal of Gastroenterology,* 84(7):756-762.

Longstreth, G. F. (1998). "Irritable bowel syndrome," in Manu, P. (Editor), *Functional Somatic Syndromes.* New York: Cambridge University Press, 58-79.

Longstreth, G. F., Fox, D. D., Youkeles, L., Forsythe, A. B., and Wolochow, D. A. (1981). "Psyllium therapy in the irritable bowel syndrome," *Annals of Internal Medicine,* 95(1):53-56.

Lucey, M. R., Clark, M. L., Lowndes, J., and Dawson, A. M. (1987). "Is bran efficacious in irritable bowel syndrome? A double blind placebo controlled crossover study," *Gut,* 28(2):221-225.

Luttecke, K. (1980). "A three-part controlled study of trimebutine in the treatment of irritable colon syndrome," *Current Medical Research and Opinion,* 6(6):437-441.

Malysz, J., Farraway, L. A., Christen, M. O., and Huizinga, J. D. (1997). "Pinaverium acts as L-type calcium channel blocker on smooth muscle of colon," *Canadian Journal of Physiology and Pharmacology,* 75(8):969-975.

Manning, A. P., Heaton, K. W., and Harvey, R. F. (1977). "Wheat fibre and irritable bowel syndrome. A controlled trial," *Lancet,* 2(8035):417-418.

Maxton, D. G., Morris, J., and Whorwell, P. J. (1996). "Selective 5-hydroxytryptamine antagonism: A role in irritable bowel and functional dyspepsia?" *Alimentary Pharmacology and Therapeutics,* 10(4):595-599.

McDonough, F. E., Hitchins, A. D., Wong, N. P., Wells, P., and Bodwell, C. E. (1987). "Modification of sweet acidophilus milk to improve utilization by lactose-intolerant persons," *American Journal of Clinical Nutrition,* 45(3):570-574.

Mitra, A. K. and Rabbani, G. H. (1990). "A double-blind, controlled trial of bioflorin (*Streptococcus faecium* SF68) in adults with acute diarrhea due to *Vibrio cholerae* and enterotoxigenic *Escherichia coli*," *Gastroenterology,* 99(4):1149-1152.

Moshal, M. G. and Herron, M. (1979). "A clinical trial of trimebutine (Mebutin) in spastic colon," *Journal of International Medical Research,* 7(3):231-234.

Myren, J., Groth, H., Larssen, S. E., and Larsen, S. (1982). "The effect of trimipramine in patients with the irritable bowel syndrome," *Scandinavian Journal of Gastroenterology,* 17(7):871-875.

Myren, J., Lovland, B., Larssen, S. E., and Larsen S. (1984). "A double-blind study of the effect of trimipramine in patients with the irritable bowel syndrome," *Scandinavian Journal of Gastroenterology,* 19(6):835-843.

Naiducci, F., Bassotti, G., Gaburri, M., Farroni, F., and Morelli, A. (1985). "Nifedipine reduces the colonic motor response to eating in patients with the irritable colon syndrome," *American Journal of Gastroenterology,* 80(5):317-319.

Newcomer, A. D., Park, H. S., O'Brien, P. C., and McGill, D. B. (1983). "Response of patients with irritable bowel syndrome and lactase deficiency using unfermented acidophilus milk," *American Journal of Clinical Nutrition,* 38(2): 257-263.

Newmark, C. S. and Raft, D. (1976). "Using an abbreviated MMPI as a screening device for medical patients," *Psychosomatics,* 17(1):45-48.

Nielsen, O. H., Jorgensen, S., Pedersen, K., and Justesen, T. (1994). "Microbiological evaluation of jejunal aspirates and faecal samples after oral administration of bifidobacteria and lactic acid bacteria," *Journal of Applied Bacteriology,* 76(5):469-474.

Noor, N., Small, P. K., Loudon, M. A., Hau, C., and Campbell, F. C. (1998). "Effects of cisapride on symptoms and postcibal small-bowel motor function in patients with irritable bowel syndrome," *Scandinavian Journal of Gastroenterology,* 33(6):605-611.

Ohnuma, T., Sridhar, K. S., Ratner, L. H., and Holland, J. F. (1982). "Phase I study of indicine N-oxide in patients with advanced cancer," *Cancer Treatment Reports,* 66(7):1509-1511.

Page, J. G. and Dirnberger, G. M. (1981). "Treatment of the irritable bowel syndrome with Bentyl® (dicyclomine hydrochloride)," *Journal of Clinical Gastroenterology,* 3(2):153-156.

Perez-Mateo, M., Sillero, C., Cuesta, A., Vazquez, N., and Berbegal, J. (1986). "Diltiazem in the treatment of the irritable bowel syndrome," *International Journal of Clinical Pharmacology Research,* 6(5):425-427.

Pontifex, A. H. and Garg, A. K. (1985). "Lead poisoning from an Asian Indian folk remedy," *Canadian Medical Association Journal,* 133(12):1227-1228.

Prior, A. and Read, N. W. (1993). "Reduction of rectal sensitivity and post-prandial motility by granisetron, a 5 HT3-receptor antagonist, in patients with irritable bowel syndrome," *Alimentary Pharmacology and Therapeutics,* 7(2):175-180.

Prior, A. and Whorwell, P. J. (1987). "Double blind study of ispaghula in irritable bowel syndrome," *Gut,* 28(11):1510-1513.

Rao, M. V. and Dutta, S. M. (1978). "Lactase activity of microorganisms," *Folia Microbiologica (Praha),* 23(3):210-215.

Schang, J. C., Devroede, G., and Pilote, M. (1993). "Effects of trimebutine on colonic function in patients with chronic idiopathic constipation: Evidence for the need of a physiologic rather than clinical selection," *Diseases of Colon and Rectum,* 36(4):330-336.

Schutze, K., Brandstatter, G., Dragosics, B., Judmaier, G., and Hentschel, E. (1997). "Double-blind study of the effect of cisapride on constipation and abdominal discomfort as components of the irritable bowel syndrome," *Alimentary Pharmacology and Therapeutics,* 11(2):387-394.

Smitherman, J. and Harber, P. (1991). "A case of mistaken identity: Herbal medicine as a cause of lead toxicity," *American Journal of Indian Medicine,* 20(6):795-798.

Snook, J. and Shepherd, H. A. (1994). "Bran supplementation in the treatment of irritable bowel syndrome," *Alimentary Pharmacology and Therapeutics,* 8(5): 511-514.

Soltoft, J., Krag, B., Gudmand-Hoyer, E., Kristensen, E., and Wulff, H. R. (1976). "A double-blind trial of the effect of wheat bran on symptoms of irritable bowel syndrome," *Lancet,* 1(7954):270-272.

Steadman, C. J., Talley, N. J., Phillips, S. F., and Zinsmeister, A. R. (1992). Selective 5-hydroxytryptamine type 3 receptor antagonism with ondansetron as treatment for diarrhea-predominant irritable bowel syndrome: A pilot study," *Mayo Clinic Proceedings,* 67(8):732-738.

Steinhart, M. J., Wong, P. Y., and Zarr, M. L. (1981). "Therapeutic usefulness of amitriptyline in spastic colon syndrome," *International Journal of Psychiatry in Medicine,* 11(1):45-57.

Su, X. and Gebhart, G. F. (1998). "Effects of tricyclic antidepressants on mechanosensitive pelvic nerve afferent fibers innervating the rat colon," *Pain,* 76(1-2):105-114.

Sutton, J. A., Kilminster, S. G., and Mould, G. P. (1997). "The clinical pharmacology of single doses of otilonium bromide in healthy volunteers," *European Journal of Clinical Pharmacology,* 52(5):365-369.

Talley, N. J. (1992). "Review article: 5-hydroxytryptamine agonists and antagonists in the modulation of gastrointestinal motility and sensation: Clinical implications," *Alimentary Pharmacology and Therapeutics,* 6(3):273-289.

Thompson, W. G., Doterall, G., Drossman, D. A., Keaton, K. W., and Kruis, W. (1989). "Irritable bowel syndrome: Guideline for the diagnosis (Working Team Report)," *Gastroenterology International,* 2(1):92-95.

Tolliver, B. A., Jackson, M. S., Jackson, K. L., Barnett, E. D., Chastang, J. F., and DiPalma, J. A. (1996). "Does lactose maldigestion really play a role in the irritable bowel?" *Journal of Clinical Gastroenterology,* 23(1):15-17.

Toskes, P. P., Connery, K. L., and Ritchey, T. W. (1993). "Calcium polycarbophil compared with placebo in irritable bowel syndrome," *Alimentary Pharmacology and Therapeutics,* 7(1):87-92.

Valori, R., Shannon, S., Reddy, N., Daniel, E. E., and Collins, S. M. (1987). "The action of trimebutine maleate on gastrointestinal motility is mediated by opiate receptors in human subjects," *Gastroenterologie Clinique et Biologique,* 11(3, Pt. 2):102B-104B.

Van Dulmen, A. M., Fennis, J. F., and Bleijenberg, G. (1996). "Cognitive-behavioral group therapy for irritable bowel syndrome: Effects and long-term follow-up," *Psychosomatic Medicine,* 58(5):508-514.

Vanherweghem, L. J. (1998). "Misuse of herbal remedies: The case of an outbreak of terminal renal failure in Belgium," *Journal of Alternative and Complementary Medicine,* 4(1):9-13.

Van Outryve, M., Milo, R., Toussaint, J., and Van Eeghem, P. (1991). "'Prokinetic' treatment of constipation-predominant irritable bowel syndrome: A placebo-controlled study of cisapride," *Journal of Clinical Gastroenterology,* 13(1):49-57.

Washington, N., Ridley, P., Thomas, C., Spiller, R. C., Watts, P. J., and Wilson, C. G. (1998). Mebeverine decreases mass movements and stool frequency in lactulose-induced diarrhoea," Alimentary Pharmacology and Therapeutics, 12(6):583-588.

Yadav, S. K., Jain, A. K., Tripathi, S. N., and Gupta, J. P. (1989). "Irritable bowel syndrome: Therapeutic evaluation of indigenous drugs," Indian Journal of Medical Research, 90:496-503.

Zighelboim, J., Talley, N. J., Phillips, S. F., Harmsen, W. S., and Zinsmeister, A. R. (1995). "Visceral perception in irritable bowel syndrome. Rectal and gastric responses to distention and serotonin 3 antagonism," Digestive Diseases and Science, 40(4):819-827.

Section IV

Abraham, G. E. and Lubran, M. M. (1981). "Serum red cell magnesium levels in patients with premenstrual tension," American Journal of Clinical Nutrition, 34(11):2364-2366.

American Hospital Formulary Service. (1997). AHFS 97 Drug Information. Bethesda, Maryland: American Society of Health-System Pharmacists.

American Psychiatric Association. (1987). Diagnostic and Statistical Manual of Mental Disorders, Revised Third Edition. Washington, DC: American Psychiatric Association Committee on Nomenclature and Statistics, 367-369.

American Psychiatric Association. (1994). Diagnostic and Statistical Manual of Mental Disorders, Fourth Edition. Washington, DC: American Psychiatric Association, 715-718.

Andersch, B. and Hahn, L. (1982). "Bromocriptine and premenstrual tension: A clinical and hormonal study," Pharmacotherapeutica, 3(2):107-113.

Andersen, A. N., Larsen, J. F., Steenstrup, O. R., Svendstrup, B., and Nielsen, J. (1977). "Effect of bromocriptine on the premenstrual syndrome. A double-blind clinical trial," British Journal of Obstetrics and Gynecology, 84(5):370-374.

Ashby, C. R., Carr, L. A., Cook, C. L., Steptoe, M. M., and Franks, D. D. (1988). "Alteration of platelet serotonergic mechanisms and monoamine oxidase activity in premenstrual syndrome," Biological Psychiatry, 24(2):225-233.

Baker, E. R., Best, R. G., Manfredi, R. L., Demers, L. M., and Wolf, G. C. (1995). "Efficacy of progesterone vaginal suppositories in alleviation of nervous symptoms in patients with premenstrual syndrome," Journal of Assisted Reproduction and Genetics, 12(3):205-209.

Bancroft, J. and Cook, A. (1995). "The neuroendocrine response to d-fenfluramine in women with premenstrual depression," Journal of Affective Disorders 36(1-2):57-64.

Bancroft, J., Cook, A., Davidson, D., Bennie, J., and Goodwin, G. (1991). "Blunting of neuroendocrine responses to infusion of L-tryptophan in women with perimenstrual mood changes," Psychological Medicine, 21(2):305-312.

Barbieri, I. and Ryan, K. J. (1981). "Danazol: Endocrine pharmacology and therapeutic applications," American Journal of Obstetrics and Gynecology, 141(4): 453-463.

Berger, C. P. and Presser, B. (1994). "Alprazolam in the treatment of two subsamples of patients with late luteal dysphoric disorder: A double-blind, placebo-controlled crossover study," *Obstetrics and Gynecology*, 84(3):379-385.

Berk, M., Mitchell, V. S., and Plein, H. (1998). "The platelet intracellular calcium response to serotonin in subsyndromal depression," *International Clinical Psychopharmacology*, 13(3):107-110.

Blake, F., Salkovskis, P., Gath, D., Day, A., and Garrod, A. (1998). "Cognitive therapy for premenstrual syndrome: A controlled trial," *Journal of Psychosomatic Research*, 45(4):307-318.

Brown, C. S., Ling, F. W., Andersen, R. N., Farmer, R. G., and Arheart, K. L. (1994). "Efficacy of depot leuprolide in premenstrual syndrome: Effect of symptom severity and type in a controlled trial," *Obstetrics and Gynecology*, 84(4):779-786.

Brush, M. G., Watson, S. J., Horrobin, D. F., and Manku, M. S. (1984). "Abnormal essential fatty acid levels in plasma of women with premenstrual syndrome," *American Journal of Obstetrics and Gynecology*, 150(4):363-366.

Brzezinski, A. A., Wurtman, J. J., Wurtman, R. J., Gleason, R., Greenfield, J., and Nader, T. (1990). "D-Fenfluramine suppresses the increased calorie and carbohydrate intake and improves the mood of women with premenstrual depression," *Obstetrics and Gynecology*, 76(2):296-301.

Burnet, R. B., Radden, H. S., Easterbrook, E. G., McKinnon, R. A. (1991). "Premenstrual syndrome and spironolactone," *Australian and New Zealand Journal of Obstetrics and Gynaecology*, 31(4):366-368.

Casper, R. F. and Hearn, M. T. (1990). "The effect of hysterectomy and bilateral oophorectomy in women with severe premenstrual syndrome," *American Journal of Obstetrics and Gynecology*, 162(1):105-109.

Casson, P., Hahn, P. M., Van Vugt, D. A., and Reid, R. L. (1990). "Lasting response to ovariectomy in severe intractable premenstrual syndrome," *American Journal of Obstetrics and Gynecology*, 162(1):99-105.

Cerin, A., Collins, A., Landgren, B. M., and Eneroth, P. (1993). "Hormonal and biochemical profiles of premenstrual syndrome. Treatment with essential fatty acids," *Acta Obstetricia et Gynecologica Scandinavica*, 72(5):337-343.

Christensen, A. P. and Oei, T. P. (1995). "The efficacy of cognitive behaviour therapy in treating premenstrual dysphoric changes," *Journal of Affective Disorders*, 33(1):57-63.

Chuong, C. J., Dawson, E. B., and Smith, E. R. (1990). "Vitamin E levels in premenstrual syndrome," *American Journal of Obstetrics and Gynecology*, 163(5, Pt. 1):1591-1595.

Collins, A., Cerin, A., Coleman, G., and Landgren, B. M. (1993). "Essential fatty acids in the treatment of premenstrual syndrome," *Obstetrics and Gynecology*, 81(1):93-98.

Dakshinamurti, K., Sharma, S. K., and Bonke, D. (1990). "Influence of B vitamins on binding properties of serotonin receptors in the CNS of rats," *Klinische Wochenschrift*, 68(2):142-145.

Davidson, B. J., Rea, C. D., and Valenzuela, G. J. (1988). "Atrial natriuretic peptide plasma renin activity, and aldosterone in women on estrogen therapy and with premenstrual syndrome," *Fertility and Sterility*, 50(5):743-746.

Deeny, M., Hawthorn, R., and Hart, D. M. (1991). "Low dose danazol in the treatment of premenstrual syndrome," *Postgraduate Medical Journal*, 67(787):450-454.

Dennerstein, L., Morse, C., Gotts, G., Brown, J., Smith, M., Oats, J., and Burrows, G. (1986). "Treatment of premenstrual syndrome. A double-blind trial of dydrogesterone." *Journal of Affective Disorders*, 11(3):199-205.

Dhar, V. and Murphy, B. E. P. (1990). "Double-blind randomized crossover trial of luteal phase estrogen (Premarin®) in the premenstrual syndrome (PMS)," *Psychoneuroendocrinology*, 15(5-6):489-493.

Diegoli, M. S. C., Da Fonseca, A. M., Diegoli, C. A., and Pinotti, J. A. (1998). "A double-blind trial of four medications to treat severe premenstrual syndrome," *International Journal of Gynecology and Obstetrics*, 62(1):63-67.

Doll, H., Brown, S., Thurston, A., and Vessey, M. (1989). "Pyridoxine (vitamin B6) and the premenstrual syndrome: A randomized crossover trial," *Journal of the Royal College of General Practitioners*, 39(326):364-368.

Eriksson, E., Hedberg, M. A., Andersch, B., and Sundblad, C. (1995). "The serotonin reuptake inhibitor paroxetin is superior to the noradrenaline reuptake inhibitor maprotiline in the treatment of premenstrual syndrome," *Neuropsychopharmacology*, 12(2):167-176.

Evans, S. M., Haney, M., Levin, F. R., Foltin, R. W., and Fischman, M. W. (1998). "Mood and performance changes in women with premenstrual dysphoric disorder: Acute effects of alprazolam," *Neuropsychopharmacology*, 19(6):499-516.

Facchinetti, F., Borella, P., Sances, G., Fioroni, L., Nappi, R. E., and Genazzani, A. R. (1991). "Oral magnesium successfully relieves premenstrual mood changes," *Obstetrics & Gynecology*, 78(2):177-181.

Facchinetti, F., Fioroni, L., Sances, G., Romano, G., Nappi, G., and Genazzani, A. R. (1989). "Naproxen sodium in the treatment of premenstrual symptoms. A placebo-controlled study," *Gynecologic and Obstetric Investigation*, 28(4):205-208.

FitzGerald, M., Malone, K. M., Li, S., Harrison, W. M., McBride, P. A., Endicott, J., Cooper, T., and Mann, J. J. (1997). "Blunted serotonin response to fenfluramine challenge in premenstrual dysphoric disorder," *American Journal of Psychiatry*, 154(4):556-558.

Freeman, E. W., Rickels, K., Arredondo, F., Kao, L. C., Pollack, S. E., and Sondheimer, S. J. (1999). "Full- or half-cycle treatment of severe premenstrual syndrome with a serotonergic antidepressant," *Journal of Clinical Psychopharmacology*, 19(1):3-8.

Freeman, E., Rickels, K., Sondheimer, S. J., and Polansky, M. (1990). "Ineffectiveness of progesterone suppository treatment for premenstrual syndrome," *Journal of the American Medical Association*, 264(3):349-353.

Freeman, E. W., Rickels, K., Sondheimer, S. J., and Polansky, M. (1995). "A double-blind trial of oral progesterone alprazolam, and placebo in treatment of severe premenstrual syndrome," *Journal of the American Medical Association,* 274(1):51-57.

Freeman, E. W., Sondheimer, S. J., and Rickels, K. (1997). "Gonadotropin-releasing hormone agonist in the treatment of premenstrual symptoms with and without ongoing dysphoria: A controlled study," *Psychopharmacology Bulletin,* 33(2):303-309.

Gangar, K. F., Fraser, D., Whitehead, M. I., and Cust, M. P. (1990). "Prolonged endometrial stimulation associated with oestradiol implants," *British Medical Journal,* 17(6722):436-438.

Goodwin, G. M., Murray, C. L., and Bancroft, J. (1994). "Oral d-fenfluramine and neuroendocrine challenge: Problems with the 30 mg dose in men," *Journal of Affective Disorders,* 30(2):117-122.

Gunston, K. D. (1986). "Premenstrual syndrome in Cape Town. Part II. A double-blind placebo-controlled study of the efficacy of mefenamic acid," *South African Medical Journal,* 70(3):159-160.

Hagen, I., Nesheim, B. I., and Tuntland, T. (1985). "No effect of vitamin B6 against premenstrual tension," *Acta Obstetrica Gynecologica Scandinavica,* 64(8):667-670.

Hahn, P. M., Van Vugt, D. A., and Reid, R. L. (1995). "A randomized, placebo-controlled, crossover trial of danazol for the treatment of premenstrual syndrome," *Psychoneuroendocrinology,* 20(2):193-209.

Halbreich, U. and Endicott, J. (1985). "Methodological issues in studies of premenstrual changes," *Psychoneuroendocrinology,* 10(1):15-32.

Halbreich, U., Petty, F., Yonkers, K., Kramer, G. L., Rush, A. J., and Bibi, K. W. (1996). "Low plasma gamma-aminobutyric acid levels during the late luteal phase of women with premenstrual dysphoric disorder," *American Journal of Psychiatry,* 153(5):718-720.

Halbreich, U., Rojansky, N., and Palter S. (1991). "Elimination of ovulation and menstrual cyclicity (with danazol) improves dysphoric premenstrual syndrome," *Fertility and Sterility,* 56(6):1066-1069.

Halbreich, U. and Smoller, J. W. (1997). "Intermittent luteal phase sertraline treatment of dysphoric premenstrual syndrome," *Journal of Clinical Psychiatry,* 58(9):399-402.

Hammarback, S. and Backstrom, T. (1988). "Induced anovulation as treatment of premenstrual tension syndrome. A double-blind cross-over study with GnRH-agonist versus placebo," *Acta Obstetrica et Gynaecologica Scandinavica,* 67(2):159-166.

Harrison, W. M., Endicott, J., and Nee, J. (1990). "Treatment of premenstrual dysphoria with alprazolam. A controlled study," *Archives of General Psychiatry,* 47(3):270-275.

Hartvig, P., Lindner, K. J., Bjurling, P., Laengstrom, B., and Tedroff, J. (1995). "Pyridoxine effect on synthesis rate of serotonin in the monkey brain measured with positron emission tomography," *Journal of Neural Transmission, General Section,* 102(2):91-97.

Hellberg, D., Claesson, B., and Nilsson, S. (1991). "Premenstrual tension: A placebo-controlled efficacy study with spironolactone and medroxyprogesterone acetate," *International Journal of Gynecology and Obstetrics,* 34(3):243-248.

Helvacioglu, A., Yeoman, R. R., Hazelton, J. M., and Aksel, S. (1993). "Premenstrual syndrome and related hormonal changes. Long acting gonadotropin releasing hormone agonist treatment," *Journal of Reproductive Medicine,* 38(11):864-870.

Hoffmann, V., Pedersen P. A., Philip J., Fly, P., and Pedersen, C. (1988). The effect of dydrogesterone on premenstrual syndrome. A double-blind, randomized, placebo-controlled study in general practice," *Scandinavian Journal of Primary Care,* 6(3):179-183.

Horwitz, R. I. and Daniels, S. R. (1996). "Bias or biology: Evaluating the epidemiologic studies of L-tryptophan and the eosinophilia-myalgia syndrome," *Journal of Rheumatology Supplement,* 46(Oct.):60-72.

Jagadeesh, S. R. and Subhash, M. N. (1998). "Effect of antidepressants on intracellular Ca++ mobilization in human frontal cortex," *Biological Psychiatry,* 44(7):617-621.

Kendall, K. E. and Schnurr, P. P. (1987). "The effects of vitamin B6 supplementation on premenstrual symptoms," *Obstetrics and Gynecology,* 70(2):145-149.

Khoo, S. K., Munro, C., and Battistutta D. (1990). "Evening primrose oil and treatment of premenstrual syndrome," *Medical Journal of Australia,* 153(4):189-192.

Kirkby, R. J. (1994). "Changes in premenstrual symptoms and irrational thinking following cognitive-behavioral coping skills training," *Journal of Consulting and Clinical Psychology,* 62(5):1026-1032.

London, R. S., Murphy, L., Kitlowski, K. E., and Reynolds, M. A. (1987). "Efficacy of alpha-tocopherol in the treatment of premenstrual syndrome," *Journal of Reproductive Medicine,* 32(6):400-404.

London, R. S., Sundaram, G. S., Murphy, L., and Goldstein, P. J. (1983). "The effect of α-tocopherol on premenstrual symptomatology: A double-blind study," *Journal of the American College of Nutrition,* 2(2):115-122.

Magill, P. J. (1995). "Investigation of the efficacy of progesterone pessaries in the relief of symptoms of premenstrual syndrome," *British Journal of General Practice,* 45(400):589-593.

Magos, A. L., Brincat, M., and Studd, J. W. (1986). "Treatment of the premenstrual syndrome by subcutaneous estradiol implants and cyclical oral norethisterone: Placebo controlled study," *British Medical Journal,* 292(6536):1629-1633.

Meden-Vrtovec, H. and Vujic, D. (1992). "Bromocryptine (Bromergon®, Lek) in the management of premenstrual syndrome," *Clinical and Experimental Obstetrics and Gynecology,* 19(4):242-248.

Menkes, D. B., Coates, D. C., and Fawcett, J. P. (1994). "Acute tryptophan depletion aggravates premenstrual syndrome," *Journal of Affective Disorders,* 32(1):37-44.

Menkes, D. B., Taghavi, E., Mason, P. A., and Howard, R. C. (1993). "Fluoxetine's spectrum of action in premenstrual syndrome," *International Clinical Psychopharmacology,* 8(2):95-102.

Mira, M., McNeil, D., Fraser, I. S., Vizzard, J., and Abraham, S. (1986). "Mefenamic acid in the treatment of premenstrual syndrome," *Obstetrics & Gynecology*, 68(3):395-398.

Mira, M., Stewart, P. M., and Abraham, S. F. (1988). "Vitamin and trace element status in premenstrual syndrome," *American Journal of Clinical Nutrition*, 47(4):636-641.

Morse, C. A., Dennerstein, L., Farrell, E., and Varnavides, K. (1991). "A comparison of hormone therapy, coping skills training and relaxation for the relief of premenstrual syndrome," *Journal of Behavioral Medicine*, 14(5):469-489.

Munday, M., Brush, M. G., and Taylor, R. W. (1981). "Correlations between progesterone oestradiol and aldosterone levels in the premenstrual syndrome," *Clinical Endocrinology (Oxford)*, 14(1):1-9.

Muneyvirci-Delale, O., Nacharaju, V. L., Altura, B. M., and Altura, B. T. (1998). "Sex steroid hormones modulate serum ionized magnesium and calcium levels throughout the menstrual cycle in women," *Fertility and Sterility*, 69(5):958-962.

Muse, K. N., Cetel, N. S., Futterman, L. A., and Yen, S. C. (1984). "The premenstrual syndrome. Effects of "medical ovariectomy," *New England Journal of Medicine*, 311(21):1345-1349.

O'Brien, P. M. S. and Abukhalil, I. E. H. (1999). "Randomized controlled trial of the management of premenstrual syndrome and premenstrual mastalgia using luteal-phase only danazol," *American Journal of Obstetrics and Gynecology*, 180(1, Pt. 1):18-23.

O'Brien, P. M., Craven, D., Selby, C., and Symonds, E. M. (1979). "Treatment of premenstrual syndrome by spironolactone," *British Journal of Obstetrics and Gynecology*, 86(2):142-147.

Parry, B. L., Gerner, R. H., Wilkins, J. N., Halaris, A. E., Carlson, H. E., Hershman, J. M., Linnolia, M., Merrill, J., Gold, P. W., and Gracely, R. (1991). "CSF and endocrine studies of premenstrual syndrome," *Neuropsychopharmacology*, 5(2):127-137.

Parry, B. L., Rosenthal, N. E., James, S. P., and Wehr, T. A. (1991). "Atenolol in premenstrual syndrome: A test of the melatonin hypothesis," *Psychiatry Research*, 37(2):131-138.

Parry, B. L., Rosenthal, N. E., Tamarkin, L., and Wehr, T. A. (1987). "Treatment of a patient with seasonal premenstrual syndrome," *American Journal of Psychiatry*, 144(6):762-766.

Pearlstein, T. (1998). "Premenstrual syndrome," in Manu, P. (Editor) *Functional Somatic Syndromes.* New York: Cambridge University Press, 80-97.

Piccoli, A., Modena, F., Calo, L., Cantaro, S., Avogadro, A., Nardo, G., and Cerutti, R. (1993). "Reduction in urinary prostaglandin excretion in the premenstrual syndrome," *Journal of Reproductive Medicine*, 38(12):941-944.

Posaci, C., Erten, O., Uren, A., and Acar, B. (1994). "Plasma copper, zinc and magnesium levels in patients with premenstrual tension syndrome," *Acta Obstetrica Gynecologica Scandinavica*, 73(6):452-455.

Puolakka, J., Makarainen, L., Viinika, L., and Ylikorkala, O. (1985). "Biochemical and clinical effects of treating the premenstrual syndrome with prostaglandin synthesis precursors," *Journal of Reproductive Medicine,* 30(3):149-153.

Rapkin, A. J., Reading, A. E., Woo, S., and Goldman, L. M. (1991). "Tryptophan and neutral amino acids in premenstrual syndrome," *American Journal of Obstetrics and Gynecology,* 165(6, Pt. 1):1830-1833.

Rausch, J. L., Janowsky, D. S., Golshan, S., Kuhn, K., and Risch, S. C. (1988). "Atenolol treatment of late luteal phase dysphoric disorder," *Journal of Affective Disorders,* 15(2):141-147.

Rosenstein, D. L., Elin, R. J., Hosseini, J. M., Grover, G., and Rubinow, D. R. (1994). "Magnesium measures across the menstrual cycle in premenstrual syndrome," *Biological Psychiatry,* 35(8):557-561.

Sampson, G. A., Heathcote, P. R. M., Wordsworth, J., Prescott, P., and Hodgson, A. (1988). "Premenstrual syndrome: A double-blind cross-over study of treatment with dydrogesterone and placebo," *British Journal of Psychiatry,* 153(Aug.): 232-235.

Sarno, A. P. Jr., Miller, E. J. Jr., and Lundblad, E. G. (1987). "Premenstrual syndrome: Beneficial effects of periodic, low-dose danazol," *Obstetrics and Gynecology,* 70(1):30-36.

Schmidt, P. J., Grover, G. N., and Rubinow, D. R. (1993). "Alprazolam in the treatment of premenstrual syndrome: A double-blind, placebo-controlled trial," *Archives of General Psychiatry,* 50(6):467-473.

Schmidt, P. J., Nieman, L. K., Danaceau, M. A., Adams, L. F., and Rubinow, D. R. (1998). "Differential behavioral effects of gonadal steroids in women with and in those without premenstrual syndrome," *New England Journal of Medicine,* 338(4):209-216.

Smith, S., Rinehart, J. S., Ruddock, V. E., and Schiff, I. (1987). "Treatment of premenstrual syndrome with Alprazolam: Results of a double-blind, placebo-controlled, randomized crossover clinical trial," *Obstetrics and Gynecology,* 70(1):37-43.

Steinberg, S., Annable, L., Young, S. N., and Liyanage, N. (1999). "A placebo-controlled clinical trial of L-tryptophan in premenstrual dysphoria," *Biological Psychiatry,* 45(3):313-320.

Steiner, M., Haskett, R. F., and Carroll, B. J. (1980). "Premenstrual tension syndrome: The development of research diagnostic criteria and new rating scales," *Acta Psychiatric Scandinavica,* 62(2):177-190.

Steiner, M., Korzekwa, M., Lamont, J., and Wilkins, A. (1997). "Intermittent fluoxetine dosing in the treatment of women with premenstrual dysphoria," *Psychopharmacology Bulletin,* 33(4):771-774.

Steiner, M., Steinberg, S., Stewart, D., Carter, D., Berger, C., Reid, R., Grover, D., Streiner, D., and the Canadian Fluoxetine/Premenstrual Dysphoria Collaborative Study Group. (1995). "Fluoxetine in the treatment of premenstrual syndrome," *New England Journal of Medicine,* 332(23):1529-1534.

Stone, A. B., Pearlstein, T. B., and Brown, W. A. (1991). "Fluoxetine in the treatment of late luteal phase dysphoric disorder," *Journal of Clinical Psychiatry,* 52(7):290-293.

Thys-Jacobs, S. and Alvir, M. J. (1995). Calcium-regulating hormones across the menstrual cycle: Evidence of a secondary hyperparathyroidism in women with PMS," *Journal of Clinical Endocrinology and Metabolism,* 80(7):2227-2232.

Thys-Jacobs, S., Ceccarelli, S., Bierman, A., Weisman, H., Cohen, M. A., and Alvir, J. (1989). "Calcium supplementation in premenstrual syndrome. A randomized crossover trial," *Journal of General Internal Medicine,* 4(3):183-189.

Thys-Jacobs, S., Starkey, P., Bernstein, D., Tian, J., and the Premenstrual Syndrome Study Group. (1998). "Calcium carbonate and the premenstrual syndrome: Effects on premenstrual and menstrual symptoms," *American Journal of Obstetrics and Gynecology,* 179(2):444-452.

Vanselow, W., Dennerstein, L., Greenwood, K. M., and De Lignieres, B. (1996). "Effect of progesterone and its 5α and 5β metabolites on symptoms of premenstrual syndrome according to route of administration," *Journal of Psychosomatic Obstetrics and Gynaecology,* 17(1):29-38.

Vellacott, I. D., Shroff, N. E., Pearce, M. Y., Stratford, M. E., and Akbar, F. A. (1987). "A double-blind, placebo-controlled evaluation of spironolactone in the premenstrual syndrome," *Current Medical Research and Opinion,* 10(7):450-456.

Walker, A. F., De Souza, M. C., Vickers, M. F., Abeyasekera, S., Collins, M. L., and Trinca, L. A. (1998). "Magnesium supplementation alleviates premenstrual symptoms of fluid retention," *Journal of Women's Health,* 7(9):1157-1165.

Wang, M., Hammaback, S., Lindhe, B. A., and Backstrom, T. (1995). "Treatment of premenstrual syndrome by spironolactone: A double-blind, placebo-controlled study," *Acta Ostetricia et Gynecologica Scandinavica,* 74(10):803-808.

Watson, N. R., Savvas, M., Studd, J. W. W., and Garnett, T. (1989). "Treatment of severe premenstrual syndrome with estradiol patches and cyclical oral norethisterone," *Lancet,* 2(8665):730-732.

Watson, N. R., Studd, J. W., Savvas, M., and Baber, R. J. (1990). "The long-term effects of estradiol implant therapy for the treatment of premenstrual syndrome," *Gynecological Endocrinology,* 4(2):99-107.

Watts, J. F., Butt, W. R., and Edwards, R. L. (1987). "A clinical trial using danazol for the treatment of premenstrual tension," *British Journal of Obstetrics and Gynecology,* 94(1):30-34.

West, C. P. and Hillier, H. (1994). "Ovarian suppression with the gonadotrophin-releasing agonist goserelin (Zoladex) in management of the premenstrual tension syndrome," *Human Reproduction,* 9(6):1058-1063.

Wikander, I., Sundblad, C., Andersch, B., Dagnell, I., Zylberstein, D., Bengtsson, F., and Eriksson, E. (1998). "Citolapram in premenstrual dysphoria; is intermittent treatment during luteal phases more effective than continuous medication throughout the menstrual cycle?" *Journal of Clinical Psychopharmacology,* 18(5):390-398.

Williams, M. J., Harris, R. I., and Dean, B. C. (1985). "Controlled trial of pyridoxine in the premenstrual syndrome," *Journal of International Medical Research*, 13(3):174-179.

Wood, C. and Jakubowicz, D. (1980). "The treatment of premenstrual symptoms with mefenamic acid," *British Journal of Obstetrics and Gynecology*, 87(7):627-630.

Wood, S. H., Mortola, J. F., Chan, Y.-F., Moossazadeh, F., and Yen, S. S. C. (1992). "Treatment of premenstrual syndrome with fluoxetine: A double-blind, placebo-controlled, crossover study," *Obstetrics & Gynecology*, 80(3, Pt. 1):339-344.

Ylostalo, P., Kauppila, A., Puolakka, J., Ronnberg, L., and Janne, O. (1981). "Bromocriptine and norethisterone in the treatment of premenstrual syndrome," *Obstetrics and Gynecology*, 58(3):292-298.

Yonkers, K. A., Halbreich, U., Freeman, E., Brown, C., Endicott, J., Frank, E., Parry, B., Pearlstein, T., Severino, S., Stout, A., Stone, A., and Harrison, W. for the Sertraline Premenstrual Dysphoric Collaborative Study Group. (1997). "Symptomatic improvement of premenstrual dysphoric disorder with sertraline treatment. A randomized controlled trial," *Journal of the American Medical Association*, 278(12):983-988.

Yonkers, K. A., Halbreich, U., Freeman, E., Brown, C., and Pearlstein, T. (1996). "Sertraline in the treatment of premenstrual dysphoric disorder," *Psychopharmacology Bulletin*, 32(1):41-46.

Young, S. A., Hurt, P. H., Benedek, D. M., and Howard, R. S. (1998). "Treatment of premenstrual dysphoric disorder with sertraline during the luteal phase: A randomized, double-blind, placebo-controlled crossover trial," *Journal of Clinical Psychiatry*, 59(2):76-80.

Conclusions

Ashby, C. R., Carr, L. A., Cook, C. L., Steptoe, M. M., and Franks, D. D. (1988). "Alteration of platelets serotonergic mechanisms and monoamine oxidase activity in premenstrual syndrome," *Biological Psychiatry*, 24(2):225-233.

Bancroft, J., Cook, A., Davidson, D., Bennie, J., and Goodwin, G. (1991). "Blunting of neuroendocrine responses to infusion of L-tryptophan in women with perimenstrual mood changes," *Psychological Medicine*, 21(2):305-312.

Carette, S., Bell, M. J., Reynolds, W. J., Haraoui, B., McCain, G. A., Bykerk, V. P., Edworthy, S. M., Baron, M., Koehler, B. E., Fam, A. G., Bellamy, N., and Guimont, C. (1994). "Comparison of amitriptyline, cyclobenzaprine, and placebo in the treatment of fibromyalgia. A randomized, double-blind clinical trial," *Arthritis and Rheumatism*, 37(1):32-40.

Carette, S., McCain, G. A., Bell, D. A., and Fam, A. G. (1986). "Evaluation of amitriptyline in primary fibrositis. A double-blind, placebo-controlled study," *Arthritis and Rheumatism*, 29(5):655-659.

Deale, A., Chalder, T., Marks, I., and Wessely, S. (1997). "Cognitive behavior therapy for chronic fatigue syndrome: A randomized controlled trial," *American Journal of Psychiatry*, 154(3):408-414.

Eija, K., Tiina, T., and Pertti, N. J. (1996). "Amitriptyline effectively relieves neuropathic pain following treatment of breast cancer," *Pain*, 64(2):293-302.

FitzGerald, M., Malone, K. M., Li, S., Harrison, W. M., McBride, P. A., Endicott, J., Cooper, T., and Mann, J. J. (1997). "Blunted serotonin response to fenfluramine challenge in premenstrual dysphoric disorder," *American Journal of Psychiatry,* 154(4):556-558.

Franzblau, S. H. (1997). "The phenomenology of ritualized and repeated behaviors in nonclinical populations in the United States," *Cultural Diversity and Mental Health,* 3(4):259-272.

Fulcher, K. Y. and White, P. D. (1997). "Randomised controlled trial of graded exercise in patients with the chronic fatigue syndrome," *British Medical Journal,* 314(7095):1647-1652.

Fulford, K. W. (1993). "Praxis makes perfect: Illness as a bridge between biological concepts of disease and social conceptions of health," *Theoretical Medicine,* 14(4):305-320.

Goldenberg, D. L., Felson, D. T., and Dinerman, H. (1986). "A randomized, controlled trial of amitriptyline and naproxen in the treatment of patients with fibromyalgia," *Arthritis and Rheumatism,* 29(11):1371-1377.

Goldenberg, D., Mayskiy, M., Mossey, C., Ruthazer, R., and Schmid, C. (1996). "A randomized, double-blind crossover trial of fluoxetine and amitriptyline in the treatment of fibromyalgia," *Arthritis and Rheumatism,* 39(11):1852-1859.

Greenbaum, D. S., Mayle, J. E., Vanegeren, L. E., Jerome, J. A., Mayor, J. W., Grenbaum, R. B., Matson, R. W., Stein, G. E., Dean, H. A., Halvorsen, N. A., and Rosen, L. W. (1987). "Effects of desipramine on irritable bowel syndrome compared with atropine and placebo," *Digestive Diseases and Science,* 32(3):257-266.

Gunn, W. J., Connell, D. B., and Randall, B. (1993). "Epidemiology of chronic fatigue syndrome: The Centers for Disease Control study," in Bock, G. R. and Whelan, J. (Editors), *Chronic Fatigue Syndrome.* Chichester, UK: John Wiley, Ciba Foundation Symposium, 173:83-101.

Halbreich, U. and Smoller, J. W. (1997). "Intermittent luteal phase sertraline treatment of dysphoric premenstrual syndrome," *Journal of Clinical Psychiatry,* 58(9):399-402.

Hannonen, P., Malminiemi, K., Yli-Kertulla, U., Isomeri, R., and Roponen, P. (1998). "A randomized, placebo-controlled study of moclobemide and amitriptyline in the treatment of fibromyalgia in females without psychiatric disorder," *British Journal of Rheumatology,* 37(12):1279-1286.

Hunter, J. C., Gogas, K. R., Hedley, L. R., Jacobson, L. O., Kassotakis, L., Thompson, J., and Fontana, D. J. (1997). "The effect of novel anti-epileptic drugs in rat experimental models of acute and chronic pain," *European Journal of Pharmacology,* 324(2-3):153-160.

Johnson, R. E. and Ried, L. D. (1996). "OTC drug use in an HMO: Comparing the elderly and younger adults," *Journal of Aging and Health,* 8(1):114-135.

Kishore-Kumar, R., Max, M. B., Schafer, S. C., Gaughan, A. M., Smoller, B., Gracely, R. H., and Dubner, R. (1990). "Desipramine relieves postherpetic neuralgia," *Clinical Pharmacology and Therapeutics,* 47(3):305-312.

Kudoh, A., Ishihara, H., and Matsuki, A. (1998). "Effect of carbamazepine on pain scores of unipolar depressed patients with chronic pain: A trial of off-on-off-on design," *Clinical Journal of Pain,* 14(1):61-65.

McQuay, H. J., Carroll, D., and Glynn, C. J. (1992). "Low dose amitriptyline in the treatment of chronic pain," *Anaesthesia,* 47(8):646-652.

Menkes, D. B., Coates, D. C., and Fawcett, J. P. (1994). "Acute tryptophan depletion aggravates premenstrual syndrome," *Journal of Affective Disorders,* 32(1):37-44.

Myren, J., Groth, H., Larssen, S. E., and Larsen S. (1982). "The effect of trimipramine in patients with the irritable bowel syndrome," *Scandinavian Journal of Gastroenterology,* 17(7):871-875.

Myren, J., Lovland, B., Larssen, S. E., and Larsen, S. (1984). "A double-blind study of the effect of trimipramine in patients with the irritable bowel syndrome," *Scandinavian Journal of Gastroenterology,* 19(6):835-843.

Pradel, F. G., Hartzema, A. G., Mutran, E. J., and Hanson-Divers, C. (1999). "Physician over-the-counter drug prescribing patterns: An analysis of the national ambulatory medical care survey," *Annals of Pharmacotherapy,* 33(4):400-405.

Sharpe, M., Hawton, K., Simkin, S., Surawy, C., Hackmann, A., Klimes, I., Peto, T., Warrell, D., and Seagroatt, V. (1996). "Cognitive behaviour therapy for the chronic fatigue syndrome: A randomised controlled trial," *British Medical Journal,* 312(7022):22-26.

Sonuga-Barke, E. J. (1998). "Categorical models of childhood disorder: A conceptual and empirical analysis," *Journal of Child Psychology and Psychiatry and Allied Disciplines,* 39(1):115-133.

Stein, D., Peri, T., Edelstein, E., Elizur, A., and Floman, Y. (1996). "The efficacy of amitriptyline and acetaminophen in the management of low back pain," *Psychosomatics,* 37(1):63-70.

Steinhart, M. J., Wong, P. Y., and Zarr, M. L. (1981). "Therapeutic usefulness of amitriptyline in spastic colon syndrome," *International Journal of Psychiatry in Medicine,* 11(1):45-57.

Stoehr, G. P., Ganguli, M., Seaberg, E. C., Echement, D. A., and Belle, S. (1997). "Over-the-counter medication use in an older rural community: The MoVIES Project," *Journal of the American Geriatric Society,* 45(2):158-165.

Stone, A. B., Pearlstein, T. B., and Brown, W. A. (1991). "Fluoxetine in the treatment of late luteal phase dysphoric disorder," *Journal of Clinical Psychiatry,* 52(7):290-293.

Talley, N. J., Zinmeister, A. R., and Melton, L. J. III. (1995). "Irritable bowel syndrome in a community; symptom subgroups, risk factors and health care utilization," *American Journal of Epidemiology,* 142(1):76-83.

Vrethem, M., Boivie, J., Arnqvist, H., Holmgren, T., Lindstrom, T., and Thorell, L. H. (1997). "A comparison of amitriptyline and maprotiline in the treatment of painful polyneuropathy in diabetics and nondiabetics," *Clinical Journal of Pain,* 13(4):313-323.

Wearden, A. J., Morriss, R. K., Mullis, R., Strickland, P. L., Pearson, D. J., Appleby, L., Campbell, I. T., and Morris, J. A. (1998). "Randomised, double-blind, placebo-controlled treatment trial of fluoxetine and graded exercise for chronic fatigue syndrome," *British Journal of Psychiatry,* 172(June):485-490.

Wikander, I., Sundblad, C., Andersch, B., Dagnell, I., Zylberstein, D., Bengtsson, F., and Eriksson, E. (1998). "Citolapram in menstrual dysphoria; is intermittent treatment during luteal phase more effective than continuous medication throughout the menstrual cycle?" *Journal of Clinical Psychopharmacology,* 18(5):390-398.

Wolfe, F., Ross, K., Anderson, J., Russell, I., and Hebert, L. T. (1995). "The prevalence and characteristics of fibromyalgia in the general population," *Arthritis and Rheumatism,* 38(1):19-28.

Young, S. A., Hurt, P. H., Benedek, D. M., and Howard, R. S. (1998). "Treatment of premenstrual dysphoric disorder with sertraline during the luteal phase: A randomized, double-blind, placebo-controlled crossover trial," *Journal of Clinical Psychiatry,* 59(2):76-80.

Index

Page numbers followed by the letter "t" indicate tables.

Molndal and Lund University, Lund,
  Sweden, 200
Monash University, Melbourne, 240
Monoamine oxidase inhibitors
  (MAOIs)
  CFS, 33-36
  fibromyalgia, 63, 72
Mononucleosis, 44, 45
Montreal General Hospital, 215, 238
Multiple chemical sensitivities, 1
Multipurpose Arthritis Center,
  Boston University, 69
Multisymptomatic presentation, 3
Muscle relaxants, use in
  fibromyalgia, 75, 109

Nacional de la Nutricion "Salvador
  Zubiran," Mexico City, 161
Naproxen
  fibromyalgia trials, 96-97
  premenstrual syndrome trial,
    242-243
National Institute of Allergy and
  Infectious Diseases, NIH,
  CFS drug treatment booklet,
  55
National Institute of Mental Health,
  Bethesda, 209, 218, 245
National Institutes of Health (NIH),
  21, 42, 43
National Sports Medicine Institute,
  57
Neurally mediated hypotension, 52
New England Medical Center, 70
New Jersey Medical School, East
  Orange, NJ, 33, 35
New York Medical College, 261
New York Psychiatric Institute, 214,
  219
Newton-Wellesley Hospital, MA, 70
Nicotinamide adenine dinucleotide
  (NADH), CFS, 38-39
Ninewells Hospital, Dundee,
  Scotland, 151

Nonpharmacological trials,
  fibromyalgia, 118-119
Nonsteroidal anti-inflammatory
  drugs (NSAIDs)
  CFS, 55
  fibromyalgia trials, 93-98
  premenstrual syndrome, 240-243
  and TCA's in fibromyalgia, 63, 75
North Charles Hospital, Baltimore,
  MD, 264
North Staffordshire Hospital, Stoke
  on Trent, UK, 228

Octylonium, irritable bowel
  syndrome trials, 141-144
Ondansetron
  fibromyalgia trial, 105-106
  irritable bowel syndrome trials,
    163-167
One-of-a-kind trials, 5. *See also*
  Unreplicated trials
Oregon Health Sciences University,
  Portland, 75, 107, 110
Osteoarthritis, 61
Over-the-counter medication,
  274-275
Oxford University, UK, 254

Pain, irritable bowel syndrome, 123,
  124
Palpation, for fibromyalgia criterion,
  61
Paroxetine, premenstrual syndrome
  trial, 198-200
Pharmacological interventions, 4, 5
  effectiveness, 272
Phenelzine, CFS treatment study,
  33-34
Physician's explanatory model, and
  therapy, 3
Pinaverium, irritable bowel
  syndrome trial, 146-147
Placebo response rate, irritable bowel
  syndrome, 124

Order Your Own Copy of
This Important Book for Your Personal Library!

The Pharmacotherapy of Common Functional Syndromes: Evidence-Based Guidelines for Primary Care Practice

_____ in hardbound at $69.95 (ISBN: 0-7890-0588-3)

_____ in softbound at $39.95 (ISBN: 0-7890-0589-1)

COST OF BOOKS_____

OUTSIDE USA/CANADA/
MEXICO: ADD 20%_____

POSTAGE & HANDLING_____
*(US: $3.00 for first book & $1.25
for each additional book)
Outside US: $4.75 for first book
& $1.75 for each additional book)*

SUBTOTAL_____

IN CANADA: ADD 7% GST_____

STATE TAX_____
*(NY, OH & MN residents, please
add appropriate local sales tax)*

FINAL TOTAL_____
*(If paying in Canadian funds,
convert using the current
exchange rate. UNESCO
coupons welcome.)*

☐ **BILL ME LATER:** ($5 service charge will be added)
(Bill-me option is good on US/Canada/Mexico orders only;
not good to jobbers, wholesalers, or subscription agencies.)

☐ Check here if billing address is different from
shipping address and attach purchase order and
billing address information.

Signature_____

☐ **PAYMENT ENCLOSED: $**_____

☐ **PLEASE CHARGE TO MY CREDIT CARD.**

☐ Visa   ☐ MasterCard   ☐ AmEx   ☐ Discover
☐ Diners Club
Account # _____

Exp. Date _____

Signature _____

Prices in US dollars and subject to change without notice.

NAME _____

INSTITUTION _____

ADDRESS _____

CITY _____

STATE/ZIP _____

COUNTRY _____ COUNTY (NY residents only) _____

TEL _____ FAX _____

E-MAIL_____
May we use your e-mail address for confirmations and other types of information? ☐ Yes   ☐ No

Order From Your Local Bookstore or Directly From
The Haworth Press, Inc.
10 Alice Street, Binghamton, New York 13904-1580 • USA
TELEPHONE: 1-800-HAWORTH (1-800-429-6784) / Outside US/Canada: (607) 722-5857
FAX: 1-800-895-0582 / Outside US/Canada: (607) 772-6362
E-mail: getinfo@haworthpressinc.com
PLEASE PHOTOCOPY THIS FORM FOR YOUR PERSONAL USE.

BOF96

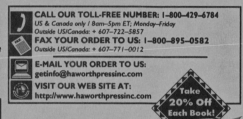